Equine Color Genetics

Equine Color Genetics

4th Edition

D. Phillip Sponenberg

Virginia-Maryland College of Veterinary Medicine
Virginia, USA

Rebecca Bellone

UC Davis
California, USA

WILEY Blackwell

Library of Congress Cataloging-in-Publication Data

Names: Sponenberg, D. Phillip (Dan Phillip), 1953- author. | Bellone, Rebecca, author.
Title: Equine color genetics / D. Phillip Sponenberg, Rebecca Bellone.
Description: 4th edition. | Hoboken, NJ, USA : John Wiley & Sons Inc., 2017.
  | Includes bibliographical references and index.
Identifiers: LCCN 2017004476 (print) | LCCN 2017005384 (ebook) | ISBN 9781119130581 (hardback)
  | ISBN 9781119130604 (Adobe PDF) | ISBN 9781119130611 (ePub)
Subjects: LCSH: Horses–Color. | Horses–Breeding. | Horses–Genetics.
  | MESH: Equidae–genetics | Pigmentation–genetics
Classification: LCC SF279 .S665 2017 (ebook) | LCC SF279 (print) | NLM SF 279
  | DDC 636.1/0821–dc23
LC record available at https://lccn.loc.gov/2017005384

Cover Design: Wiley
Cover Image: Courtesy of Francesca Gorizia Gianino

Set in 10/12 pt WarnockPro-Regular by Thomson Digital, Noida, India

10 9 8 7 6 5 4 3 2 1

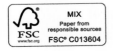

The Best Colour
Tradition, they say
Can teach us a lot,
So here is what horsemen
On colour have thought.

A bay is hardy
A chestnut is fast
And you can't kill a buckskin
He'll just last and last.

A gray is gentle,
A sorrel is hot,
A dun is a horse
You'll be happy you bought.

"White eyes" are flighty,
White feet may crack,
While some won't rely on
The feet of a black.

Some pintos are lucky,
Like the Medicine Hats,
But all horsemen agree –
The best colour is fat.

Marjorie C. Lacy

Contents

Preface to the Fourth Edition

This is the fourth edition of a guide to equine color identification and genetics. The first edition was published in 1996, the second in 2003, and a third in 2009. Each one built on advances in knowledge of equine coat color genetics, which have been accelerating at an ever more rapid pace. The understanding of many genetic mechanisms at work in horses and donkeys has greatly increased since the third edition. So too has the understanding of the biochemical and molecular processes underpinning pigment cell biology in many mammalian species. These advances have produced a much more complete explanation of horse color, and have sparked more extensive coverage in this edition. To make this knowledge available to those who will want to apply it in breeding horses, the explanation of important molecular processes as well as the terms frequently used in genetic studies has been expanded. In most instances the increased knowledge has simplified the understanding of horse colors, in other cases it has pointed to areas where further investigation is needed in order to make sense of various colors and patterns.

Many of the photographs have been updated, with the goal of providing better examples of various colors, shades, and patterns. Several photographs of odd combinations have also been located, and those have added to the completeness of the visual documentation. Many other figures have been included to more adequately illustrate some of the notoriously complicated concepts. Francesca Gianino deserves our special thanks for sharing her talent, creativity, and time in crafting these illustrations.

This work is the result of fruitful collaborations over many years, and bears the imprint of all those wonderful professional and personal relationships that have enriched our lives over the years. The generosity of the community that is interested in the details of horse color is remarkable, and is especially on display in many of the photographs that were offered as illustrations for the various details in the text. These are acknowledged in Table 13.8, where the details of the horse, breed, owner, and photographer for each photograph are indicated. In addition, special thanks go to Sheila Archer, Bianca Waud, Tosso Leeb, and Lesli Kathman for fascinating discussions and insights, all of which have improved our clarity in describing their important work. This, in turn, has greatly added to this book. Many other breeders, scientists, and other colleagues have likewise contributed various insights and details.

We have attempted to make this book complete and accurate. Any omissions or errors are entirely our own, and we hope the reader enjoys our efforts to explain the intricacies of horse color.

The authors dedicate this book to two scientists whose work and input shaped their own careers. Decades ago, Stefan Aðalsteinsson encouraged and provided key insights to

Phil Sponenberg, both on color genetics and breed conservation. His keen insights, humor, and encyclopedic knowledge of animal breeds and genetics were always inspirational. Dr Teri Lear had a similar influence for Rebecca Bellone. Teri was an avid horse lover and an exceptional equine cytogeneticist whose work signficantly contibuted to our understanding of equid chromosomes. Her love for both horses and people made the field of horse genetics a rich and deep experience, beyond the mere science that is so important. Both of these giants contributed to the field of genetics, to our careers, and both are greatly missed.

1

Introduction

This book is intended to be a complete discussion of horse and donkey colors. It includes details of color identification as well as their genetic control. The goal is to include all color variations occurring throughout the world and to fit these into a framework that is based on traditional American nomenclature as well as on the genetic phenomena controlling the color variations.

Identification and definition of horse color are important for several reasons, and each of these reasons demands a different organization and presentation of the material. Reasons for accurate horse color classification include identification of individual horses for legal purposes, health records, and breed registrations. In addition, breeders who are interested in producing or avoiding specific colors of foals find that accurate identification of colors in their breeding stock is essential to their success.

The organizational structure of this book combines a strictly visual approach (what color the horse appears to be) with the genetic control (how that color was produced by the interactions of the genes involved). Each section starts off with the visual approach and then delves into the genetic aspects. Unfortunately, a few specific details of horse color are better understood by first explaining the underlying genetic mechanisms that give rise to the colors rather than from any other point of view. In those few cases genetic mechanisms are presented first with the visual aspects following.

The genetic approach to understanding horse color is becoming increasingly common as deoxyribonucleic acid (DNA)-based tests for many of the genes causing the colors are now available. The results of these tests help breeders to better understand the colors and the genetic basis of their production, as well as the range of colors a specific horse can produce. While genetic testing has been generally helpful, it has also revealed a few confusing issues. Some horse colors, when classed only by visual appearance, appear to be a single group, but this single group includes the results of several very different genetic formulas. This occurs with **black** horses, and also with some of the light colors such as **champagne** and **pearl**, as well as **silver dapple** and **mushroom**. These different genetic formulas are presented at length in the corresponding sections of the book and are examples of the complexity of the genetic systems that produce a horse's final color.

New instances of multiple genetic formulas leading to visually identical colors are regularly coming to the attention of researchers in this field, and these can easily cause confusion to owners of horses with some of the variants. These colors present a very real challenge because a single outward appearance can spring from very different genetic mechanisms. In most cases it is fortunate that only one of the several possible genetic mechanisms for a confusing set of colors is common, and the few others that are possible

Equine Color Genetics, Fourth Edition. D. Phillip Sponenberg and Rebecca Bellone.
© 2017 John Wiley & Sons, Inc. Published 2017 by John Wiley & Sons, Inc.

are much more rare. Consequently, discussion of the colors can still proceed from the basics of the most common mechanisms, even though the more rare mechanisms that lead to similar visual results must also be considered for completeness. Those that are known are presented here.

Importantly, even though some mechanisms are common and others rare, when a rare mechanism is present it becomes the only one of importance in understanding how a specific horse or donkey will produce color in a breeding program. In a very real sense, "rare" is only really an issue at the population level. At the level of the individual horse the only thing that is important is the specific blend of individual genetic variants, regardless of their frequency in a population.

Choosing a set of nomenclature for horse colors presents an interesting array of challenges. Historical approaches were of necessity based solely on visual classification. These older, traditional systems were detailed and technical and have served well for centuries. They were based on a rich lore of horse-specific information and were generated by people closely familiar with horses and their variation. This traditional approach deserves great respect for having served well for so long.

From a strict and non-equine viewpoint, nearly all horse colors could simply be described as a shade of brown or black or a mixture of those two. People with no equine background do indeed tend to lump most horses as "**brown**," because to the inexperienced eye they indeed are. One step beyond the "most horses are **brown**" approach is the traditional equine-specific nomenclature based on various details related to visual appearance. While traditional nomenclature varies region to region, it has served well for identifying horses by color. It has also served as the framework under which genetic investigations were first accomplished.

In recent years, an approach based more on genetics has come into vogue for understanding and classifying horse color. This approach can often simplify nomenclature. This is especially true when similar phenotypes are caused by mutations in the same gene. However, the genetic approach can also complicate nomenclature, as novel genes or mutations are given new names that have no equivalent in the more traditional system. This can muddy the identification of horse colors.

The presence, for some colors, of multiple genetic mechanisms causing visually similar results presents very real problems for developing a consistent nomenclature based on genetic information alone. Nomenclature can either be visually based or genetically based, but choosing either one of these as the primary organizer of nomenclature will inevitably cause problems for situations in which the other basis is a more compelling consideration. Still, the historic, visually based approach is the only one that is likely to succeed in field situations where genetic details are only rarely known. In contrast, the genetically based approach can be more useful in classing and defining the color of breeding horses when their owners are preferentially interested in producing specific colors of foals. This guide generally uses a visually based approach, but the more genetically based approach is referred to when appropriate.

Colors are discussed in a sequence that first examines dark colors because these tend to be the most common colors in most breeds and most regions. An understanding of less common (generally lighter) colors is then built as a progression from the dark colors. Each section first defines and classifies a color or group of colors by the visual approach and then delves into the details of what is known about the genetic control.

The addition of white hairs can be superimposed on any background color, and each pattern of these white hairs or patches is examined after all basic colors are considered. The patterns of white hairs are organized in the same fashion of first classifying each pattern by its visual appearance, followed by an explanation of the underlying genetics.

Donkey colors are the subject of a separate discussion following the section on horse colors. The donkey color discussion is organized in a manner similar to that of the horse color section, but is shorter. Much less is known about donkey color than is known about horse color, although this body of knowledge has recently begun to expand. Subtle details of donkey color are understood more readily when considered in the light of horse color identification and genetics, which also makes a shorter discussion appropriate.

Mule colors are omitted, except for a few examples. This is due to mule colors being somewhat less well understood than those of horses and donkeys, while at the same time being generally consistent with the expected interactions of the genes controlling color in the two parent species.

A series of summary tables is presented in Chapter 13, after the text and illustrations. Table 13.1 is a list of color names that are included in the text, serving as an attempt at a reasonably complete single list of horse color names and their main distinguishing features. Table 13.2 is a similar list for the patterns of white hairs. Table 13.3 lists the various genes affecting horse color and their actions. This includes both the loci and alleles. Table 13.4 is similar to Table 13.3, but is devoted to the genes associated with patterns of white. Table 13.5 lists genotypes of the different colors so that breeders can more adequately understand them and predict the possible color outcomes from mating various colors of horses. Table 13.6 outlines the various alleles present in different breeds. It can be used by breeders to develop the potential array of colors in various breeds. Table 13.7 is a large and cumbersome table that outlines the potential results of mating various parental colors. Table 13.8 has the details for horse names, breeds, and sources of photographs and other figures.

1.1 Basic Horse Color Identification

One purpose for understanding horse color is to be able to identify horses accurately. Accurate identification of horse color is a key ingredient in understanding the genetic or biologic basis of color and is the foundation upon which genetic investigations are built. Even a casual observer soon realizes that horses have a wide variety of colors. A standardized classification is necessary to begin communicating subtle differences between some specific horse colors. Any standardized system of color nomenclature depends on observers viewing a horse's color in the same general way.

Different languages and cultures each have distinct approaches to describing and classifying colors of horses. These distinctions are due to differences in deciding which specific characteristics of color are most important. Different classification systems each proceed logically from a few key characteristics, although these characteristics vary from system to system. The approach of each language has merit, even though the internal logic differs from one to another. Languages and cultures tend to vary enough that a concise one-to-one correlation of color names is usually impossible between languages, as certain details that are important in some languages are simply lacking in others.

An ideal system of horse color nomenclature would be one in which each unique color name (phenotype) corresponds to a specific genotype (genetic makeup) and each specific genotype results in a unique color or phenotype. An absolutely perfect one-to-one correspondence between genotypes and phenotypic nomenclature is lacking in all systems that are in use. Sometimes the lack of correspondence is for biologic reasons, but more frequently it arises from cultural or historic reasons.

Even though all systems fail to accomplish a tight one-to-one correspondence of terminology and genetic foundation, it is important to acknowledge that all nomenclature systems have a cultural and historic backdrop and that each has merit for specific details. For example, the one color group designated as **chestnut** in English is seen as three different colors (**alazán**, **ruano**, and **tostado**) by some Spanish-speaking traditions.

Attempts to force a genetically based nomenclature onto descriptions of horse color are becoming increasingly common. Though these systems may have great utility for horse breeders interested in producing specific colors, it is also true that many horse owners and enthusiasts find them confusing. These newer systems have failed to be adopted for general use because older and time-tested systems of nomenclature based on visual appearance have been successfully used for millennia and are difficult to replace.

As already noted, some single colors result from distinct and different genetic mechanisms, and therefore a one-to-one correspondence of genotype and color is impossible without genetic testing. As an example, many combinations of different dilution mechanisms are notoriously consistent in producing beige horses with pale brown manes, tails, and lower legs, and yet each of these horses comes to its similar color through a different genetic combination. These pale horses, though all a similar color, will each produce a very different array of colors in their foals. Devising unique names for each unique genetic combination can be useful to breeders but ignores the fact that the horses being described are all remarkably similar colors when seen out in the field. This is especially true if the horses are viewed at a distance.

The similar visual results of multiple genetic mechanisms are doubly confusing if nomenclature separates them and demands documentation of genes and alleles for each horse before it can be classified by color. A strategy for compensating for the lack of a one-to-one correspondence between nomenclature and genetics is to note the multiple genotypes included under a color name wherever possible. Likewise, the reverse problem of a single genotype giving rise to colors that are assigned different color names can be noted. These confusing situations are fortunately rare, so that a general trend toward one-to-one correspondence of color name to genotype is indeed the case. Those cases in which multiple mechanisms exist usually consist of one very common mechanism and one or two additional, but very rare, ones.

A few concepts form the sound foundation from which horse color can be understood, regardless of the system of nomenclature in use. The first important concept to understand in horse color identification is that background colors of horses occur independently of dilutions, and are also independent of any white markings horses may have. White hairs occur as a result of hair lacking pigment granules, so white patches, markings, or individual white hairs result from absence of color rather than being a true color in themselves. An incorrect belief, held by many people, is that various colors are superimposed on a white horse in much the same way that an artist applies paint to a white canvas. Any white areas, they believe, simply did not receive color. This incorrect idea, therefore, holds that horses are basically white. However, the truth is just the opposite; white is superimposed on and covers up areas genetically destined to be specific colors. The important detail is that the genetic actions determining the color of the pigmented areas generally operate independently of those determining the extent and location of the white areas.

It is very important that white be understood to be superimposed over some color that would otherwise have been present. All horses have the genetic capability to produce pigment over all the body. This capability has been changed on some horses (or on portions of some horses) by a superimposed genetic directive to impede the production of color, leaving white hairs or areas. The basic color of a horse must therefore be considered by first ignoring any white areas. Horses that are entirely white (or nearly so) will of course make this approach impossible. However, the tactic of first ignoring white does work well for most horses and is essential in deciding the basic color of a horse. For this reason, patterns of white are discussed in the chapters following those on basic colors because the two categories (color and patterns of white) are genetically distinct.

Another important concept is the definition of the "points" of a horse. In horse color terminology the points are the mane, tail, lower legs, and ear rims. The importance of the concept of the points is that their color usually determines the name given to the overall color combination on a horse. Specific combinations of point color and body color determine most horse color names.

The two main groups of horse colors are those with black points and those with nonblack points. Nonblack points are usually red or cream, but occasionally are a brown color. The division of points into black and nonblack is important for identification and also has important genetic implications. Specific combinations of point color with body color yield the final color name; so, once point color is appreciated, it becomes fairly easy to identify most horse colors.

Black and nonblack points are usually easy to distinguish from one another (Figures 1.1 and 1.2). In some instances black manes and tails become faded or sunburned to brown, and in these cases the lower leg is the most accurate indicator of point color. In most horses with black points the black carries to the hoof and involves at least the pastern. In most horses with nonblack points the pastern and coronary region are lighter than the remainder of the lower leg, so this region is very useful in deciding whether a horse has black or nonblack points. Distinguishing between the two groups of point color is usually simple because horses with confusing point color are rare.

Point color can be confusing on foals (Figure 1.3). Foals of all colors frequently have very pale points, even on those colors that have black points as adults. Even though experienced observers can usually predict adult coat color from characteristics of the foal coat, exceptions are numerous and frequent enough that everyone should be cautious in predicting adult color from foal coat color. Betting on the final color from a foal's coat is a good way to lose money, especially in breeds with wide color variation!

Also potentially confusing are horses with extensive white markings, because they can have their point color completely masked by the absence of pigment in these markings (Figure 1.4). In these cases mane and tail color become the most important indicator of point color, but even then it can still be difficult to accurately assess point color. It is essentially impossible to determine point color accurately on some horses with extensive white markings.

Various combinations of point colors and body colors are given different names in different geographic regions, and no single system or language is complete for naming

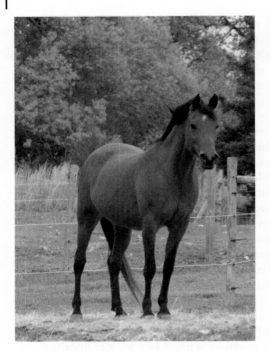

Figure 1.1 **Bay** horses have black points, which include the mane, tail, ear rims, and the lower portions of the legs. *Source:* courtesy of Dyan Westvang.

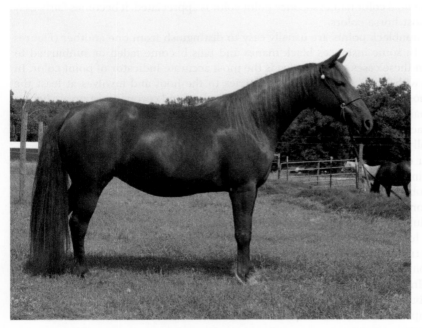

Figure 1.2 **Chestnut** horses have nonblack points. This horse has red points that are similar to the body color; however, point color can vary widely in horses with nonblack points. *Source:* courtesy of Dyan Westvang.

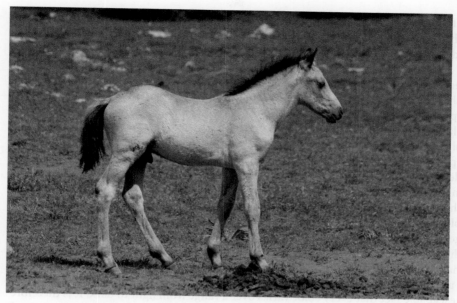

Figure 1.3 Foals of colors with black points, like this **dun**, usually do not have black points at birth but only develop them later. This is one reason adult colors can be difficult to predict from foal colors, even for experienced observers. *Source:* courtesy of Nancy Cerroni.

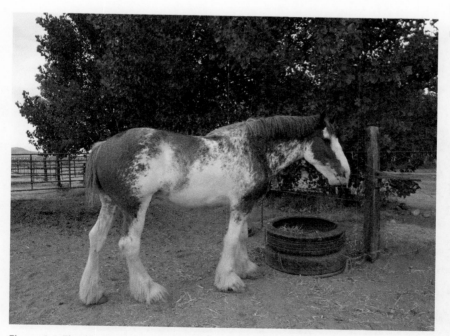

Figure 1.4 This **bay** horse has extensive white markings that obscure the lower leg color, leaving the mane and tail as the only accurate indicator of point color. On this horse, even the mane and tail are mixed with white hairs, although the basic black point color is still clearly evident. *Source:* courtesy of Jeannette Beranger.

the details of all of these combinations. The approach taken in this guide is consistent with the usual approach in the western USA. The westerners in the USA developed a fairly detailed vocabulary for describing horse color. This vocabulary functions well for nearly all color variations possible on horses. In addition, it usually corresponds well to the underlying genetic mechanisms. A few rare colors or combinations have no names in English. In such cases, other cultures or languages have been consulted for names and concepts that will help in understanding these rare colors and how they occur. While other languages and cultures have been considered, the final nomenclature is usually an English equivalent so that English speakers can more readily understand and use the concepts adopted from these sources.

A detail that can sometimes lead to confusion is that horses can vary in color from season to season or year to year (Figures 1.5 and 1.6). Horses are generally darkest when they shed their thick winter coats in the spring. Sun, wind, and rain can then act to bleach the color, although some horses remain unaffected by such weathering. Horses also can change shade of color due to their state of nutrition, condition, and general health. Healthy, well-fed, and well-conditioned horses are usually darker than are those less fortunate horses lacking the same benefits.

An additional detail that becomes a problem confronting an observer of horse color is the inescapable fact that every color varies over a range from light to dark. It is therefore always possible to find some individual horses that are at the boundary of two defined colors. This is simply a consequence of the complexity of the genetic control of horse color, coupled with the uncertainties and inconsistencies of the environment. A

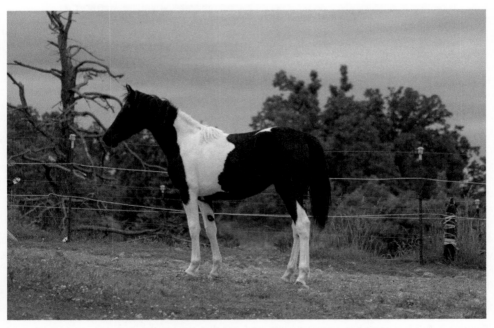

Figure 1.5 This is a **black tobiano** horse early in spring after shedding the winter coat, when colors are usually at their darkest and most distinct. *Source:* courtesy of Dyan Westvang.

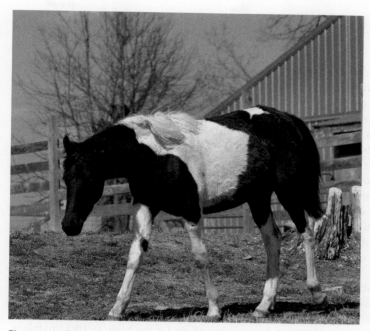

Figure 1.6 This is the same horse as in Figure 1.5, but in winter when the longer coat is much lighter. *Source:* courtesy of Dyan Westvang.

thorough understanding of the genetic control of horse color can be helpful in such instances because an observer is then at least able to understand how the color arose, and this can help answer the question of color terminology if only through the back door. The overall process of correctly identifying horse color begins with the descriptive stage. Descriptive knowledge helps in the understanding and appreciation of the biologic (genetic) control of color. Finally, knowledge of genetic control circles back to enhance the appreciation of descriptive categories and subtleties.

Horse color is generally believed by most breeders to be only a cosmetic detail. But many horse owners, and indeed entire horse-using cultures, have long attributed specific characteristics to horses of specific colors. Such beliefs are generally dismissed as fiction, but a kernel of truth may well lie behind a few of them. A small collection of European research has verified that horses of specific colors do tend to react somewhat predictably in certain situations and that these reactions vary from color to color. A general trend seems to be that horses of darker colors are livelier than lighter ones, but the breeds in which this was determined were not noted, so the range of colors is likewise uncertain. While any behavioral connections to horse color are far from proven, these tidbits of folklore will be noted as the different colors are discussed. Even though relationships of behavior and color are speculative, they are an interesting part of the art of horse breeding and horse keeping. The interaction of color and behavior is treated briefly in Hemmer's (1990) *Domestication: The Decline of Environmental Appreciation*, listed in the Bibliography.

1.2   Basic Principles of Genetics, Genomics, and Molecular Biology

A thorough understanding of the genetic control of horse color takes study and hard work. The reward is an enhanced appreciation of horses and the biology behind their beauty, as well as more accurate descriptions of horses for registration purposes. An understanding of genetics is almost essential for breeders interested in producing specific colors of foals. An overview of some principles of genetics as well as some definitions of genetic terms is a good starting point for this endeavor.

A horse's color results from the interaction of several generally independent processes (or factors). About 14 of these have been documented to date, and account for nearly all variations in horse color. Most of these processes are known to involve a specific gene. Others have only been characterized visually, such as **mushroom**, but have not yet been characterized genetically. Interaction of so many factors unfortunately means that the control of color is inherently complicated; it cannot be made completely simple. The interaction of all of the factors results in the many different shades and types of horse colors.

For most colors, each specific combination of interacting components results in a unique color. A few colors are exceptions to this rule. The genetic basis of the colors, therefore, neatly explains most of the colors by accounting for the complex interactions that cause them. These interactions can be understood best if the basic factors are taken one at a time. In this way the number of complex interactions can be broken down into fewer key components, and the colors can be understood sequentially by adding the effects of each of the processes in turn. The genetic basis for most of the 14 processes controlling color has been documented by a variety of scientific studies, resulting in a fairly complete understanding of them. However, the theoretical basis for some of the processes is currently only an educated guess.

Genes are responsible for all biochemical processes that occur in living organisms. They are defined as units of heredity and they carry the information from one generation to the next by storing the information inside the nucleus of each cell. Genes code for the necessary information to make life processes happen, as explained in more detail later. Genes themselves are composed of DNA. DNA is made up of building blocks that are linked together to form a long chain. These building blocks are known as nucleotides, and they come in four types. For simplicity these are referred to by the abbreviations A (for adenine), T (for thymine), C (for cytosine), and G (for guanine). Each gene has a unique sequence of these four building blocks of DNA, allowing it to store the information to perform a specific function in the cell. This information typically codes for proteins. The stored information in the form of DNA (nucleic acid) can be translated into a new language for proteins (made of amino acids rather than nucleic acids). Proteins perform most of the functions in the cell, so the DNA code directly affects cell function.

It is the precise order and combination of the DNA nucleotide building blocks that makes one gene different from the next. Any given gene can have slight modifications in the order of the building blocks. These alternative forms of genes are known as alleles. Alleles differ from one another in many possible ways. The alleles are referred to as polymorphisms, meaning "many forms." A simple example is the situation in which one nucleotide differs between two alleles of a given gene. For example the short sequence of nucleotides TAGACAT could be changed to TACACAT (genes have nucleotide sequences of hundreds or more than thousands of nucleotides, so this short sequence is not an entire gene). In this example "C" replaces the third "G." This difference is called a single nucleotide polymorphism, or SNP for short. This variation can be translated differently from DNA to protein, much the way "TAG A CAT" means something different than "TAC A CAT." Modifications in the order of the nucleotide building blocks change the function of the gene because the resulting protein has a different sequence of amino acids, all caused by changes in the original genetic code. When the genetic code is altered in this fashion the result is called a "missense mutation." This is a change in the DNA sequence that results in substituting one amino acid for another in the final protein product.

Other changes include insertions of extra nucleotides into the sequence, which shifts the way the code is read and therefore the final product. Another type of change occurs when portions of the code are deleted. The missing segments likewise change the final message, and therefore the final protein that is made from the message.

Most genes in organisms that have cells with a nucleus (including horses) are organized by alternating different sorts of DNA sequences. These are known as "exons" and "introns." The sequences that actually code for the protein product are the exons; as a result, the changes in those regions can change the final protein product, and therefore also change its biologic function. The exons are interrupted by the introns, which are sequences that do not code for the final protein. While the introns do not code for the protein product, many of the introns do have important regulatory functions that instruct the cell as to how to put the exons together. The consequence of this is that mutations in the intron sequences can still have consequences for the final action of the gene. Two examples, discussed in more detail later, are *brindle 1* (Chapter 3) and *sabino 1* (Chapter 7).

In horses, as in all mammals, genes occur on chromosomes. A simple way to imagine this is that chromosomes are long stretches of DNA. The DNA is folded up with proteins known as histones to fit inside the nucleus of the cell. Horses have two copies of every chromosome for a total of 32 pairs (Figure 1.7). Each pair of chromosomes contains specific genes.

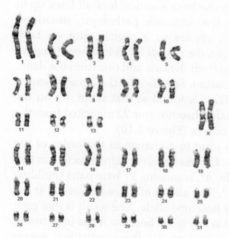

Figure 1.7 The microscopic chromosomes in a cell can be photographed, cut apart, and then arranged in their pairs. The resulting array is called a karyotype. Horses have 32 pairs of chromosomes. *Source:* courtesy of Dr. Teri Lear.

The complete set of an organism's genes is referred to as its genome. The genome represents the DNA from one set of the chromosomes. The first horse genome (from a **grey** Thoroughbred mare) was sequenced in 2009. An entire horse genome contains approximately 2.7 billion DNA nucleotide building blocks.

The most modern techniques reveal that chromosome organization is very complicated, but they can still be loosely thought of as strings of genes. The genes are something like beads of information, and thinking of them this way facilitates understanding the basics of their function as genetic units passing from generation to generation.

Chromosomes occur in pairs; an individual gets one of the pair from the sire and the other from the dam. When an individual reproduces, it contributes a random half of its chromosomes (one of each pair) to its offspring. The other half of the resulting offspring's genetic makeup comes from the mate. This halving of genetic material from parents and pairing in offspring is the mechanism by which the genetic code works its way through generations and populations, and is also the source of variation from parents to offspring as the combinations are reshuffled in each generation. This separation and rejoining is the basis of heredity and explains how two offspring from the same two parents can look different—they each received a different "half" of the genetic material from the parents.

It is essential to understand the concept of halving and subsequent rejoining into pairs at each generational step in order to appreciate the impact of genetics on horse color (Figure 1.8). The recombination of pairs at each generation is the basis of how genetics operates. The components of the pairs are constrained by the specific variants in the parents, and only those parental variants will be available for contribution to the offspring. Recombining of genes from generation to generation is frequently called "segregation" because the genes can appear in different combinations at each generational step.

Each gene occupies a specific site on a specific chromosome. This site is called a locus (plural, loci), and frequently genes are described by their locus names. Locus simply means an address for a gene; it is a specific physical place that a gene occupies. For example, the gene responsible for appaloosa patterns is located at a specific locus on horse chromosome 1 (Figure 1.9).

Both members of a pair of chromosomes in a horse have identical loci, all lined up in the same sequence. The only exceptions are a few, generally pathologic, situations. Usually, the term locus, even though singular, applies to a specific site on both chromosomes of an individual animal. For example, the *Agouti* locus in a horse implies the specific genetic site on two chromosomes (one from the sire, and one from the dam), each coding for the same piece of genetic information. Specifically, the *Agouti* locus is found at a specific site on horse chromosome 22. It is found at that same site on the chromosome 22 inherited from the sire as well as the chromosome 22 inherited from the dam, and indeed is at that same location in all horses (Figure 1.10).

When a gene occurs in more than one form (due to a change in the order of the nucleotides), the different forms are called alleles. For example, the *Agouti* locus has two well-characterized alleles (Figure 1.11). One allele, A^a, is missing 11 base pairs (building blocks) when compared with the other allele, A^A. The alleles of a gene all occur at the same locus, although each chromosome can only have one allele. The result is that each horse has, at most, a total of two different alleles at any locus because it has only two of each chromosome. The wide variety of horse colors results from individual horses

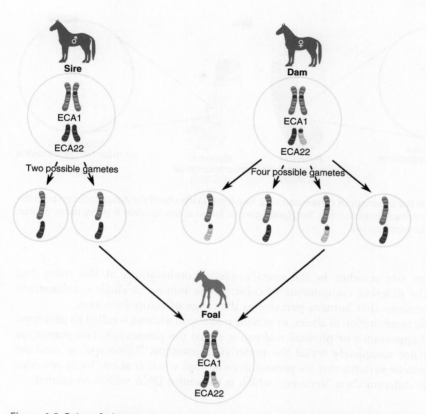

Figure 1.8 Pairs of chromosomes separate at random during the formation of egg and sperm, and these pairs then rejoin during fertilization. This separation and rejoining is the basis of heredity. This figure shows only one possible result, and illustrates how new combinations can be formed as a consequence of the process of reshuffling the chromosomes. *Source:* courtesy of Francesca Gianino.

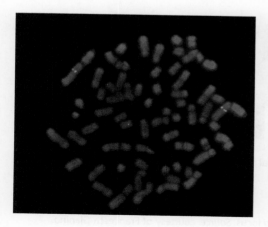

Figure 1.9 This is a horse karyotype as it appears before cutting the image and pairing up the chromosomes. The green dye indicates the locus for appaloosa pattern (*LP*), and lights up the same specific site on both copies of chromosome 1. *Source:* courtesy of Dr. Teri Lear.

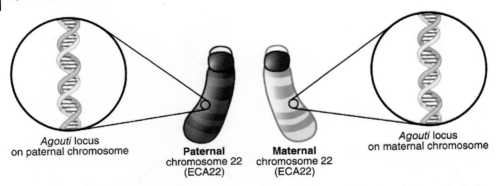

Figure 1.10 This is a schematic of chromosome 22, highlighting the site of the *Agouti* locus on both the maternal and paternal chromosomes. The *Agouti* gene is found at this location in every horse. *Source:* courtesy of Francesca Gianino.

differing from one another in the specific allelic combinations at the many loci controlling the different components of color. These numerous allelic combinations cause the variations that humans perceive as the range of colors in horses.

The specific combination of alleles, or genetic makeup of a horse, is called its genotype. The external appearance or physical makeup is called the phenotype. The phenotype may or may not completely reveal the underlying genotype. "Genotype" is used for the specific genetic variants that are present in an animal, whether at one locus or many. This is subtly different than "genome," which is the entire DNA within an animal.

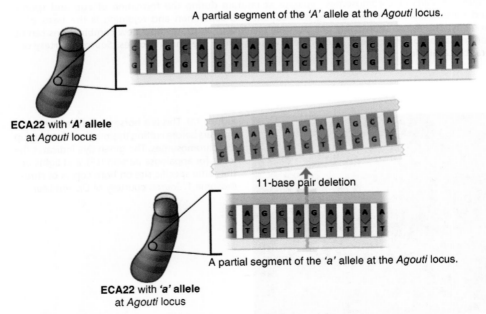

Figure 1.11 The two known alleles at the *Agouti* locus. *Source:* courtesy of Francesca Gianino.

The condition of having two identical alleles at a locus (one on each chromosome) is called "homozygous." When the alleles are different, the situation is called "heterozygous." This terminology (homozygous/heterozygous at a locus) reflects back to the concept of "locus" as encompassing a specific site on both of two chromosomes that codes for the same gene and the fact that an individual horse only has two of each chromosome. As a result, the only options at a locus are to have two identical copies of the gene (homozygous) or one copy of each of two different alleles of the gene (heterozygous).

Alleles at a genetic locus interact in a variety of ways. Some alleles are not expressed phenotypically unless both copies of the gene in an individual are the same (homozygous). These are recessive alleles (or genes, the two terms are sometimes used interchangeably). Dominant alleles, in contrast, are expressed identically whether in one copy (heterozygous) or two copies (homozygous). The main concept is that a dominant allele masks the phenotypic expression of a recessive allele when the two are paired together in the heterozygous condition. As a result, colors associated with recessive alleles can appear to pop up out of nowhere because they can be carried along, unexpressed phenotypically, as long as they are paired with a dominant allele. They can be carried along this way for several generations.

Recessive alleles are perceived as surprises when they become expressed by virtue of being paired in the homozygous offspring of two individuals that carry them. In this case, the carrier parents do not show the effect of these alleles because they are being masked by a dominant allele. Dominant alleles cannot be carried along in a hidden state in this manner. If a dominant allele is present, it is expressed phenotypically. As a result, the presence of dominant alleles shows up in each generation and they are therefore are not the source of surprises except very rarely, such as in the case of a spontaneous mutation. Mating of recessive to recessive can yield no surprises because nothing is hidden, and the phenotype therefore betrays the genotype completely, or nearly so.

It is important to understand that the character of an allele as dominant or recessive is inherent in the functional capability of the allele itself. This does not change over time, nor does it change in various situations. Many people are under the mistaken impression that dominant alleles are necessarily common and that recessive alleles are necessarily rare. The issue of allele frequency is totally separate from the issue of dominance and recessiveness. Some recessive alleles, such as *chestnut*, are indeed common to the point of being uniform throughout some breeds of horses, such as the Suffolk or the Haflinger. The uniformity of the *chestnut* allele in the Suffolk in no way changes its character as a recessive allele, so that crosses of Suffolks to black Percherons result in few if any chestnut foals, because the black points of the Percheron will dominate the *chestnut* allele of the Suffolks. Likewise, some dominant alleles, such as *white*, are incredibly rare or nonexistent in most breeds and yet are routinely passed as dominant alleles in those few families in which they occur.

Some alleles are described as incompletely dominant, which means that two, one, or no copies each results in a separate appearance. Each situation can be detected phenotypically by examining external appearance. Incompletely dominant systems are the easiest to understand, because no surprises can result, such as occur with hidden recessive alleles. With incompletely dominant alleles the two different homozygous genotypes, as well as the heterozygous genotype, each have a distinct phenotypic appearance.

Another interaction of genes is called epistasis. This refers to the ability of specific allelic combinations at one locus to mask the expression of alleles at another locus. Epistasis is another example of the complexity of genetic interactions. It is similar to the relationships of dominant and recessive alleles, but concerns two or more loci instead of only one. The locus that is masked by an epistatic gene (or allelic combination) is referred to as being hypostatic, while the locus or gene combination causing the masking is called epistatic. Hypostatic genes can pop up as surprises, much as do recessive genes when masked by dominant ones. Specific examples in the discussion of the colors will illustrate this phenomenon and will help in the understanding of what can be a subtle and confusing concept.

Genetic loci can be considered as separate little biochemical factories. Each locus controls some unique aspect of the color that is finally produced and seen. It is convenient to consider the control exercised by each locus as a decision mechanism. At most loci the choice is either "situation A" or "situation B." Thinking about the loci as responsible for separate decisions helps in understanding that each locus presents a choice, and the sum of all the choices will affect the resulting color. If each locus is considered to make a separate component of the final appearance, it is easier to understand how color arises as the final result of specific combinations of choices.

As an illustration, consider horse color to be like a cup of coffee. The first choice is to have dark roast or light roast, which determines the base color. The next choice is to add cream, or not, which will either dilute the base color or leave it dark. Finally, any sweeteners can be added, just like adding white patterns to a horse. Much in the same way that the final cup of coffee is dependent on which choices were made at each of the decision steps, a horse's final appearance is the result of the combination of all the options encoded in the alleles of the genes. By understanding the components it is possible to appreciate the interactions that led to the color that is present on the horse. Because each locus has only two (or a few) choices, the components are fairly easy to understand once they are identified and appreciated as basic components of a final combination. The concept of each locus doing a separate job is the key to understanding the genetic basis of horse color. By viewing genetics in this way it is possible to appreciate how the various colors can be built in successive steps from the various component parts.

Genetic nomenclature is subject to a number of conventions, and these are variable in much of the literature. A standard format is used throughout this guide, and follows the guidelines of the Committee on Genetic Nomenclature of Sheep and Goats, which has been expanded to now include other domesticated animals. Names of loci have an initial capital letter to distinguish them from names of alleles, which are all in lowercase letters. Both loci and alleles are in italic type. *Dun* is a locus, *black* is an allele. The symbols for loci are abbreviations of the names and are in italics, with an initial capital letter. Allele symbols are added to locus symbols as superscripts to separate them from the locus symbol. The symbol "+" is used to denote the probable wild-type allele at a locus.

For example, Dn^+ is the *wild-type* allele at the *Dun* locus. The wild type is inferred from the probable original color of horses before their domestication. Inferring the wild-type color is important for genetic nomenclature, but has become more difficult because the sequencing of DNA from fossil remains has indicated multiple color variants were present in horses before the time of domestication. While the list is incomplete,

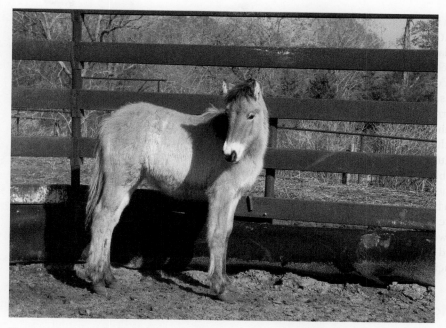

Figure 1.12 This light **zebra dun** with the **mealy** overlay is likely the original color of horses. *Source:* courtesy of Jeannette Beranger.

Siberian Pleistocene animals included **bay**-based horses and a few others. Some evidence points to the *leopard* allele being present before domestication. Similarly, the *black* allele and the *non-dun* allele have also been found in at least some pre-domesticated horses. While assigning a single wild-type color is increasingly difficult, it is most likely that a light yellow, shaded version of **dun** was the most common wild-type color, similar to the color of today's Przewalski's horse and present only rarely in most horse breeds (Figure 1.12). This color is taken as the single wild-type color in this work, despite its limitations.

Symbols for alleles other than *wild type* are standardized so that dominant alleles have an initial capital letter, while those for recessive alleles have a lowercase letter. This convention is used even though names of both dominant and recessive alleles, when spelled out and not referred to by abbreviated symbols, have an initial lowercase letter. As a result, *dominant black* is an allele proposed at the *Extension* locus, and has the symbol E^D.

Another convention is the abbreviation of genotypes by using dashes to fill in behind dominant alleles when the second of the pair is unknown or unimportant for determining phenotype. For example, A^A— (*bay* at the *Agouti* locus) can be used for $A^A A^A$ and $A^A A^a$, which both appear the same phenotypically. $A^a A^a$ (a homozygous genotype with two *black* alleles at the *Agouti* locus) has no abbreviation, because a recessive genotype masks nothing, although sometimes a single A^a is used as a phenotypic abbreviation for $A^a A^a$.

A further problem in nomenclature is becoming increasingly frequent as the biochemistry and molecular mechanisms of the gene products become established. It is now common for the older symbols to not match the loci documented by results of molecular investigations. Most of the newer locus names and symbols are based on mouse nomenclature, because the molecular genetics of mice has been so much more extensively characterized than has that of any other species. For example, the *Agouti* locus encodes for the protein called the agouti signaling protein (ASIP). The result is that this locus, traditionally represented as the *A* locus, is also represented as the *ASIP* locus in modern studies. In this text the molecular loci are noted, while the older symbols are still retained because long use has made these widely accepted and understood. To change them in order to match the molecular aspects would increase confusion, rather than reduce it, because so many of those interested in horse color first encountered the earlier abbreviations and are now familiar with them.

Another convention used throughout this guide is the printing of names of horse colors in bold type. This reduces confusion between a discussion of a color in general and a specific name for a horse color. Black, for example, is a general name for a color in nature, while **black** is specifically the color of a **black** horse. Other peculiarities of eye color and hair are also printed in bold type because these also have specific connotations when their use concerns horses.

1.3 Pigment Cell Function and Genetic Control

A fundamental principle to understand about horse color is that color in horses is due to the presence of pigments in the hair. Two major pigments account for all colors of mammals (including horses). One of these is eumelanin (YOO mel a nin), which is responsible for black or slate blue. In a very small number of horses eumelanin is brown (flat, chocolate brown) rather than black. This chocolate brown type is similar to the color that is common in retriever or spaniel dogs. The switch between black and brown eumelanin is an "either/or" phenomenon for the whole horse: a horse can form either black or brown, but not both. This is an important detail, even though the colors based on brown are so rare.

The other pigment is pheomelanin (FEE oh mel a nin), which produces colors ranging from reddish brown or tan to yellow. Pheomelanin can vary in shade on a single horse, and on many individual horses pheomelanic areas do indeed vary from dark to light. Most horses have both pheomelanic and eumelanic areas on them and are therefore combinations of black along with red- or yellow-pigmented areas. Dark pheomelanin sometimes can resemble brown eumelanin and is much more common than eumelanin as a source of any brown areas on horses. Pheomelanin usually retains at least some of its reddish color, even when very dark, and this reddish tinge helps to distinguish pheomelanic areas from eumelanic areas.

White hairs result from a lack of pigment granules, and these are essentially hairs without color. Skin that lacks pigment granules is characteristically pink, and it gets its pink tone from the presence of blood in small, superficial blood vessels.

Color in horses is possible because pigment cells, called melanocytes, act to put pigment granules into cells that become hair and skin. The presence and function of these cells determines the amount, type, and character of pigmentation. Melanocytes migrate to the skin in embryonic life. They originate along the neural crest, a specific group of embryonic cells that also give rise to the spinal cord and brain. The importance

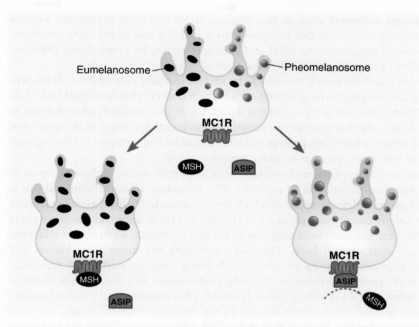

Figure 1.13 Pigment cells are capable of producing two types of pigment, which is regulated by the activation or inactivation of a cell surface receptor (MC1R). When MSH is bound to the receptor, it activates the receptor and the cell then produces eumelanin (black or brown pigment). When ASIP is bound to the receptor, then the receptor is blocked, cannot be activated, and the cell produces only pheomelanin (red or yellow pigment). *Source:* courtesy of Francesca Gianino.

of this detail is that the pigmentary system and the nervous system are closely allied in embryologic life, and some specific genes affect both of these systems instead of only one or the other.

Melanocytes can produce either pheomelanin or eumelanin (Figure 1.13). The determination of which pigment is formed is accomplished by a receptor that is on the surface of melanocytes. This receptor is the melanocortin 1 receptor, or MC1R for short, and is activated by a protein known as melanocyte-stimulating hormone (MSH). This hormone is produced by the pituitary gland, located at the base of the brain. In the absence of activation by MSH, cells form pheomelanin. When the receptor is activated, the result is eumelanin formation.

The switch between eumelanin and pheomelanin production can be influenced at several different steps. One switch is the presence or absence of MSH (the protein hormone that activates the receptor just described). This is a fairly rare switching mechanism in animals, and is unimportant in horse color because MSH is thought to be constantly available to all cells of horses.

A second switch is at the level of surface receptors. These are produced by genetic codes at the *Extension* locus as well as a few other loci. In other words, the *Extension* locus codes for MC1R. Some mutations, such as *dominant black*, produce a receptor stuck in the "on" position in many species. This is called a gain-of-function mutation. The result is an entirely eumelanic, usually black, phenotype. In this situation the receptor is always activated, even in the absence of MSH. Other mutations, such as *chestnut*, result in a totally inactive receptor (this is called a loss-of-function mutation) that is incapable of responding to MSH and therefore results in a completely pheomelanic (red/yellow) phenotype in most cases.

A third way to affect the switch is to block the surface receptor externally. This leads to an inability of the receptor to be activated even though the receptor is normal and MSH is present. This mechanism is typical of the *Agouti* locus and results in pheomelanin in those areas of the body that express the agouti protein (causing a blocked receptor) and eumelanin in others where this protein is lacking (unblocked receptor). The regional distribution of the agouti protein is under genetic control.

The internal workings of the melanocyte are as important as the surface receptor in determining the final production of pigment. The formation of eumelanin and pheomelanin involves several steps, some of which are common to both pigments and some of which are unique to only one pigment or the other. This is important because some mutations affect the production of only one of the two pigments, while others affect the production and character of both. The loci controlling the internal packaging and production of pigment in horses are increasingly being characterized at the molecular level. As a result, past uncertainty concerning homologous loci (those with identical function) in other species is slowly being resolved. This contributes to deeper understanding of the specific mechanisms leading to the various colors of horses.

The pigments are formed in small packages called melanosomes. These can be moved from the melanocyte to surrounding hair and skin cells. The packaging and distribution of melanosomes is another potential site of variation, which can result in different visual appearances of colors that are caused by identical pigments. These changes are under genetic control at yet other loci distinct from those already mentioned.

Mutations can occur in the surface receptors themselves (*Extension* locus), or the proteins that bind directly to them (*Agouti* locus). The consequence of these surface changes is stimulation or blockage of these receptors, which results in changes in the type of pigment produced (eumelanin versus pheomelanin). In contrast to these surface changes, changes in the internal machinery of the melanocyte usually result in changes in the amount of pigment that is produced or how it is packaged. The consequences of internal changes usually then determine the degree of dilution of pigment rather than changes in the specific pigment type. These include loci controlling *Dun*, *MATP* (*Cream and Pearl*), *Champagne*, *PMEL17* (*Silver Dapple*), and *Mushroom*. The difference between the two sites ("surface" versus "internal to the cell") is basically one of "which" (surface) versus "how much" (internal).

White patterns are controlled at yet other loci that affect the migration, survival, or function of melanocytes. A handful of loci consistently cause white patterns in several species. One of these is the receptor for endothelin B, which is affected by the *frame* mutation. Other good candidates for white-pattern mutations include the mast cell growth factor locus (the *KIT* locus). This locus appears to be affected by many mutations and is thought to be the locus responsible for several different white patterns such as *roan*, various *sabino* mutations, and *dominant white*, among others. This locus is also very close to the allele for *tobiano*. The homologies of white-pattern alleles with those of other species are still not fully documented in horses.

By mid-2016, 40 polymorphisms in at least 14 genes had been identified that contribute to or are associated with horse color variation. While the resulting biochemical mechanisms have been extensively studied for some of these, the functions of others are only speculative. Some of these discoveries were aided by the sequencing of the reference horse genome that was published in 2009. Additionally, sequencing the genomes of horses from a variety of different breeds has allowed for the development of new tools that help to identify chromosomal regions and mutations associated with different phenotypes. These include coat color as well as disease and performance traits. These new tools, along with new sequencing techniques, will undoubtedly hasten the pace of characterization of the genes involved in different color phenotypes, and will also reveal novel genetic mechanisms involved in producing them.

2

Basic Dark Horse Colors: Bay, Chestnut, Black, and Brown

2.1 Bay, Chestnut, and Black

2.1.1 Definition and Classification

Dark horse colors are generally the most common colors in any breed, and the most common of these are usually referred to as "dark" or "hard" colors. Most observers include **bay**, **black**, **brown**, and **chestnut** as the "hard colors." Occasionally **grey** is classified among these, but because **grey** is a pattern of white hairs it will be considered separately with other patterns of white. The three colors (which are really two colors and one pattern) **bay**, **chestnut**, and **grey** account for the coat color phenotype of the vast majority of horses. The simplest way to untangle the complexity of a horse's coat color is to first determine the base as **bay**, **chestnut**, **brown**, or **black**, and then identify the various modifications superimposed on these basic four. Understanding the relationship of these four is the basis for comprehending all of the other colors, because one of these lies at the base of almost all other colors.

Bay (Figure 2.1) describes horses with black points and reddish brown body color. **Bay** is the most frequent horse color. **Bay** horses are very widespread and are common in all but a handful of breeds. All breeds in which **bay** does not occur have been defined more or less as encompassing other specific colors, and **bay** is simply not one of those colors. Examples are the Friesian (**black**), Percheron (**black** or **grey**, rarely **chestnut**), Haflinger (**chestnut** and **sorrel**), and Suffolk Punch (**chestnut**) breeds. Selection in all of these breeds has eliminated the **bay** color that is otherwise so common in horses. In contrast, at least one breed consists of **bay** horses only: the Cleveland Bay.

Folk wisdom holds that **bays** are sanguine. They are reputed to be quiet and inconspicuous and tend to be durable and rather average, steady horses. If true, these characteristics could well account for the widespread distribution of this color! Some Polish investigations in the Arabian breed suggest that **bays** mature more slowly than **chestnut** horses, but that **bays** tend to have longer racing careers, although other more recent research findings refute this relationship.

Chestnut (Figure 2.2) is another common dark color, usually second in frequency to **bay** in most breeds of horses. **Chestnut** horses are some shade of red and have nonblack points. The basic **chestnut** shade is essentially red all over, in contrast to the black points on **bay** horses. **Chestnut** is common in most breeds of horses, although it is rare in the Highland, Connemara, and Percheron. It is eliminated, or nearly so, in the Friesian,

Equine Color Genetics, Fourth Edition. D. Phillip Sponenberg and Rebecca Bellone.
© 2017 John Wiley & Sons, Inc. Published 2017 by John Wiley & Sons, Inc.

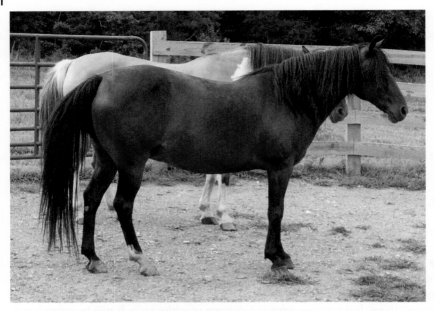

Figure 2.1 **Bay** is typically a red-based body with black points. The white marks on the legs can obscure the black points, although if these are minimal (as on this mare) the underlying point color is usually obvious.

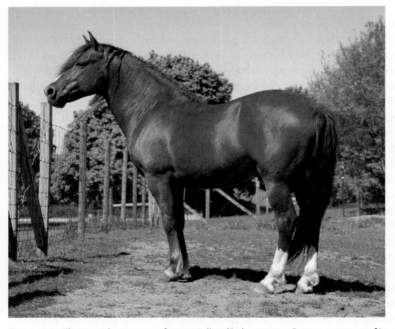

Figure 2.2 **Chestnut** horses are often an "all red" phenotype. *Source*: courtesy of Laura Hornick Behning.

Cleveland Bay, Exmoor, and, at least temporarily in the recent past, the Andalusian. In these breeds it has generally been eliminated by selection, but a few **chestnuts** still do rarely occur from time to time. Some breeds, such as the Haflinger or the Suffolk Punch, are all **chestnut** (although spelled "**chesnut**" by breeders of the Suffolk Punch breed) as a result of past selection for a restricted color range.

Folk wisdom holds that **chestnuts** are choleric. Some observers indicate that **chestnut** horses are flightier than **bays** and tend to react more strongly to external stimuli than do **bays**. They are also more vigilant and watchful than are horses of other colors. They mature more quickly than **bays**. A few early studies provided tantalizing evidence that at least in Polish Arabians the **chestnut** horses had better average race performance at younger ages. More recent studies have refuted these tendencies, though, and found that the color of Thoroughbreds and Arabians has no effect on racing performance. The recent studies have been more carefully done and failed to indicate any difference in temperament among the different coat colors. This part of traditional lore may in fact not be founded on true tendencies.

Black horses have black bodies and black points (Figure 2.3). **Black** is generally less frequent than **bay** or **chestnut** in most breeds. Many horse fanciers are fairly stingy in their use of the term **black** and reserve it for those horses that have absolutely no brown or red hairs anywhere on the body. Such brown or red hairs, when they occur, are usually on the muzzle or in the flanks, and many observers consider **black** horses with even a few of these lighter hairs as a type of **brown** instead of truly **black**. This may be somewhat too stringent from the genetics point of view, but it is the generally accepted approach of many horse fanciers. Even horses that are truly **black** vary somewhat in the depth of the

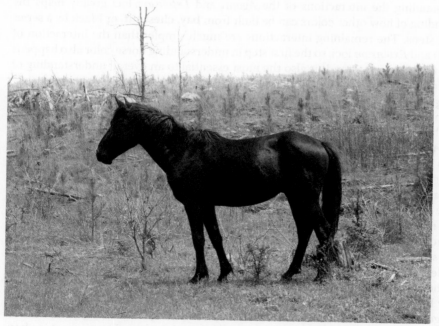

Figure 2.3 This **black** stallion has the typical uniform appearance of most **black** horses. *Source:* courtesy of Jeannette Beranger.

color. Spanish observers get around the problem of defining **black** by resorting to "dark" (*prieto* in Mexico, *oscuro* in Argentina) for describing this color.

Black horses are rare in many breeds of horses, even though the color does occur in most breeds. Exceptions include breeds for which a narrow range of colors has become the standard: Haflinger, Fjord, Cleveland Bay, and Suffolk Punch. The frequency of **black** varies both with fashion and with breed. Some breeds, such as the Percheron, are usually **black**, although other colors do occur. Other breeds, like the Friesian, are consistently **black** because the rare foals that are not **black** are denied registration. **Black** horses are also common in the Shire breed. **Black** horses are fairly common in some other breeds, especially those based either on Spanish breeding or on heavy horse breeding. This contrasts with their rarity in most breeds in which Arabian or Thoroughbred ancestry predominates.

Black horses are reputed by folk wisdom to be melancholic and are "sleepier" than horses of the other hard colors. **Black** horses do hold an almost mystic fascination for many people, as characterized by the popular series of children's books about a **black** stallion (including *The Black Stallion*) by Walter Farley.

2.1.2 Genetic Control

The genetic control of the **bay**, **chestnut**, and **black** colors of horses is the result of interaction at two genetic loci: *Agouti* and *Extension*. It is possible to build most other horse colors step by step from these three dark colors, so they are a good starting point for discussion of horse color genetics. The two loci control the expression of these three basic colors.

Understanding the interactions of the *Agouti* and *Extension* loci greatly helps the understanding of how other colors can be built from **bay**, **chestnut**, or **black** by a series of logical steps. The remaining interactions are much simpler than the interaction of the *Agouti* and *Extension* loci, so the first step in understanding horse color also happens to be the trickiest to master. It is also the most essential to an overall understanding of horse color.

The *Agouti* locus is named after a South American rodent, which explains its rather unusual name. The *Agouti* locus controls the relative distribution of black and red areas on those horses that are capable of forming black pigment. Another way of stating this is that the *Agouti* locus determines the basic color of horses with black points. Although this is an oversimplification, it is certainly true for the vast majority of horses.

The *Agouti* locus codes for the protein called ASIP, the name coming from mouse nomenclature. Mouse nomenclature is increasingly used across all species due to more complete investigations of mouse genetics than is typical of most other species. Because its use is not yet completely uniform the locus is variably referred to as *Agouti* or *ASIP*.

The most common allele at the *Agouti* locus is a dominant allele. It restricts black to the points, resulting in **bay** horses. The recessive allele results in a uniformly **black** horse. These alleles can be symbolized in the usual genetic shorthand as A^A for *bay* and A^a for *black*. The various combinations are then $A^A A^A$ or $A^A A^a$ resulting in **bay** horses and $A^a A^a$ for **black**. The usual shorthand shortens this even further by lumping $A^A A^A$ and $A^A A^a$ together as A^A— because the second member of the pair is unimportant to the visible color and cannot be determined by visual inspection alone. Figuring out if a **bay** horse has a **black** recessive allele historically required knowing the color of parents, or offspring, or both. Currently, a DNA-based genetic test is available that is a specific assay for the presence or absence of the *black* allele. The test functions by detecting the specific mutation, *black*, which is due to an 11 base-pair deletion within the *ASIP* locus (Figures 1.11 and 2.4). **Black** is a rare color in most breeds, so most **bay** horses are $A^A A^A$ and not $A^A A^a$.

The ASIP blocks the melanocyte surface receptor from activation by the MSH. The protein acts as an antagonist to MSH, preventing interaction of the hormone with the receptor. Body areas in which the agouti protein is expressed cannot respond to stimulation by MSH, and therefore can form only pheomelanin (tan or red pigment). Areas lacking the agouti protein have receptors that are unblocked, can respond to MSH, and as a result form eumelanin (black pigment). The distribution of areas with the protein is generally symmetrical, so that the resulting distribution of pheomelanin and eumelanin is consistently symmetrical. At the biochemical level, a horse of genotype $A^a A^a$ produces an ASIP that is not functional, and as a result it is unable to block the MSH receptor. Such animals can produce only black pigment. This is illustrated in Figure 2.4.

It is logical that the more red/tan *Agouti* patterns (**bay**) are dominant to those less red/tan (**black**) because a single copy of an allele forming the ASIP is sufficient to block the action of the MSH in any regions in which it is expressed.

The *Extension* locus interacts with the *Agouti* locus to provide the three basic horse colors. The recessive *chestnut* allele (E^e) results in uniformly red horses without black points. This causes **chestnut** horses, and $E^e E^e$ results in **chestnut** regardless of which alleles are present at the *Agouti* locus. This is a key concept in understanding horse coat color genetics: the recessive $E^e E^e$ genotype at the *Extension* locus completely masks the *Agouti* genotype. That is, the $E^e E^e$ combination is epistatic to the *Agouti* locus. The *Agouti* locus is therefore hypostatic, because it is the one whose expression is masked. A useful shorthand for **chestnut** is $—, E^e E^e$, which indicates that the *Agouti* genotype is unimportant to the visible phenotype.

The *Extension* locus codes for the MSH receptor itself. The mouse locus is *MC1R* (an abbreviation of *melanocortin 1 receptor*) and it is sometimes referred to by this name in the horse. The effects of mutations at this locus are easily understood if it is remembered that they influence the receptor involved in switching between eumelanin and pheomelanin production. In all species, recessive alleles at this locus generally arise from mutations that make the receptor totally inactive. In horses, the E^e allele is the result of a single base change in the DNA sequence that results in an amino acid change in the MSH receptor. This change causes the receptor to be inactive. Melanocytes in horses that are homozygous for this allele cannot respond to MSH, which basically makes any blockage by ASIP irrelevant. The result of this defective receptor is a totally pheomelanic animal, which is **chestnut** in horses unless further modified by other loci.

The function of the *Extension* locus helps to explain why the $E^e E^e$ genotype is epistatic to the *Agouti* locus. The receptor is defective, so it does not matter whether the ASIP is present or not because the melanocytes can only produce pheomelanin. It is logical that this action is recessive, because a single copy of the wild-type allele would code for a normal receptor. The presence of any level of normal receptor would easily override the abnormal receptors because the normal receptors are sensitive to the MSH and can trigger the internal cellular cascade leading to eumelanin production. These normal receptors would also be sensitive to the ASIP, the result being that control of color then

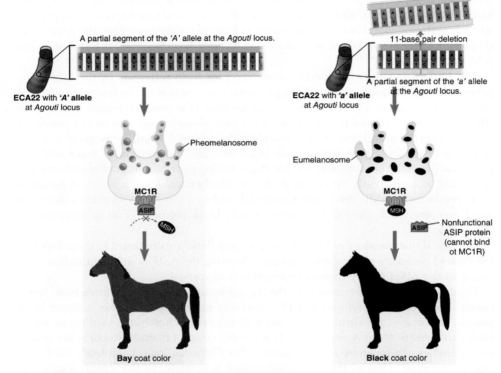

Figure 2.4 *ASIP* alleles control pigmentation. Pigment cells are capable of producing two types of pigment (eumelanin and pheomelanin). The switch between these is regulated by the activation or the inactivation of a cell surface receptor (MC1R). Cells express the ASIP in some body regions if at least one copy of the dominant allele is present (A^A). In these horses, ASIP is able to bind to the receptor, block it, and the cell then produces red/yellow pheomelanin pigment. Alternatively, if the horse only has the recessive allele $A^a A^a$, no functional ASIP is produced, the receptor is not blocked, and the horse is therefore only capable of making black pigment (eumelanin). *Source:* courtesy of Francesca Gianino.

resides with the *Agouti* locus. The cells of heterozygotes (E^+E^e) are expressing both the normal and abnormal receptor, but the active one is fully subject to stimulation by the hormone as well as to blockage by the signaling protein, as shown in Figure 2.5.

The neutral, or *wild-type*, allele allows a normal MSH receptor, with the consequence that color is then determined by the *Agouti* locus. Therefore, horses with a **bay** color ($A^A—,E^+—$), or one based on **bay**, have the wild-type *Extension* allele. Most **black** ($A^a A^a$, $E^+—$) horses also have this allele, although a few are exceptions to this rule and are discussed in more detail later in Section 2.4.

The *Agouti* and *Extension* loci can be imagined to function like switches. The *Extension* locus is important as the first major switch controlling horse color. The most common *Extension* alleles function as a switch for "**chestnut**" versus "**not chestnut**." The *Agouti* switch is important for those horses that are not **chestnut**, and choices at this locus are most commonly "if not **chestnut** then **bay**" versus "if not **chestnut** then **black**," as shown in Figure 2.6.

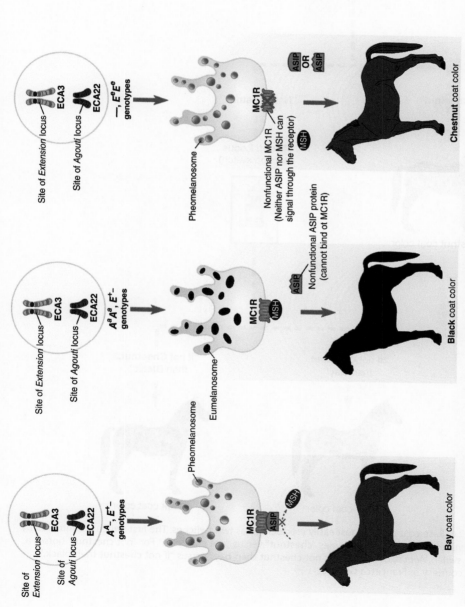

Figure 2.5 *MC1R* and *ASIP* alleles in pigmentation. When the dominant allele of *MC1R* is present (E^+) the receptor is able to respond to both ASIP and MSH, and is therefore capable of producing both types of pigment. Which pigment is produced then depends on the genotype at the *ASIP* locus. If, instead, the horse only has the recessive *MC1R* allele (E^eE^e), the receptor is not functional and therefore only red-based pheomelanin pigment is produced regardless of the genotype at the *Agouti* locus. *Source:* courtesy of Francesca Gianino.

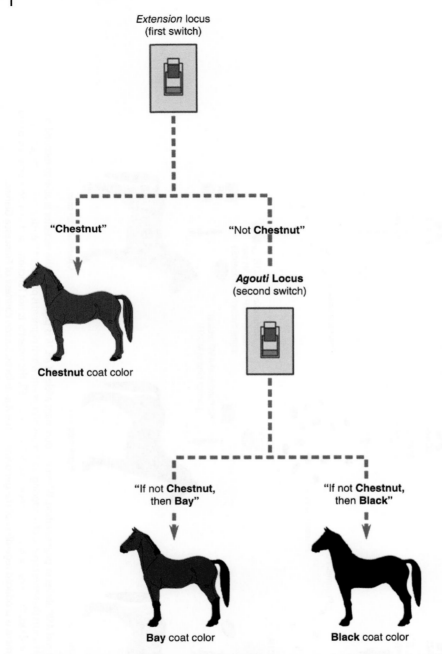

Figure 2.6 Base coat color is most easily represented as two switches. The first switch is controlled by the *Extension* locus, which determines "chestnut" versus "not **chestnut**." For "not **chestnut**" horses a second switch, *Agouti*, determines "if not **chestnut** then **bay**" versus "if not **chestnut** then **black**." *Source:* courtesy of Francesca Gianino.

The presence of the *chestnut* allele can be established by a DNA test that is based on the character of the *chestnut* mutation as a single base-pair substitution at the *Extension* locus. Many breeders find this test useful in predicting color breeding outcomes. The test is specific for the *chestnut* allele, and the absence of the *chestnut* allele is usually assumed to assure the presence of the *wild-type* allele. This is accurate for most breeds and most situations, except that a second recessive allele also occurs at this locus. This second recessive allele makes the assumption wrong that if E^e is absent then E^+ is present. The intricacies of DNA testing are more complicated if this second, rare allele is present.

This second single base-pair substitution at the *Extension* locus is symbolized E^a, and leads to a **chestnut** phenotype that is indistinguishable from the usual **chestnut** color. This recessive mutation has so far only been documented in a few breeds, including Black Forest horses, a draft horse breed from Germany. The significance of this allele, even though it is rare, is that a very few **chestnut** horses can be E^aE^a and would therefore test negative for the usual E^e allele. Also confusing can be **chestnut** horses that are E^eE^a because they will test heterozygous for the E^e allele despite their **chestnut** phenotype. In most breeds the assumption is that any heterozygote is E^+E^e, so the results of genetic testing in breeds with both E^e and E^a can be misleading.

The usual jargon associated with results of this DNA test can lead to confusion. Most people use "red factor" for the *chestnut* allele and "black factor" for its absence (which, in most breeds, means that E^+ is present). This nomenclature can be confusing because most "black-factored" horses are indeed **bay** and not **black**. The "red factor" designation for the recessive allele is reasonably accurate, but "black-factored" is only accurate when point color is considered. In most breeds such horses are not truly **black**, but instead are more likely to be **bay** or one of its derivatives. Many breeders optimistically and naively consider that "black factor" horses can routinely produce **black** foals, when in fact very few can do so due to the *bay* allele at the *Agouti* locus being so common. The most accurate analysis is to test for the presence of recessive alleles at both the *Agouti* and the *Extension* loci, instead of relying on test results from only one or the other for complete prediction of color production.

The interactions of the *Extension* and *Agouti* loci are the most complicated of the genetic interactions in horse color genetics, but are also the most critical to understand because they involve the three most common colors of most breeds. The three colors **bay**, **black**, and **chestnut** are the bases for building other colors and must be understood before remaining colors can begin to make sense. The general tendency of extensive red/tan being dominant at the *Agouti* locus while being recessive at the *Extension* locus is the single most important concept to grasp for an understanding of the interactions of these two important loci.

A few confusing issues can be encountered in some of the past literature concerning the **chestnut** horse color, and some of these issues must be discussed to lay to rest some theories that have been rejected. In the past, the entire **chestnut** group of colors was attributed to the recessive *brown* allele (B^b) at the *Brown* locus (in mice this is the *TYRP1* locus, for tyrosinase-related protein 1). This theory was widely published. The confusion it has caused can be avoided by realizing that the *Extension* locus is the true cause of **chestnut** and colors based on it. The difference between the mechanisms of the two loci is the important detail. The *Brown* locus controls an enzyme called tyrosinase-related protein 1. Changes in this enzyme result in eumelanin being brown instead of black due to an alteration in melanosome structure. The important detail here is that eumelanin is changed but pheomelanin remains unchanged.

If **chestnut** were a *Brown* locus phenomenon then **chestnut** would result from eumelanin and would be chocolate brown in character. This is clearly not the case because it is a pheomelanic red. Additional evidence against the *Brown* locus as a cause for **chestnut** colors is the phenomenon that the expression of **chestnut** is epistatic to the *Agouti* colors (**bay** and **black** and their derivatives). The *Brown* locus has no such epistatic relationship to *Agouti*. The *Extension* locus is the true source of control of **chestnut** colors, as evidenced by their characteristic pheomelanin pigmentation (red) and their epistasis to the *Agouti* locus colors. Linkage relationships (discussed in more detail in Chapters 6 and 7 for **roan** and **tobiano**) also clearly indicate that the *Extension* locus is responsible for **chestnut** colors. As final evidence, molecular investigations of the *MC1R* gene also support the *Extension* locus in this role.

Some publications attempt to revive the *Brown* locus as important in the genetic control of **liver chestnut**, but even for this color the *Brown* locus does not appear to be the site of genetic control. No evidence has arisen in horses to support the contention that the *Brown* locus contributes to basic color variation. While mutations have been found at this locus, none of them has correlated with a change in color, so none of these has been documented as being responsible for changes in the basic colors of **bay**, **brown**, **black**, or **chestnut**.

While the *Brown* locus can be dismissed as contributing to basic horse color, a problem remains in that **brown** is a term that is legitimately used to denote specific horse colors. However, **brown** horses are not the brown of other animals that results from *Brown* locus mutations. Specifically, they are not the flat, uniform chocolate brown so typical of retriever or spaniel dogs. **Brown** as a horse color is discussed in more in Sections 2.3 and 3.2. The important concept with regard to the *Brown* locus is to realize that this locus is not known to be involved in determining horse base coat color. This is true even though a few horse colors go by the name **brown**. The **brown** horse color name was in use long before genetics became a science and has left behind this unfortunate nomenclature problem.

2.2 Two Subtypes of Bay: Wild Bay and Bay

At least two different subtypes of color occur within the larger **bay** classification (Figures 2.7 and 2.8). These two subtypes do not have separate names in English, but are considered to be separate colors in some other languages. One of these subtypes is the more common **bay** in which black on the legs extends up to the knees and hocks or even above them. In the other subtype, which is much less common, black extends only up to the pastern or fetlock. On the cannon area it extends only partially, leaving interplay of red areas and black areas. This subtype of **bay** with low black stockings is fairly rare in most breeds of horses and is the original **wild bay** counterpart of **bay**, although in truly wild horses it was further modified to their final pale color.

Control for the difference between **wild bay** and **bay** most likely resides at the *Agouti* locus. The *Agouti* locus in mammals other than horses has a consistent trend in that

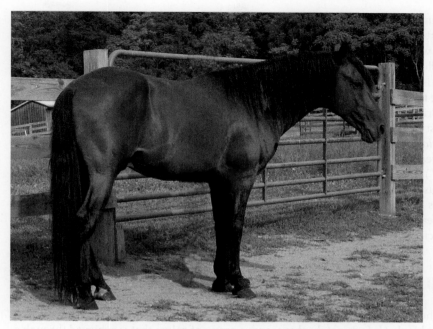

Figure 2.7 A typical **bay** phenotype of a red body and black points, with the black of the points extending to the knees and hocks.

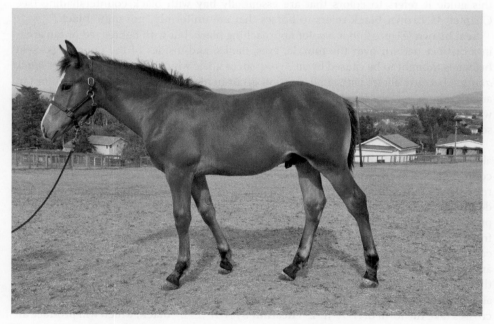

Figure 2.8 The **wild bay** phenotype has black points that extend less than those on more usual **bays**. *Source:* courtesy of Kleary Field.

more dominant alleles cause more extensive red areas, while more recessive alleles result in more extensive black areas. If a similar trend exists in horses (and this is certainly consistent with the relationship of **black** and **bay**), then the two subtypes of **bay** are probably alleles at the *Agouti* locus. Common **bay** is expected to be recessive to **wild bay** because it is less extensively red. The **wild bay** subtype has a much more restricted occurrence than the common **bay** type and does not occur in all breeds. This **wild bay** is the wild, original type color at this locus, and so it should be symbolized A^+.

The most important and well-documented alleles at the *Agouti* locus are certainly *bay* (A^A) and *black* (A^a), and their relationship is fairly straightforward. The *wild bay* allele does not really confuse this, because it only splits the **bay** group into two subtypes (A^A and A^+). It is also important to realize that the common DNA-based genetic testing at this locus is only testing for presence or absence of the *black* (A^a) allele. The usual inference is that if A^a is absent, then *bay* (A^A) is present. If multiple alleles do reside at this locus, each leading to a slightly different extent of black areas versus red areas, then the intricacies become more complicated than a single two-way switch.

2.3 Seal Brown

Brown, in horse color terminology, is used to refer to colors that are darker than **bay** and lighter than **black**. Unfortunately, this covers a group of colors that is achieved through a handful of different genetic mechanisms. Most of these can be separated on visual inspection with fairly reasonable accuracy. These include the distinct colors of **brown**, **brown-black**, and **seal brown**. **Brown** is discussed further in Section 3.2, but as used in this guide it refers to colors that are essentially **bay** with black countershading (see Chapter 3). **Brown-black** refers to horses that are uniformly "not quite **black**."

Seal brown (Figure 2.9) is a color approaching black, but with lighter red or tan areas in a distinct pattern over the muzzle, eyes, flanks, and insides of the upper legs. **Seal brown** is thought to be caused by an *Agouti* locus allele which is symbolized A^t for *black and tan* because alleles with similar action occur in many species, and lead to minor tan areas in the same locations as the **seal brown** color of horses. A DNA test for this allele was once available but has been discontinued, and the specific underlying genetic sequence has never been published.

The common interactions of the *Agouti* and *Extension* loci are important as the base of almost all horse colors and are summarized in Table 2.1. These interactions can be confusing. For example, although both **chestnut** and **black** can be considered to be recessive to **bay**, when they are mated together they indeed can produce **bay**, which is dominant to both. The underlying biology is explained further in Figures 2.4 and 2.5. The production of **bay** foals from crossing **black** to **chestnut** is actually common and results from the fact that it is impossible to detect by phenotype alone which *Agouti* alleles are carried by a **chestnut** horse unless the horse's DNA is tested directly. In most instances and in most breeds, **chestnut** horses carry the A^A or *bay* allele because **bay** horses (and therefore the A^A allele) are so much more frequent than are **black** horses (and the A^a allele). As a consequence of the frequencies of these alleles, most **chestnut** by **black** crosses take the form of $A^A A^A, E^e E^e$ **chestnut** by $A^a A^a, E^+ E^+$ **black**, which will produce an $A^A A^a, E^+ E^e$ **bay** foal every time.

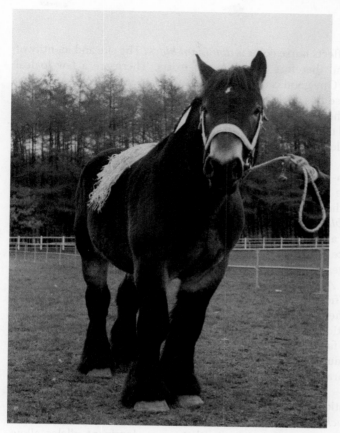

Figure 2.9 This **seal brown** horse has the black coat with the typical light areas over the eyes, muzzle, and belly that characterize this color. *Source:* courtesy of Laurent Rottiers.

Table 2.1 Interactions of the common alleles at the *Agouti* and *Extension* loci. E^a, in those few breeds in which it occurs, mimics the action of E^e.

Agouti genotype	Extension genotype	Color phenotype
A^+-	E^+-	**Wild bay** (rare in most breeds)
A^A-	E^+-	**Bay** (common in most breeds)
A^t-	E^+-	**Seal brown** (rare in most breeds)
A^aA^a	E^+-	**Black** (variable by breed)
A^+-	E^eE^e	**Chestnut** (rare)
A^A-	E^eE^e	**Chestnut** (common)
A^t-	E^eE^e	**Chestnut** (usually rare)
A^aA^a	E^eE^e	**Chestnut** (usually rare)

2.4 Dominant Black

A relatively rare allele that affects horse color is *dominant black*. The site and identity of this allele are uncertain, and therefore no DNA test exists. There are a few logical candidate loci for this allele. One good candidate gene is an allele at the *Extension* locus, *dominant black* (E^D), because this allele at this locus functions as a cause of uniformly **black** animals in several other species. Another candidate is the *Beta Defensin* locus, which has been documented to have an allele with similar function in dogs. Whatever the locus of residence of this allele, it causes a **black** (or nearly so) horse regardless of the *Agouti* genotype. Evidence in the Arabian breed indicates that *dominant black* is responsible for some **brown-black** and some **black** Arabians. This allele is also present in other breeds, such as the Appaloosa, but only as a rarity.

Dominant alleles at either the *Extension* or the *Beta Defensin* loci are good candidates for *dominant black*, but would have different mechanisms to produce that color. The dominant alleles at *Extension* "lock" MSH receptors into the "on" position even in the absence of MSH binding with the receptor. This signals the cell's internal machinery to be geared for eumelanin production exclusively, regardless of the *Agouti* genotype. The *Agouti* block, which is external to the cell, is therefore circumvented internally. The dominant alleles at *Beta Defensin*, in contrast, have an action that is external to the cell. They provide for a signal that binds to MC1R, and forces it into the "on" position as well as making these receptors unresponsive to any other external cues. The final result is a similar completely black phenotype, so determining if the color is due to a block internal to the cell or external to it cannot be determined by visual appearance alone. The result is **black**, and in common parlance a **dominant black** horse.

Dominant black is epistatic to the *Agouti* locus colors, much as is the *chestnut* allele, even though *dominant black* is dominant while *chestnut* is recessive. The *Extension* locus follows a consistent pattern of activity in that more dominant alleles allow expression of black areas, and more recessive alleles restrict expression of black areas. This is somewhat opposite to the action of *Agouti* alleles, although the underlying biology of these two loci makes it plain why this is so. The action of the allele to lock the MSH receptor in the "on" position makes it clear why this is a dominant allele. Any receptor locked in the "on" position will override any others that are present, so that a single copy of the allele is all that is needed to assure production of black pigment, with expression in the phenotype.

Black horses caused by *dominant black* do have some subtle differences from the more common A^a mechanism (Figures 2.10 and 2.11). The *dominant black* allele is somewhat "weaker" or "leakier" than the *Agouti* black, and as a result many horses with *dominant black* are a **brown-black** or **dark brown** instead of a true **black**. Many *dominant black* horses are born a color similar to **bay** and then darken to **black** at a year or two old. This color change can easily confuse horse owners who have not seen this color before, especially because some horses do not become **black** until they are a few years old. The dominant black allele varies in expression from a very **jet black** to a lighter **brown-black** color, and this difference does not seem to depend on the remaining genotype. That is, it appears that the **brown** versus **black** status of these horses does not reveal anything about their underlying *Agouti* genotype. A^A-,E^D- (assuming that *dominant black* is at *Extension*) is frequently **brown** (a "nearly **black**" or "**brown-black**"

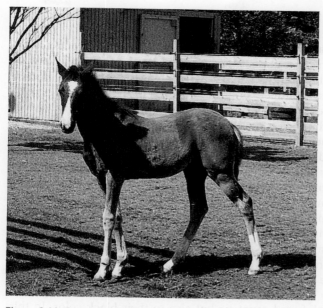

Figure 2.10 **Dominant black** foals usually have a "nonblack" appearance. This color of this foal's coat is more typical of horses that are **bay** at maturity. Most **black** foals are much more of an ash color and lack the redness of this foal. *Source:* courtesy of Dyan Westvang.

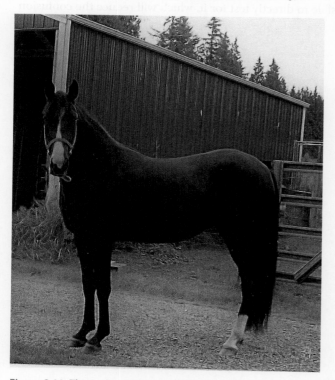

Figure 2.11 This is the same horse as Figure 2.10, showing a mature color that is nearly **black**. This is typical of **dominant black**, which is often lighter than **jet black**. *Source:* courtesy of Dyan Westvang.

type), although it can be truly **black** as well. The genotype A^aA^a,E^D— is **black**, but, of course, rare.

The **blacks** and **brown-blacks** caused by *dominant black* should produce **bays** occasionally as a recessive, which would not be expected if **browns** and **blacks** were caused by the *Agouti* locus alleles. For example, a cross of a **black** A^aA^a,E^+E^+ by a **black** or **brown-black** A^AA^A,E^DE^+ can routinely produce **bay**: A^AA^a,E^+E^+.

The *dominant black* allele (regardless of the specific locus involved) is rare or absent in most breeds. The extent to which the genotype A^A—,E^D— is classified as **black** is an important issue. If most of these horses are classified as **brown-black**, and therefore registered as **bay** in most breeds, then the E^D allele really does not upset the expectation that **black** is recessive. If a few of the A^A—,E^D— horses are registered as **black**, though, the result will be **bay** foals in some instances in which they are not expected. This occurs only rarely in most of the common breeds, although selection in favor of **black** horses in many breeds may be increasing the frequency of the *dominant black* allele.

The results of genetic testing have led to a few problems of nomenclature for these dominant **black** horses. In many cases the results of the loci that can be tested are consistent with a **bay** horse because any horse lacking A^a and E^e is assumed to be A^A—,E^+—, which should be bay. In the case of **dominant black**, though, the observer is faced with a phenotypically **black** animal. Many people then resort to calling these **black bays**, as a nod to their inferred genotype but also to their **black** color. In this case the attempt to include the genotype in the color name is misleading, because these horses are visually **black** and not **bay** at all. Once the allele causing **dominant black** is documented it should be possible to directly test for it, which will reduce the confusion that surrounds this color.

3

Modifications Affecting Most Colors

All horse colors are variable over a range that includes the depth of the color as well as other features. These variations are caused by modifications of a color within a basic color group and are important because they are the foundation of many of the details of horse color. As a result of modifications, not all **bay** horses are the same color, neither are all **chestnut** nor all **black** horses. Modifications are important in distinguishing more finely drawn subcategories within these basic colors to allow for more accurate identification of horse color. Three of the most common modifications can affect any basic color. These are **shade**, **sooty**, and **mealy**. Other modifications are more specific and act on only one or a few basic colors rather than on all of them.

3.1 Shade

3.1.1 Definition and Classification

One general modification of a horse's basic color is that of "shade." This is the phenomenon that describes variations within a basic color group resulting from light to dark shades of body color. Modifications caused by shade are most notable on red background colors, such as **bay** or **chestnut**. Red pigment can vary from light and close to yellow, to dark and almost purple, brown, or nearly black. While similar variation in depth is sometimes noticed on **black** horses, it is more subtle and is not as important for distinguishing among **black** horses as it is on **bays** and **chestnuts**. Name changes resulting from dark, middle, and light shades on the basic colors of horses are summarized in Table 3.1.

On **bay** horses the shade of body color can vary from a very dark red to a washed out yellow color that still retains a red tinge. Different shades of **bay** have different names. The rare but beautiful **blood bay** is a clear dark red that tends to a purple-red (Figure 3.1). Extremely dark **bays** can be nearly **black** and are called **mahogany bay** and are a flatter color that is less red than **blood bay** (Figure 3.2). **Bay** or **red bay** is the term used for the more common brownish red medium shade of **bay**. Some of these medium shades are browner, and some are redder. The very reddest medium shades sometimes are called **cherry bay**. **Sandy bay**, **honey bay**, and **light bay** describe those **bay** horses whose bodies are a lighter, yellow shade of red (Figures 3.3 and 3.4). A very few bays have a pronounced golden tone to the body color and are called **golden bays**.

Equine Color Genetics, Fourth Edition. D. Phillip Sponenberg and Rebecca Bellone.
© 2017 John Wiley & Sons, Inc. Published 2017 by John Wiley & Sons, Inc.

Table 3.1 Effect of shade on base colors.

Base color	Dark shade	Medium shade	Light shade
Bay	Blood bay	Bay	Sandy bay
	Mahogany bay	Red bay	Golden bay
		Cherry bay	Light bay
Chestnut	Liver chestnut	Red chestnut	Light chestnut
	Dark chestnut	Copper chestnut	Golden chestnut
			Yellow chestnut
Black	Jet black	Black	Summer black
	Raven black		

One problem with having many shades of **bay** is that horses can change shade somewhat with season of the year. While subdivisions of **bay** are helpful for identification in the field, they can often be too fine a split for use in permanent identification, such as registration descriptions.

Chestnut horses likewise can vary in shade. The darkest red shades are called **liver chestnut** (Figure 3.5). A rich dark red is often called **red chestnut** (Figure 3.6). The middle shade of red generally is called simply **chestnut** (Figure 3.7). The lighter reds can

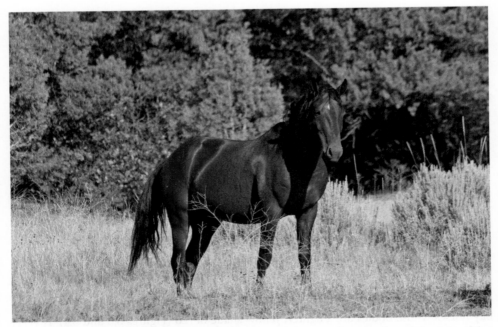

Figure 3.1 **Blood bay** is at the darker end of the shades of bay, but still retains the red character of the color that is typical of **bay** horses. *Source:* courtesy of Dan Elkins.

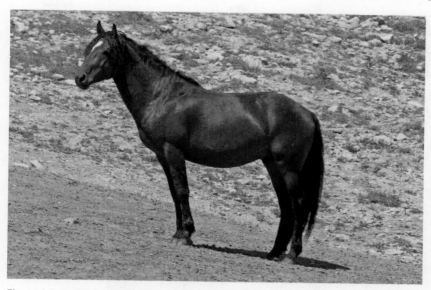

Figure 3.2 Darker **bay** horses are often called **mahogany bay** and are usually less distinctly red than **blood bay**. *Source:* courtesy of Nancy Cerroni.

tend toward a yellow shade and are called **light chestnut** or **sandy chestnut** (Figure 3.8). In the Suffolk breed all horses are some shade of **chestnut** (spelled **chesnut** by Suffolk owners and breeders), and the range is divided into seven categories: **liver, dark, red, gold, copper, light,** and **yellow**.

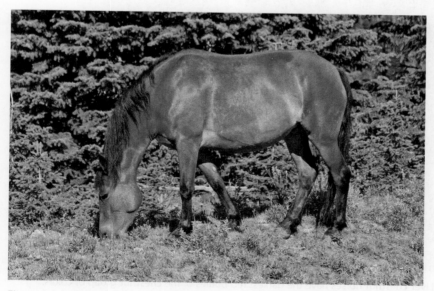

Figure 3.3 Light **bay** has the reddish color typical of **bays**. *Source:* courtesy of Dan Elkins.

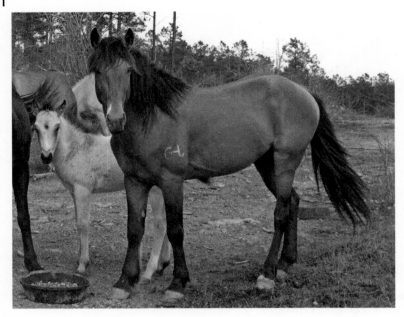

Figure 3.4 The lightest **bays** are honey colored, and retain little of the red tint typical of the color. The freeze brand on this horse has grown white hairs, as is typical of this method of horse identification. *Source:* courtesy of Jeannette Beranger.

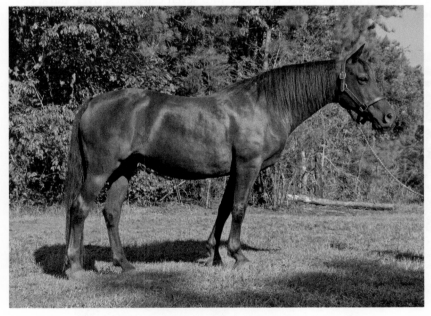

Figure 3.5 **Liver chestnut** horses have the darkest red bodies of the **chestnut** group of colors. *Source:* courtesy of Laura Hornick Behning.

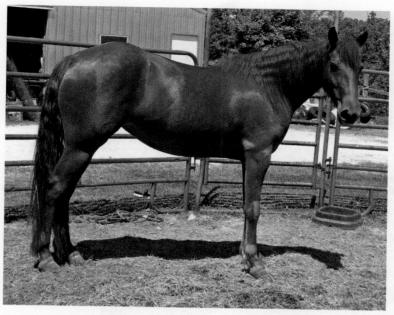

Figure 3.6 **Red chestnut** is among the richer and darker shades of the common **chestnut** color. *Source:* courtesy of Dyan Westvang.

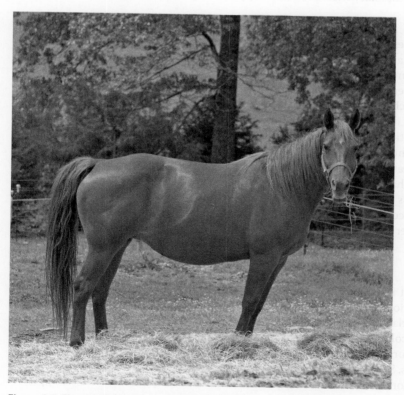

Figure 3.7 The middle range of **chestnut** is a common color in several breeds. Many of these have a uniform color throughout the body and points. *Source:* courtesy of Dyan Westvang.

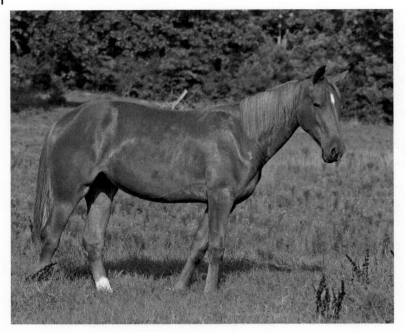

Figure 3.8 Lighter **chestnut** horses have a distinctly yellow or gold appearance. *Source:* courtesy of Dyan Westvang.

Within the **chestnut** group the **liver chestnuts** have long been highly esteemed. Both Bedouin Arabs and Spanish conquistadors held **liver chestnuts** in high regard for general ability and endurance.

Striking differences as the result of shade are not as obvious on **black** horses as they are on **bays** and **chestnuts**. Some **black** horses never seem to fade in the sunlight and are called **jet black** or **raven black** (Figure 3.9). Others tend to get a rusty tinge during certain times of the year and are then a flatter color, but are still **black**. In Austria these are called **summer black** (*Sommer Rappe*), which reflects the fact that many **black** horses fade at least somewhat in the heat and sunlight of summer (Figure 3.10). While the effects of shade are noticeable on some derivations of **black**, they are hardly noticeable unless the **black** background color has been modified in some way by other loci. To further confuse the issue of shades of **black**, some horses are **jet black** in some years, and rustier and lighter in other years.

3.1.2 Genetic Control

The shade effect is under complex, multifactorial genetic control, so that relationships between the various shades are not straightforward. At least in the Franches-Montagne breed in Switzerland, the darker shades of colors are recessive to the lighter shades. The depth of body color is also subject to environmental influences in addition to genetic influences, so horses that are well fed and very physically fit tend to be darker than less fortunate horses. Some breeds, such as the Morgan, have been selected for dark shades in all the basic colors, and these are fairly consistent across the entire breed. An opposite

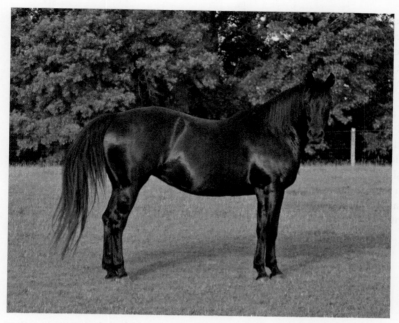

Figure 3.9 **Jet black** horses are rare in most breeds and are usually found in horses at the peak of their prime and in good nutritional condition. *Source:* courtesy of Laura Hornick Behning.

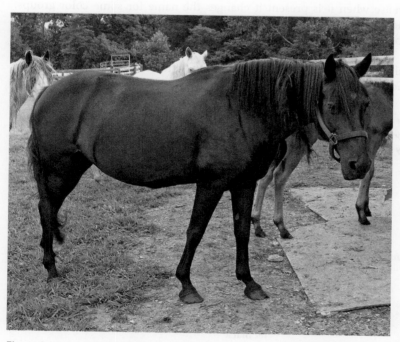

Figure 3.10 **Summer black** has a reddish tinge to the body, but retains the black points typical of **black** horses.

example is the American Belgian, in which very light yellowish red body color is typical on the many **chestnuts** and the few **bays** in the breed.

The shade effect, even if it is not a single locus, can still be understood as a switch, with the choices being "dark," "middle," or "light." The switch for shade is not documented at the DNA level, in contrast to those involved with base coat color discussed in Chapter 2. It is important to point out that shades of horse color are arbitrarily split into these three categories. The actual situation is that shades of color are innumerable, and the categories blend imperceptibly into one another. This makes studying the genetic control of the differences very difficult, because accurate and repeatable classification of the fine variations is hard to achieve. The concept of shade as a switch among a few choices greatly simplifies classification of the color of many horses, even though the classification can get muddier because shade varies along a continuous array, and an abrupt border really does not occur between dark and middle or middle and light shades of the various colors.

3.2 Sooty

3.2.1 Definition and Classification

Another general modification of body color is the presence of black hairs among the body hairs. This modification is called **sooty** or **smutty**. The consequences of the **sooty** modification on the base colors are summarized in Table 3.2. **Sooty** is an important modification because when it is present it changes the name for some color groups. On **bay** horses the **sooty** effect is most commonly expressed over the top of the horse so that the back, shoulder, and croup can almost look black whereas the horse is redder on the lower body, belly, and upper leg. This effect is called black countershading, or "**sooty**," and results in an animal that is dark on top and lighter beneath. The presence of black countershading can be very minimal or very extensive. When it is very extensive

Table 3.2 Effect of **sooty** on base colors. The final appearance depends not only on the base coat color, but also on the relative degree of the **sooty** effect, which can be quite variable.

Base color	Sooty variant
Blood bay	**Dark brown**
Red bay	**Brown (mahogany bay)**
Sandy bay	**Light brown**
Liver chestnut, nonsooty type	**Liver chestnut** **Black chestnut**
Red chestnut	**Liver chestnut**
Sandy chestnut	**Liver chestnut**
Jet black	**Jet black**
Black	**Jet black**
Summer black	**Black**

the resulting horse can be nearly black. When minimal, it is easy to overlook the presence of the black hairs. The darkest manifestations on **bays** are easily confused with **seal brown**.

The nomenclature of the colors resulting from the combination of **sooty** and **bay** is confusing. Most horse fanciers include **bays** with black countershading in the usual **bay** group of colors. A different approach is used by some people who rely on the presence or absence of black hairs to distinguish **bay** from **brown**. The logic of this second approach is that any reddish horse with black points and lacking **sooty** countershading is **bay**, and any reddish horse with black points and black hairs in the body coat is called **brown**, and not **bay**. A more common name for these **sooty**, black countershaded **bays** is **mahogany**, as in **mahogany bay** (Figure 3.2). To add to the confusion, those who use black countershading to distinguish **bay** from **brown** also use the **mahogany bay** designation for darker noncountershaded bays.

As a general rule, better accuracy is achieved by distinguishing **brown** from **bay** by the presence of **sooty** countershading. Because this is a more accurate approach, it is the preferred method, even though it is less frequently used than the method that lumps both countershaded and noncountershaded animals into the **bay** group. This guide considers all **sooty bays** as **brown**, largely because this is a useful convention that helps in understanding the genetic control and origin of these colors as well as several other colors derived from them (Figures 3.11 and 3.12).

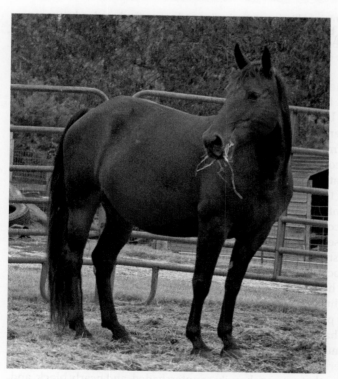

Figure 3.11 **Sooty** or black countershading is a convenient way to separate **brown** from **bay** horses. This is a logical way to designate the differences in these dark colors. The black countershading on this horse therefore classifies it as **brown**. *Source:* courtesy of Dyan Westvang.

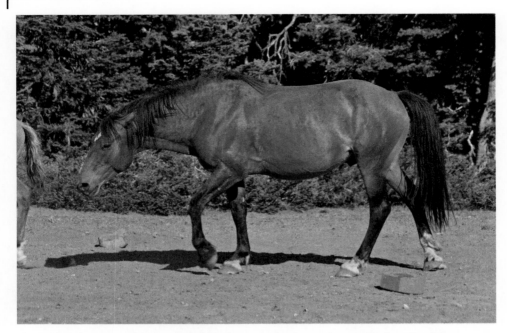

Figure 3.12 Some horses have minimal black countershading and are easily classed as **bay** even though a more accurate name is **brown**, which reflects the underlying genetic potential of the horse. This horse is classified as a light **brown**, although it is easy to appreciate that many observers would simply call this color **bay**. *Source:* courtesy of Dan Elkins.

Brown, as a horse color term, is confusing, and horse owners and breeders use the term in a few different ways. In general, all dark colors with black points that are lighter than **black** but darker than **bay** are called **brown**. The **brown** classification is really a hodgepodge of dark colors and shades that occur between **black** and **bay**. Many horse breeders do not use the term **brown** at all, preferring to lump all **browns** with **bays**. Some breeders say that the color name **brown** "is used only by people with one horse or with two hundred." The point of this comment is that **brown** is more likely to be used by inexperienced observers, or those owning so many horses that identifying the animals requires many subdivisions of color. The **brown** classification is very useful for achieving an understanding of horse color genetics, and it should be more widely used than it is presently. Most **brown** horses result from the **sooty** effect on an otherwise **bay** horse, which can help in the understanding of many colors that are derived from these **bay** and **brown** by alleles at other loci.

The sootiness of **brown** horses can vary from slight to extreme, and the resulting horses are likewise very light to nearly **black**. **Bays** (restricting that color term to its narrow sense in the system presented here) lack the **sooty** black overlay. **Light brown** has minimal **sooty** countershading and is nearly as light as most **bays**, but these still have the characteristic **sooty** countershaded overlay of black hairs dorsally, which places them in the **brown** category rather than in the **bay** category. At the dark extreme, the **brown** group of colors includes those that are very heavily countershaded, and nearly **black**, and for these horses this system and the more widespread approach that defines **brown** as "nearly **black**" then agree. These horses can closely mimic **seal brown**. **Brown** includes a

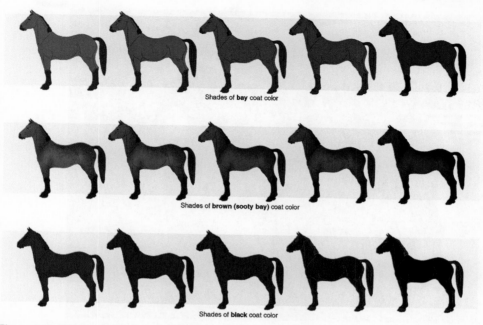

Shades of **bay** coat color

Shades of **brown (sooty bay)** coat color

Shades of **black** coat color

Figure 3.13 **Shade** and black countershading interact to result in a number of different final colors.

wide range of colors because both the extent of the **sooty** hairs and the depth of the shade of the basic red body color are highly variable. These two sources of variation combine to yield a wide range of final appearances.

The approach of using **sooty** countershading to distinguish **brown** from **bay** is less commonly used than the "nearly **black**" definition, but it does have the advantage of more neatly and objectively separating **brown** from **bay** and therefore makes the genetic control of many colors easier to understand and study. The changes in **bay**, **brown**, and **black** horses are diagrammed in Figure 3.13.

Brown-black horses, in most systems of identification, are those that are not quite black enough to be considered **black**, nor light enough to be **bay**. These are usually not **sooty**, but are more likely to be genetically *black* at *Agouti* or *dominant black* at whatever locus houses that allele. In either case they are more subtle than the usual **brown** that results from the **sooty** overlay on a **bay** background color.

Seal brown horses, as mentioned earlier in this chapter, are nearly black but with conspicuous lighter regions in the flanks, muzzle, and around the eyes. In some cases, **dark brown** horses with the **sooty** mechanism could be confused with **seal brown** horses. In general, though, **brown (sooty bay)**, **seal brown**, and **brown-black** horses can all be distinguished well enough from one another to serve as useful classifications of horse color.

Black countershading can occur on **chestnut** horses, despite their recessive *Extension* genotype that should prevent black hairs. Sootiness on **chestnut** horses tends to be less conspicuous than the **sooty** countershading on **brown (sooty bay)** horses. The resulting dark shades of **chestnut** are usually lumped together with the dark, nonsooty **chestnut** colors as **liver chestnut**. The **liver chestnut** classification therefore includes dark **chestnut** colors that achieve their darkness through two separate mechanisms including

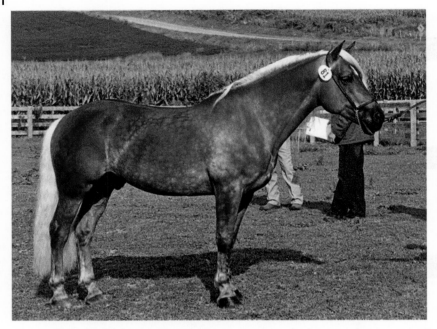

Figure 3.14 **Sooty** overlay on lighter **chestnut** colors is easily distinguished due to the contrast of the black hairs with the lighter base coat. *Source:* courtesy of Ruth Schwab.

shade and **sooty** (Table 3.2). One mechanism simply deepens red pigment to a dark color (this is the **shade** effect). The other adds black hairs and achieves overall darkness from this mechanism (the **sooty** effect). On lighter **chestnut** horses the **sooty** effect is easily noted (Figure 3.14).

In some breeds, **chestnut** horses with black countershading in the coat are called **black chestnut** if they are very, very dark (Figure 3.15). Black countershading on **chestnut** horses is less conspicuously dorsal than it is on **browns**. The black hairs are usually more evenly spread over the entire body. They tend to not affect the lower leg, which allows the basic redness of the coat color to show through. This phenomenon is helpful in the very darkest horses, because their **chestnut** classification can still be determined by the point color of the lower leg.

The effects of sootiness on **black** are barely distinguishable from those of shade, primarily because they are not readily observable unless the **black** base color has been otherwise modified.

3.2.2 Genetic Control

The genetic control of the **sooty** effect is not simple, nor is it well documented. The sootiness of colors with black points (**brown**) is probably genetically different from the sootiness of colors with nonblack points (**chestnut**). Phenotypic evidence for this is that sootiness on the **chestnut**-based colors is uniform, in contrast to the dorsal distribution of sootiness on black-pointed colors.

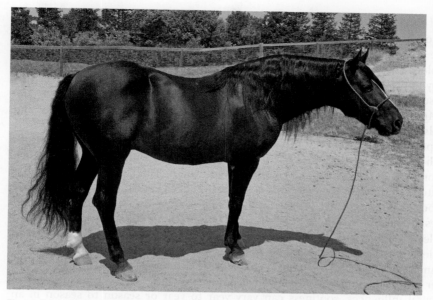

Figure 3.15 **Black chestnut** horses arrive at their final distinctive color through an interaction of sooty and **dark shade**. The lower leg in most cases betrays their true chestnut color. Most of them also have nearly black manes and tails, contributing to the near blackness of the final color. *Source:* courtesy of Robin Collins.

One unproven theory that might explain the genetics of the countershading on black-pointed colors is to postulate another allele at the *Extension* locus. Such an allele, E^B, for *extension brown*, would reside above the *wild-type Extension* allele, E^+, in dominance. Such an allele would differentiate between **browns** ($A^A—,E^B—$) and **bays** ($A^A—,E^+—$) if one is using the logic that all black-pointed red horses with black countershading are **brown** and only those with noncountershaded body coats are **bay**. Such an allele is consistent with the experience of those few breeders who have kept track of counter-shading as a separate trait, although such breeders are few and far between so that no statistical analysis has been done on this detail.

If the number of alleles available as candidates at the *Extension* and *Agouti* loci is greater than A^A, A^a, E^+, and E^e, then understanding the interactions becomes more complicated, although the general range of dominance at the *Extension* locus is as follows: E^D (if *dominant black* resides here) dominates E^B (if there is such an allele), which dominates E^+, which dominates E^e, and E^a (each of these last three is well documented). Some of these alleles are common (E^B, E^+, and E^e), and two are very rare (E^D and E^a). Likewise, at the *Agouti* locus, A^+ dominates A^A, which dominates A^t, which dominates A^a, with A^A being the most common and A^a also being routine in many breeds.

Regardless of the existence or absence of additional alleles at *Agouti* or *Extension*, it remains true that if one lumps into the color **bay** all of the reddish, black-pointed horses, and if one lumps into **black** all those that are black or nearly so, the result is that **black** is indeed recessive to **bay** with very few exceptions. Because most people deal with horse color in broad classifications, this approach generally works well. The finer details within the classifications are explained by adding these other, hypothetical alleles. *Dominant* *black* could easily confuse the issue, and while this might be important in a few breeds, it is rare in most breeds and therefore usually unimportant. The frequency of the *dominant black* allele may be increasing in several breeds in which **black** has recently become a popular color. The *dominant black* allele is important in those few situations where breeders try to produce consistently **black** horses because it can result in **bay** or **brown** foals as a surprise from two **black** parents if it is present in the breed involved. The recessive *Agouti* locus **blacks**, when mated together, cannot produce such **bay** and **brown** foals as surprises to the breeder.

The proposed E^B allele does not explain the sootiness that can occur on the nonblack-pointed (**chestnut**) colors, because E^B would produce colors with black points, which by definition excludes **chestnut** and colors derived from it. The **sooty** effect (for either black-pointed or nonblack-pointed horses) has not yet been shown to be due to a single gene. For both color classes it is at least somewhat genetic in origin based on breeders' experiences. In most breeds the sootier **chestnut** colors seem to be somewhat dominant over the clearer colors, but this does not necessarily imply a single gene in all cases.

In addition to being undocumented genetically, **sooty** is also subject to modification by environmental influences. Most horses fed on very rich forages will express sootiness to a greater degree than if they were fed feeds of lower quality. Owing to its response to environmental influences, sootiness can vary year to year or season to season in an individual horse. Even though the genetic control of sootiness is poorly understood, it is useful to consider it as a single switch whose choices are "clear" (or "nonsooty") versus "sooty." This simplifies the understanding of many horse colors. Sootiness does vary in extent, but usually horses can be considered to either have it or lack it in the overall appearance of the color.

An additional detail of the *Agouti* locus depends on how finely the different shades of **bay** are split (**mahogany**, **blood**, **red**). Many splits between these categories may ultimately reveal that these are all caused by several closely related alleles at the *Agouti* locus. Because these colors are all lumped together as **bay**, it is difficult to determine whether the genetic differences between them are due to alleles at the *Agouti* locus or due to modifiers at other loci. It would be consistent with other mammals, however, if the control of at least some of these differences were at the *Agouti* locus, as are (almost certainly) the differences between **wild bay**, common **bay**, **seal brown**, and **black**. The interactions of the more hypothetical *Agouti* and *Extension* locus alleles are summarized in Table 3.3. These additional alleles simply mean that instead of a two-way switch, as is

Table 3.3 Likely results of interactions of the known and proposed alleles at the *Agouti* and *Extension* loci.

Extension genotype	Agouti genotype			
	A^+	A^A	At	A^a
E^D	**Brown-black or black**	**Brown-black or black**	**Black**	**Black**
E^B	**Wild brown**	**Brown**, less accurately mahogany bay	**Seal brown**	**Black**
E^+	**Wild bay**	**Bay**	**Seal brown**	**Black**
E^e and/or E^a	**Chestnut**	**Chestnut**	**Chestnut**	**Chestnut**

the case at most loci, the *Agouti* locus and the *Extension* locus are each a four-way switch. Each individual horse, though, can have at most two choices at each locus, so all variations in genotype occur as differences in these pairs.

3.3 Mealy

3.3.1 Definition and Classification

The **mealy** modification causes pale red or yellowish areas on the lower belly, flanks, behind the elbows, inside the legs, on the muzzle, and over the eyes (Figures 3.16 and 3.17). The **mealy** effect can occur on any background color. This effect varies from very extensive, in which case it causes a dramatic paleness to the ventral body color, to minimal, in which it is very subtle and easily missed as contributing to the overall color of a horse. In English it is usually referred to as "**mealy**," "**mealy mouth**," "**mealy muzzle**," or "**toad eye**," but it frequently escapes mention in horse descriptions. In South American Spanish the **mealy** effect is called *pangaré* and is more consistently considered in horse descriptions than is the case in English.

Horses that are **black** but have the **mealy** effect superimposed are usually called **seal brown**. The **seal brown** horses that are the result of the **mealy** effect usually have more extensive light areas than do those resulting from the proposed *Agouti* locus *black and tan* allele, although these two do overlap. Both **seal brown** and **brown** occur in most

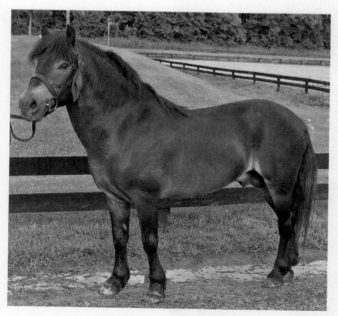

Figure 3.16 Exmoor ponies are uniformly **mealy** superimposed over a fairly limited range of base colors that includes **bay** and **brown**. The interactions yield a variety of closely related final colors depending on the extent of the **mealy** areas, the extent of sooty countershading, and the shade of the base color. *Source:* courtesy of Exmoor Ponies of North America.

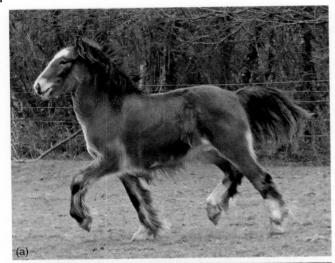

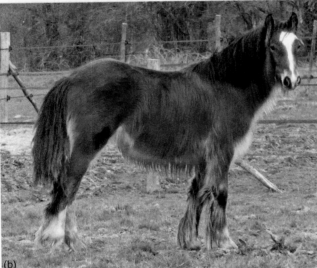

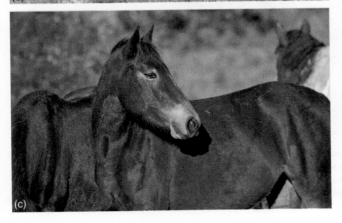

Figure 3.17 The **mealy** modification can be quite pronounced on some horses. When superimposed on **bay** it is unlikely to be confused with **seal brown** (caused by the *black and tan* allele).
Source: a and b courtesy of Laurence Viala, c courtesy of Neil Chapman.

breeds in which **bay** and **black** also occur. **Seal brown** and **brown** are frequently lumped together with **bay**. **Seal browns** and very darkly countershaded **browns** can look almost identical and serve as a reminder that occasionally it is difficult to assess a horse's genotype accurately by visual inspection of phenotype alone. Usually, the light areas resulting from the **mealy** effect are somewhat more yellow than the light areas remaining from the **sooty** effect, and they are often more extensive than the usual **seal brown** that results from the *black and tan* allele at the *Agouti* locus (see Chapter 2).

The **mealy** effect is important in the **chestnut** group of colors in some breeds. Traditionally, draft horse breeders tend to reserve the term **sorrel** for **chestnut** horses with the **mealy** effect superimposed (Figures 3.18 and 3.19). They then use the term **chestnut** for all **chestnut** shades with uniform body color. In contrast, the breeders of other breeds, notably the American Quarter Horse, use the term **sorrel** for lighter **chestnut** shades, with or without the **mealy** effect. The shades that are **red chestnut** and lighter are likely to be called **sorrel** by American Quarter Horse breeders.

The result of these different approaches to the definition of **sorrel** is that draft horse fanciers acknowledge **liver sorrels**, because they limit **sorrel** to horses with multiple shades of red on the body and **chestnut** to those lacking such shading. The shading of body color is accomplished by the **mealy** effect, and so the differences in nomenclature between **sorrel** and **chestnut** in the draft horse sense are based on a genetic difference. The American Quarter Horse approach is based mainly on **shade**, which is not well documented as a simple genetic phenomenon. A third approach, which is less common than these other two, is to use **sorrel** only for lighter shades with a flaxen mane and tail.

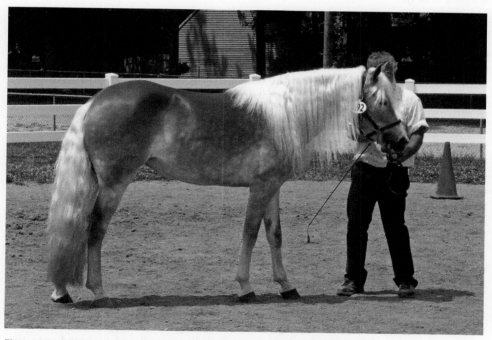

Figure 3.18 In some horse breeds the **mealy** effect is used to separate **sorrel** from **chestnut**. The **mealy** effect is pronounced and obvious in Haflingers and some draft breeds. *Source:* courtesy of Ruth Schwab.

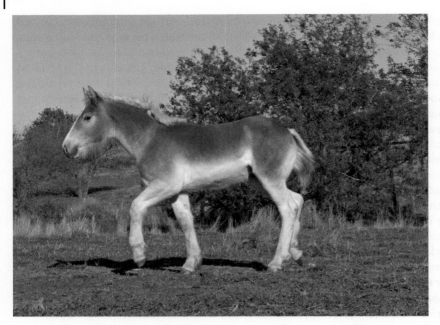

Figure 3.19 The **blond sorrel** of the American Belgian combines a very light **shade** with the **mealy** variant, all on a **chestnut** genetic background. The final color is distinctive, and nearly unrecognizable as fundamentally **chestnut** even though it is indeed derived from that base color. *Source:* courtesy of Jeannette Beranger.

The two different approaches of the draft horse and American Quarter Horse fanciers supply the two major meanings of the term **sorrel**, and these meanings are entirely distinct. Fortunately, most **sorrels** in the draft horse sense are lighter shades of color, so the end result for most cases is that the term **sorrel** is used to describe lighter colored **chestnut** horses, even though a traditional draft horse owner uses entirely different logic to arrive at that color designation than does an American Quarter Horse owner.

Sorrel, in the draft horse sense, is a fairly rare color in most breeds. It is common in some draft breeds, notably the American Belgian, in which **chestnut** is rare but **sorrel** very common. A similar situation is present with the Haflinger breed, which has both **chestnuts** and **sorrels** (**chestnut** with the **mealy** effect) and no other colors. In many other breeds the **sorrel** color, in the sense of the **mealy** effect causing varying colors on the body, is reasonably rare.

The **mealy** effect on other colors, such as **bay** or **brown**, is acknowledged only rarely by any special nomenclature in English. Some horse owners and breeders refer to the result of the **mealy** pattern on these background colors as **mealy bay** or **mealy brown**. It is only when it is superimposed on **black** to yield one type of **seal brown**, or on **chestnut** to yield **sorrel**, that the basic color name changes.

While **mealy** is a reasonably widespread effect, its presence is usually overlooked in English-speaking traditions. It is present in all Exmoor ponies as a breed characteristic. It is likely to have been a component of the original wild-type color of horses because it contributes to final colors that are well camouflaged to blend into the environment.

Table 3.4 Combinations of the **mealy** effect with various colors.

Base color	Base color genotype	Mealy variant (Pa^+)
Bay	$A^+\!-\!E^+\!-$	Mealy bay
Brown	$A^+A^+E^B\!-$	Mealy brown
Black	$A^aA^aE^+\!-$	Seal brown
Chestnut	$-\!-\!E^eE^e$	Sorrel

3.3.2   Genetic Control

The **mealy** effect is due to a dominant allele that has the symbol Pa^+, because it was first documented in Spanish research by the name **pangaré**. Recent studies have identified the locus for *Pangaré*, although the specific mutation had not been reported at the time this was written. The recessive allele is non**mealy** or Pa^{np} (for *nonpangaré*). This locus is easily viewed as a switch between "non**mealy**" and "**mealy**." On some dark horses, such as **blacks** and **bays**, the **mealy** effect can be confused with **sooty**. The two effects can result in very similar colors at the darker end of the **bay** or **brown** range, although the light areas resulting from **mealy** are characteristically lighter and more yellow than those resulting from **sooty**, which are usually more red. Combinations of **mealy** and various base colors are summarized in Table 3.4.

The genetic control of **seal brown** can be confusing. It is one of those cases where similar final colors result from combining various alleles at completely different loci. The *black and tan* allele at the *Agouti* locus is the cause of most **seal browns**. This color can be closely mimicked by **sooty** superimposed over **bay**, and also by **mealy** superimposed over **black, brown**, or darker shades of **bay**. All of these are dark colors with the distinctive lighter areas typical of **seal brown**.

Some of the confusion concerning the **mealy** effect probably arose from the lack of recognition in English nomenclature of **mealy** combinations on any but a black background color. This situation illustrates the need for good, complete, and accurate nomenclature because it allows for better record keeping, which ultimately leads to accurate explanations for the genetic control of colors.

3.4   Mane and Tail Color on Chestnut and Sorrel

3.4.1   Definition and Classification

Body color and mane color both vary in **chestnuts** (and **sorrels**), and many combinations are possible. The darkest manes and tails on these colors are nearly black, but the lower leg remains red and so these horses generally can be distinguished easily from **bays** (Figures 3.20 and 3.21). The nearly black manes and tails merge with those that are dark brown, and then merge into the ones that are red (Figure 3.22). All of these darker shades of mane and tail seem to be a characteristic of only the mane and tail, with the lower leg remaining the expected red of **chestnuts**.

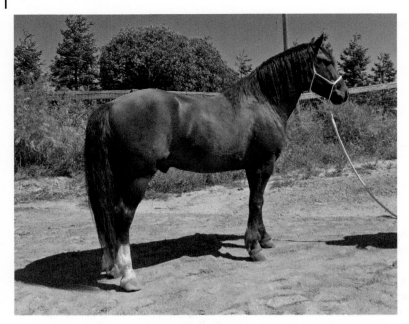

Figure 3.20 Very dark manes on **chestnut** horses are confusing, especially when they are nearly black. The color of the lower legs of these horses is a more accurate indicator of point color than is the mane. *Source:* courtesy of Robin Collins.

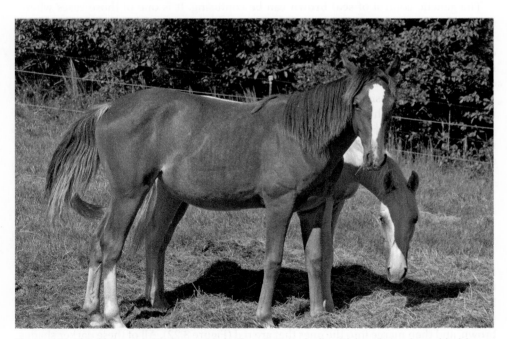

Figure 3.21 This filly's nearly black mane and tail contrast markedly with her obviously nonblack lower legs. Many observers confuse this combination with **bay**, even though it is a variant of **chestnut**. *Source:* courtesy of Dyan Westvang.

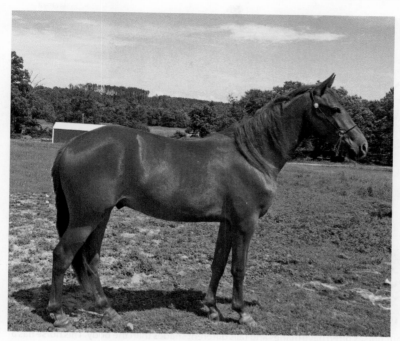

Figure 3.22 Many **chestnut** horses have the same shade of red on mane, tail, and body. *Source:* courtesy of Dyan Westvang.

At the lighter end of variation it is common for the mane to be lighter than the tail, which can either be darker, similar to, or lighter than the body (Figures 3.23 and 3.24). Some manes and tails are mixtures of nearly white hairs and dark hairs. These are called **silver**. Depending on the relative amount of light and dark hairs, **silver** manes and tails can either be quite dark or quite light. The lightest manes and tails are called **flaxen**, and in some cases these are nearly white (Figure 3.25). The very lightest manes and tails seem to occur together, and most of these horses also have a similar pale color on the lower legs. Some people refer to the lighter-maned varieties as **sorrel**, but this has not become as standard as the American Quarter Horse or draft horse uses of the term **sorrel**.

In North America, **chestnuts** are generally named by the shade of body color only, while ignoring mane and tail color. An exception is those horses with **flaxen** manes and tails, which are commonly called **flaxen liver chestnut**, **flaxen chestnut**, or **flaxen sorrel**, and so on. The lightest shade of **flaxen sorrel** is common in the American Belgian and is a yellow shade that reveals hardly any redness at all. This shade is called **blond sorrel** by breeders of American Belgians and results from a combination of **chestnut**, light **shade**, **mealy**, and **flaxen**. These all contribute to the overall paleness of the **blond sorrel**. **Blond sorrel** is often a lighter color than the darkest **palominos**, and is a good example of the complexity of the intricate interactions of multiple factors leading to final colors.

South American Spanish has terms for the **chestnut** group that divide the colors by point color and only secondarily by body color. In South America, *tostado* describes

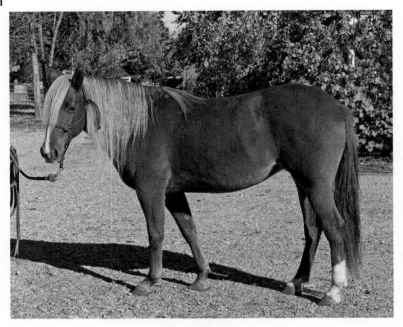

Figure 3.23 **Chestnut** horses often have manes and tails different shades than the body. This horse has a mane distinctly lighter than the body, while the tail is darker. *Source:* courtesy of Jeannette Beranger.

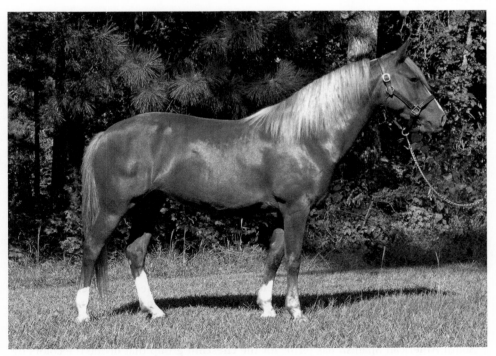

Figure 3.24 This is a **chestnut** horse with both mane and tail lighter than the body color. *Source:* courtesy of Laura Hornick Behning.

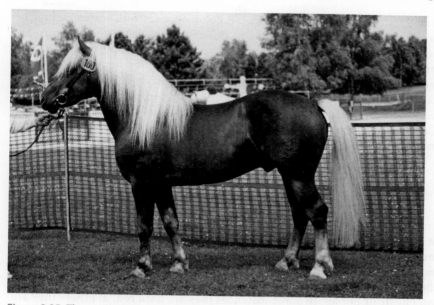

Figure 3.25 The very lightest manes and tails on **chestnut** horses are called **flaxen**, and can occur with any shade of **chestnut** body color. **Flaxen chestnut** (as in this figure) and **flaxen sorrel** are especially common in the Haflinger and other breeds that have undergone selection specifically in favor of this variant. *Source:* courtesy of Evelyn Simak.

those with darker manes and tails, *alazán* is used for those with red manes and tails, and *ruano* or *pelo de vaca* for those with flaxen manes and tails.

No single language seems to divide **chestnuts** and **sorrels** by manes, tails, and body colors to give the many distinct combinations possible. The usual approach in English is to denote the shade of **chestnut** (such as **liver chestnut**, **red chestnut**, **sandy** or **light chestnut**, and **sorrel** in some breeds) and then separately add **flaxen** if the mane and tail color are very light. Added accuracy comes from using the draft horse approach to the **sorrels**, but because these horses usually have lighter manes and tails, the point color is less important for these than for **chestnuts**.

Point color on the **chestnut** horses of many breeds varies through the entire range of possibility. The lighter **flaxen** manes are especially common in some draft horse breeds, while they are rare in breeds such as the Thoroughbred.

3.4.2 Genetic Control

Mane and tail colors on **chestnuts** (and **sorrels**) do not appear to be controlled by a single gene, even though some reports have been published stating that **flaxen** manes and tails are the result of a single recessive allele (reported as P^f for *flaxen*). Recent evidence suggests that it is more accurate to consider the determination of mane and tail color of **chestnuts** and **sorrels** as a polygenic trait (influenced by more than one gene). Many horses have mixed manes and tails in which dark, red, and light hairs all occur, which no doubt confounds genetic research into mane and tail color of **chestnut** horses because accurate classification into neat categories is impossible.

Unfortunately, the control of mane and tail color on **chestnut** horses cannot be viewed as a switch between mutually exclusive choices because all of the intermediate shades do occur. Most mane and tail colors of the **chestnut** group of colors can be grouped into the categories of **dark**, **red**, **light**, and **flaxen**. This simplistic approach lumps together some very different colors, but is a practical and reasonably accurate solution to a complicated issue. **Silver** manes and tails complicate definitions and nomenclature, because the intermixture of light and dark hairs varies from minimal to extensive, and the relative darkness of the dark hairs also covers the entire range possible on **chestnut** horses.

3.5 Bend Or Spots

Another common aspect of color on **chestnut** (and its derivatives) is the presence of random dark spots on the **chestnut** background color (Figure 3.26). These are called **Bend Or** (sometimes **Ben d'Or**) **spots**, after a Thoroughbred horse by that name, although these spots occur in all breeds. Indeed, most chestnuts have one or more of these dark spots. **Bend Or spots** can occur on other colors but are most common on **chestnut** horses. In some instances they are dark red, in others they are dark brown or black. They vary in number from being few to many. **Bend Or spots** vary from very large and unmistakable, to small and inconspicuous. **Bend Or spots** are scattered widely over the bodies of some horses. Whether these spots are under genetic control is unknown; however, they occur in most or all breeds with **chestnut** horses.

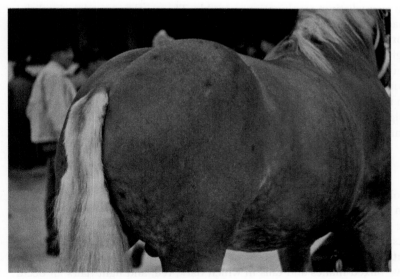

Figure 3.26 **Bend Or spots** are distinctive darker spots that occur on many **chestnut** horses. *Source:* courtesy of Evelyn Simak.

3.6 Dapples

Horses of most colors that are in good nutritional and physical condition are frequently **dappled**. Dappling is usually a network of dark and light areas in which the centers are lighter than the peripheries (Figure 3.27). Rarely is this interplay reversed, with the centers being dark and the peripheries being lighter (Figure 3.28). The dappling phenomenon can occur on any color. It is not necessarily consistent year to year or season to season and is therefore a detail of color that can be transient and not useful as a part of a permanent description of a horse.

    Dapples are most commonly noted on **sooty** colors due to the contrast of the black hairs with lighter ones, but can and do occur on all colors, including pale ones. **Dapples** can even be present as a subtle textural difference on **black** horses.

3.7 Brindle and Chimeras

Brindle is a rare horse color. **Brindle** in most mammals refers to vertical stripes on any background color. In most species the stripes are black, or one of the derivatives of black. Most horse owners are more liberal in the use of **brindle** and include any vertical striping pattern over any background color. Brindling tends not to affect the points, and these remain solid black or red. Brindling is considered to be a modification of a background color. It is usually seen on a **brown** (**sooty bay**) background, which results in a **bay brindle**, but it also can be seen on backgrounds of other colors. **Brindle** frequently

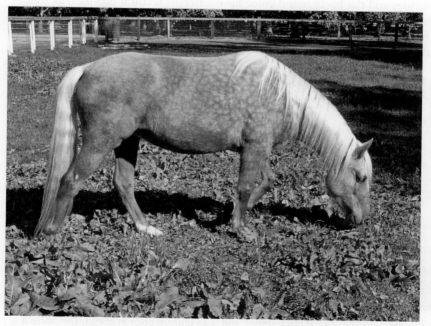

Figure 3.27 **Dapples** can occur on any color, and are a network of lighter and darker areas. Most dapples have lighter centers and darker peripheries.

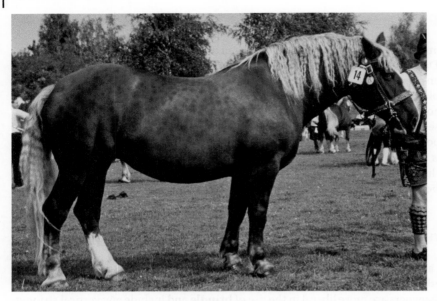

Figure 3.28 In rare cases the shading of **dapples** is reversed, so the centers are darker than the periphery. *Source:* courtesy of Evelyn Simak.

seems to require **sooty** black countershading for its expression and reorganizes **sootiness** into vertical stripes instead of a more uniform sprinkling of hairs. On many **brindle** horses the stripes and the background color have different textural qualities, as well as variations in color (Figures 3.29 and 3.30).

   Brindle has been seen as a rare variant in a variety of countries and horse breeds, but is so rare that generalities about its breed occurrence or genetic control have made it

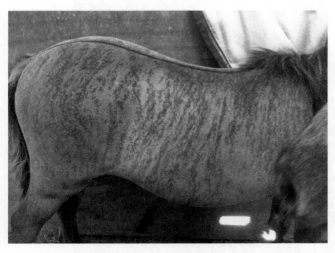

Figure 3.29 **Brindle** is usually vertical black stripes, and is an unusual color in horses. This horse is a **brindle grullo** with the black stripes superimposed over the expected slate body color, while the **dorsal stripe** of the **grullo** color is also retained. *Source:* courtesy of Chanel Bradley.

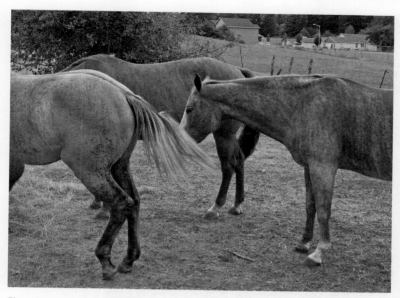

Figure 3.30 **Brindle** horses, in contrast to other species, can have different combinations of stripe and background color. The texture of the hair of the stripes can also be different from that of the background color. *Source:* courtesy of Denise Charpilloz.

difficult to study. Other mammals on which brindling occurs include dogs and cattle, and in these two species brindling is due to dominant genes. Results from the mating of **brindle** horses point to a similar dominant genetic phenomenon in horses, but the need for black countershading means that horses require both the genetic machinery for brindling as well as a specific background color that allows its expression. The exact combinations required for the final **brindle** appearance are therefore somewhat rare, and that can make the production of **brindle** horses seem somewhat haphazard.

Three separate biologic mechanisms have been described for **brindle**-type patterns in horses, and only two of these can be transmitted genetically to offspring. The first of these is associated with a skin disorder similar to *incontinentia pigmenti* in humans. This condition causes lesions to develop on the skin soon after birth; the regrowth in the affected areas is abnormal, which results in the **brindle** pattern. This is caused by a mutation located on the X chromosome, with a dominant mode of inheritance. As a result, only females develop the condition, because the mutation is lethal to male embryos and they die during development in the uterus. A single base change in the *inhibitor of kappa light polypeptide gene enhancer in B-cells* gene (*IKBK*) located on the X chromosome is thought to cause this condition. This is a rare disorder, and has only been reported in a single family of horses.

The second genetic mechanism has been documented in a family of American Quarter Horses that produced **brindle** horses consistent with an X-linked (sex-linked) dominant allele but without the underlying skin lesions of the *IKBK* mutation. This has been named *brindle 1* (*BR1*) (Figure 3.31). The phenotype varies, and horses have irregular coat texture and color in a typical striped pattern. Some of the horses were reported to have sparse manes and tails. The cause is a single base change in the

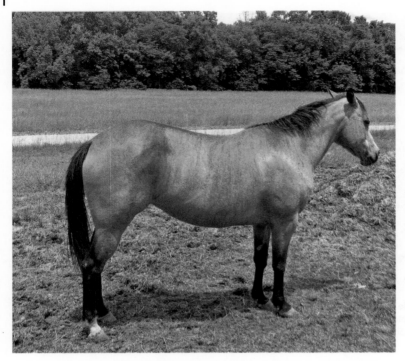

Figure 3.31 This is a **brindle** horse with the X-linked genetic mechanism. *Source:* courtesy of Janelle Osborne.

membrane bound transcription factor peptidase, site 2 (*MTFPS2*) gene, which is located on the X chromosome. This mutation removes parts of exon 10 and exon 11 from the final protein in a proportion of the gene products. Similar to the calico phenotype in cats, it is possible that random inactivation of the X chromosome leads to this **brindle** phenotype in females. Expansion of pigment cells that contain the nonmutated active form of the gene are the normal background color, while the **brindle** stripes have the other X chromosome activated, the one with the mutated copy of the *MTFPS2* gene. Further investigation may reveal the precise functional mechanism for these stripes, but they are likely due to differences in hair growth with hyperpigmentation.

A third mechanism for causing the striped appearance of one color laid over a second distinct background color occurs in animals that are chimeras (Figure 3.32). Chimeras result from the fusion of two embryos early in gestation, with a mixture of cells from the two different embryos into one final embryo (Figure 3.33). In these cases the striping of the **brindle** pattern results from the mixing of two embryos of different color, with the stripes of one color being from one embryo and the stripes of the other color from the second embryo. Chimeras are unable to pass along their **brindle** color to the next generation because their germ cells are each from only one embryo of the chimeric combination, and never from both.

The final appearance of **brindle** horses from each mechanism (genetic mutation or chimera) is similar, so the two types cannot typically be distinguished by visual

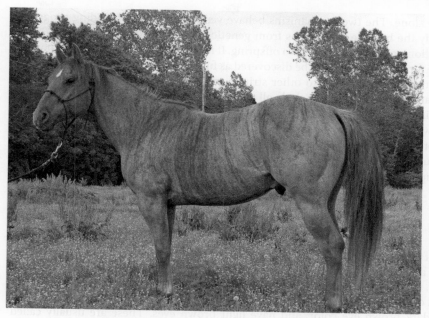

Figure 3.32 Most chimeric horses have a **brindle** pattern. *Source:* courtesy of Janelle Osborne.

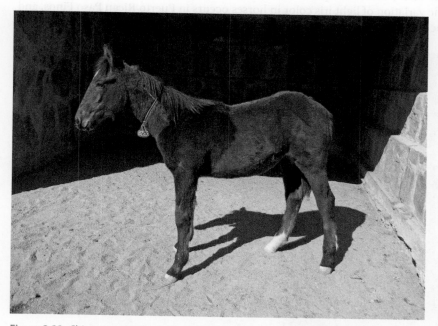

Figure 3.33 Chimerism might also be a factor in horses with an unusual interplay of somewhat random patches or stripes of color. *Source:* courtesy of Fran Ackley.

appearance alone. The two mechanisms behave very differently in breeding programs, because only the **brindle** that comes from genetic mutations, such as the *MTFPS2* or *IKBK* mutations, can be transmitted to offspring. It is possible that other novel mutations responsible for **brindle** color will be discovered as further investigations are undertaken.

The relationship of **brindle** to other striped patterns, usually with white stripes, is uncertain, and many observers include all of these as **brindle** patterns. A link between black striping and white striping is not present in other species. However, Sharon Batteatte, who has long had an interest in breeding **brindle** horses, has noticed that **brindle** horses can sometimes also produce white striping (or uneven **roan**) patterns. This intriguing result suggests that **brindle** in horses may be more closely related to a general striping phenomenon than it is in other species.

3.8   Eye Color

The eyes of horses are usually a dark brown color (Figure 3.34), and usually the sclera is pigmented as well, with the exception of **leopard** complex patterned horses (described in Chapter 8), which tend to have a white unpigmented sclera. The result is that eye color is usually not carefully scrutinized because variations are so rare. Some horses do vary from the usual dark brown eye color, and have light brown eyes. These are usually called **amber** or **hazel**. While these can occur with a variety of body colors, they are especially common on horses with alleles that dilute the base coat color, for example some horses with one dose of *cremello* (C^{Cr}) and somewhat more consistently in horses with a **champagne** (Ch^{C}) color or a **pearl** (C^{pr}) color.

A specific variation of light iris color in horses occurs in Puerto Rican Paso Finos, and is not associated with any base color dilution. These eyes are called **tiger eyes** or **goat**

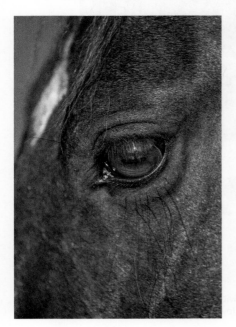

Figure 3.34 Most horses have dark brown eyes. *Source:* courtesy of Neil Chapman.

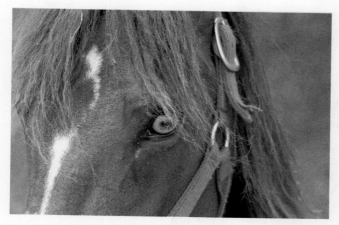

Figure 3.35 **Tiger eyes** are yellow, or light amber, and have been shown to be genetically inherited in Puerto Rican Paso Fino horses. *Source:* courtesy of Jo-Ann Ferré Crossley.

eyes for their characteristic yellow, amber or brighter orange color (Figure 3.35). In the Puerto Rican Paso Fino this **tiger eye** phenotype is due to a recessive allele that has been mapped to horse chromosome 1, and genetic loci from this chromosome are being investigated to identify the specific mutation causing this change.

Some horses, of many different colors, have eyes that are best described as **grey**. These are lighter than the normal dark eyes, but still dark and not easily confused with other eye colors. A few horses have light **amber** or **hazel** eyes, which can almost be **green**. These are more typical of **champagne** or **pearl** colors than any other color.

Blue eyes also occur and can either be dark or very pale (Figures 3.36 and 3.37). These are called **wall**, **blue**, **china**, **glass**, **watch**, or **white** eyes, depending on the shade

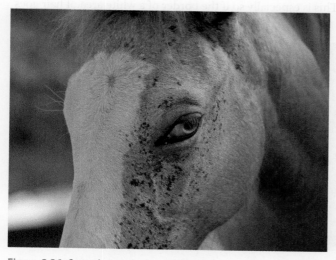

Figure 3.36 Some horses have variably dark blue, grey, and light blue areas in their eyes. *Source:* courtesy of Neil Chapman.

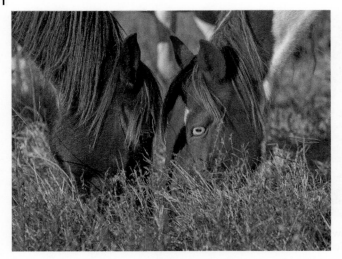

Figure 3.37 Light blue, or **glass eyes**, are unusual in horses without white markings. The horse on the right has a blue eye likely caused by the mutation that is also causing the white pattern. *Source:* courtesy of Neil Chapman.

and also on terminology that varies among localities. Blue eyes are consistent in horses with two doses of $C^{Cr}C^{Cr}$. They also occur very commonly in eyes that are surrounded by unpigmented (pink) skin. Most of the control over areas of unpigmented skin lies with genes coding for white patterns on the base colors, discussed further in Chapter 7.

A few horses with a dark base color and very little white marking have **blue** eyes, and the genetic mechanism behind these is very poorly understood. Horses with extensive white patterns sometimes have eyes that are a combination of blue areas and either dark or hazel areas (Figure 3.38). This is especially so if the border of a white area of hair goes

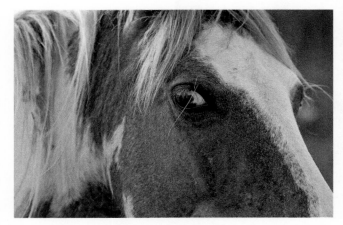

Figure 3.38 Horses with white marks on the head are the most likely to have eyes that have blue and brown areas mixed together. *Source:* courtesy of Neil Chapman.

through the eye socket. In many cases the blue portion of the eye is in the white area, but it is also fairly common for this relationship to be reversed so that the blue portion is adjacent to the pigmented area of skin.

All of the different colors of eyes seem to function just about equally well, although folk wisdom persistently holds that pale eyes are weaker than dark eyes.

3.9   Foal Color

The final adult color of foals can sometimes be tricky to predict. Foals are generally born a fairly pale shade, and then darken to the adult color when they shed the foal coat (Figure 3.39). **Black** horses, for example, are usually ashen grey as foals. An exception to this general rule is that foals of the **champagne** group of colors are frequently born darker than their color at maturity (Figure 3.40). The point color of foals is nearly always very pale, regardless of the final adult color. Some changes in the color of horses can be expected even up to a year or two of age (Figure 3.41). The adult color of most foals can be accurately predicted in those breeds in which a narrow range of dark adult colors occurs (**bay**, **chestnut**, **black**, and **grey**). But even in those breeds some foals will have adult coats that could not have been accurately predicted from the foal color.

The adult color of many foals is impossible to accurately determine. It is especially difficult to predict the adult color of foals in breeds in which some of the light colors are

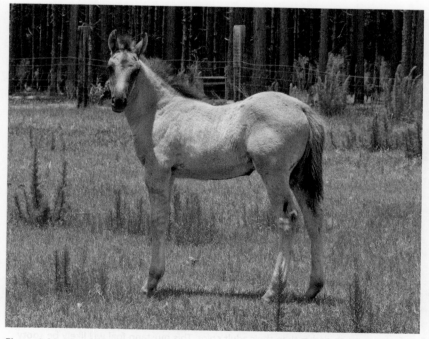

Figure 3.39   Most foals, like this **dun** foal, are born considerably lighter than their final adult color. *Source: courtesy of Jeannette Beranger.*

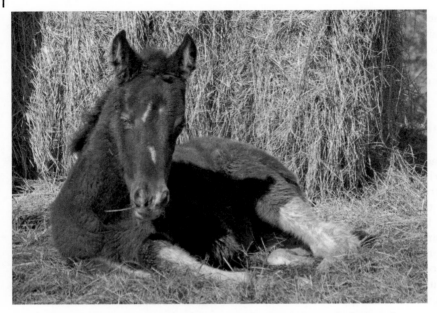

Figure 3.40 **Champagne** foals, of all shades, tend to be darker as foals than they are as mature horses. This **classic champagne tobiano** foal will be much lighter once shed out of its foal coat. The telltale light eyes and skin, though, are readily apparent even as foals. *Source:* courtesy of Vonda Hamilton.

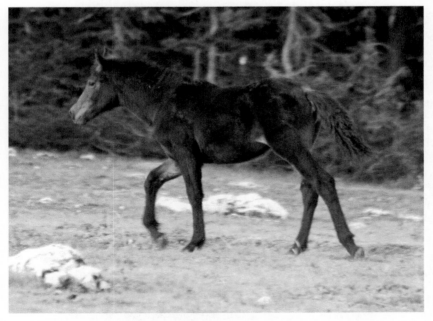

Figure 3.41 Few foals are much darker than their adult color. This mustang foal will likely be **sooty buckskin** at maturity. *Source:* courtesy of Dan Elkins.

common, such as **linebacked duns**, **cream**-related colors, **silver dapple**, **champagne**, and **pearl**. The foal coats of many of these colors are very similar to one another and mask the subtle distinctions that will later appear. For accurate identification it is generally wisest to wait until the foal coat is shed. The color of some horses does not stabilize until 2 or 3 years have passed. This is especially true if **dominant black** is present in the breed. A very few horses slowly and continually change color throughout life. Fortunately for those who study horse color genetics, such horses are rare.

4

Dilutions of the Basic Dark Colors

Many, but not all, of the colors derived from the darker colors **bay**, **chestnut**, **black**, **brown**, and **seal brown** are pale colors. As a group these colors are usually known as "dilute colors," and they fascinate many horse breeders. In many breeds these pale colors are experiencing an upswing in popularity, and it is increasingly important to classify them correctly as well as to understand their genetic control. Advances in the genetic understanding of the mechanisms behind these colors have proceeded rapidly, and many of the underlying causes and relationships of these colors are now well understood.

The incidence of the light colors differs from breed to breed, and also from region to region. The relative importance of these colors and their nomenclature have varied considerably both by time and place. In many traditions these colors have historically been rare, so they have tended to be grouped together, and the subtle but important differences between them have not always been appreciated. Confusion has long been typical of the understanding of this whole group of interesting colors.

Horse fanciers in some regions have for centuries used the term **dun** in a very general sense to refer to all pale, or dilute, colors of horses. This usage can be confusing because a closer look reveals a multitude of very distinctive dilute colors and shades. Confusion, especially historically, arose from the tendency to group all of these together (under the term **dun**) in breeds and regions in which these colors were rare, but to carefully and accurately designate each color separately in regions or breeds where these colors were more common. To further add to the confusion, **dun** is also often used for a specific single color within this group, and the specific color designated by this term is not always the same one from breed to breed. This makes it impossible to always know when "specific **dun**" or "general **dun**" is what is meant.

Light colors tend to be rare in those regions where the horse tradition is based on breeds of horses primarily of British origin (the eastern USA) and are more common in regions where the tradition involves breeds based on Spanish influences (the western USA). As a result of these two traditions the names of these colors vary. This guide adopts the more detailed terminology typical of the western USA and attempts to correlate the external phenotype to the underlying genotype. Genetic combinations are reflected in a unique name for each color to the extent that this is reasonably accurate and understandable. Owing to similarities of some of these colors this approach is not always successful, and those situations will be noted as they occur.

The recent upsurge of interest in and popularity of these colors in several breeds has also increased appreciation of them and their classification. In some breeds these colors

Equine Color Genetics, Fourth Edition. D. Phillip Sponenberg and Rebecca Bellone.
© 2017 John Wiley & Sons, Inc. Published 2017 by John Wiley & Sons, Inc.

have become common to the point of now being routine. This trend has especially been prominent in several breeds of gaited horses, such as Tennessee Walking Horse, Missouri Fox Trotter, Rocky Mountain Horse, and Mountain Pleasure Horse. This increase in frequency of the colors has greatly multiplied the color possibilities officially recognized by the registries for these breeds.

The dilute colors include at least seven groups. The two most common are **linebacked duns** (those that have **primitive marks**, including stripes on knees and hocks and stripe down the back) and **cream**-related colors. Two other groups are more limited in occurrence: **champagne** and **silver dapple**. **Pearl** and **mushroom** horses are currently rare in most breeds, but may well increase as selection favors them and increases their numbers. Finally, a very rare type of dilution has been documented in Arabian horses, although the cause is yet unknown. A few other breeds have other candidates for rare dilutions.

4.1 Linebacked Dun

4.1.1 Definition and Classification

An important group of pale colors includes **linebacked duns**, which generally consist of colors that have **primitive marks** (Figures 4.1, 4.2, 4.3, 4.4, and 4.5). These marks are darker than the base color and always include a stripe down the back (called the **list**, **dorsal stripe**, **lineback**, **backstripe**, or **eel stripe**). The **dorsal stripe** on many

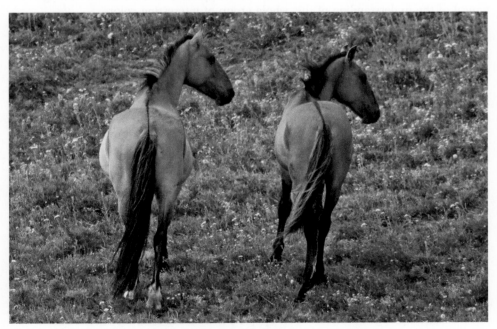

Figure 4.1 Dorsal stripes on **duns** vary from thin and delicate to much wider. *Source:* courtesy of Nancy Cerroni.

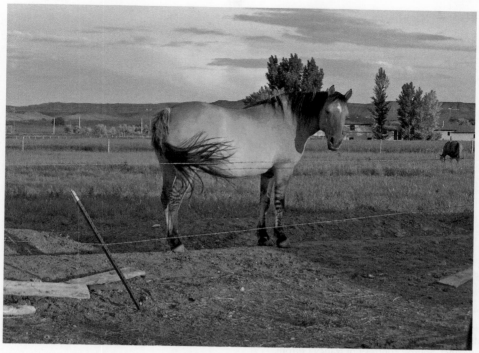

Figure 4.2 Striping on the legs of **dun** horses is usually behind the knees and to the sides of the hocks, and varies from extensive to nearly absent. The stripes are most likely to be subtle or missing on darker horses with very extensive black points.

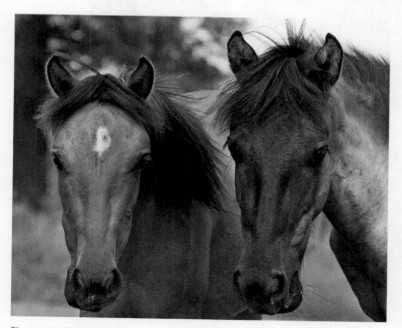

Figure 4.3 The delicate black stripes on the **dun** horse of this pair is called **spider webbing,** and is a fairly rare manifestation of **primitive marks**. The black region on the head of the **grullo** is typical of most horses of this color, and also occurs on a few **duns** as well. *Source:* courtesy of Neil Chapman.

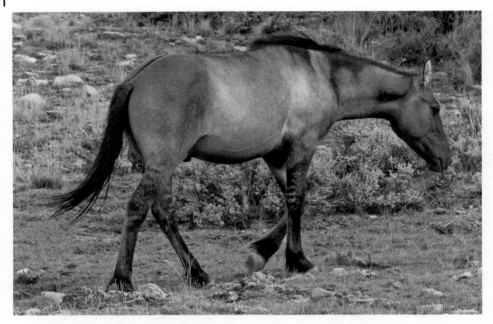

Figure 4.4 This **grullo** has multiple wither and neck stripes as well as a few more subtle transverse stripes off of the dorsal stripe. On some horses these are crisp and clear, whereas on others they are blurred and indistinct. *Source:* courtesy of Nancy Cerroni.

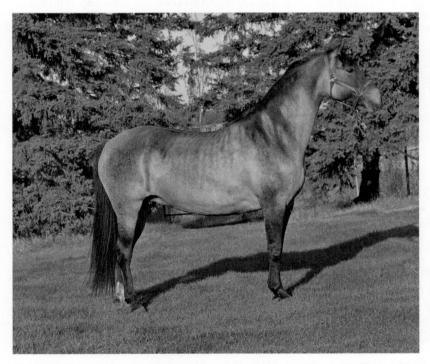

Figure 4.5 This mare is a combination of **dun** and **buckskin**, as well as **sooty**. The result is a heavily striped horse, with the typical yellow character of a **buckskin** underlying the overall color. As is common with darker **duns**, the **zebra stripes** on the legs are covered by black areas. *Source:* courtesy of Cindy Dietz.

linebacked duns carries into the mane and tail, resulting in manes and tails with dark centers and pale edges. Other **primitive marks** include bars on the sides of the hocks as well as behind, above, or below the knees (known as **zebra** or **tiger stripes**). Also included as **primitive marks**, although less frequent than **zebra stripes** or **dorsal stripes**, are stripes over the withers (**cross, withers stripe**) and sometimes concentric dark rings or fine stripes on the forehead or front of the face (**cobwebbing** or **spider-webbing**). Some observers include darker ear rims in the group of **primitive marks**. Darker ear rims are, in fact, present on most horse colors but are overlooked on darker colors because the contrast with body color is so subtle. Dark ear rims, therefore, are not an integral part of the group of **primitive marks**, even though they are more dramatic on **linebacked duns** than they are on other colors.

Primitive marks vary in extent and can occur in different combinations. The **backstripe** is a consistent feature and is the reason that horses with colors of this group are called **linebacked duns**. The other types of striping that are included as **primitive marks** are much more variable than the **backstripe**. When **primitive marks** are present in an extreme degree a horse can exhibit very many stripes. Extremely rarely are horses striped enough to resemble zebras in the number and intensity of stripes. These usually have a colored background rather than the nearly white background that is typical of zebras. The stripes on these tend to follow the general pattern of striping on zebras, varying in orientation depending on the body region. This contrasts with the consistently vertical character of striping on **brindle** horses.

Although the **primitive marks** are usually associated with **linebacked duns**, they can also occur on the non-dilute darker colors such as **bay** or **chestnut**. This is especially true of the **dorsal stripe**. The marks are fairly common in a low grade of expression on most colors if the hair coat is clipped short. In most of these cases the **backstripe** does not extend completely from tail to mane, which it almost invariably does on true **linebacked duns**. This detail bewilders many observers who confuse these somewhat weakly expressed **backstripes** with the prominent and obvious ones on **dun** horses.

The presence of **primitive marks** on non-dilute colors has led to great confusion over the character and classification of **dun** horses. However, genetic results, detailed later, indicate that the **linebacked** variant of dark non-dilute colors does have a genetic difference from both **linebacked duns** and dark horses lacking the **dorsal stripe**. The result is that not all horses with **primitive marks** are **duns**, which always have the combination of relatively pale colors and **primitive marks**. To add to the confusion of the classification of these colors, the **dorsal stripe** is especially likely to occur transiently on foals.

Dun, in the system of classification presented here, specifically refers to the lighter base colors that also have **primitive marks**. The array of traits that **dun** horses have (light color and **primitive marks**) is a single package, and no **dun** horses display the typical pale **dun** color without also having the **primitive marks**. Equally, nomenclature has historically grouped the dark colors as single colors, despite the presence of a **dorsal stripe** on some of them. All colors of the **dun** group do have some **primitive marks**, and these marks and the lighter background colors serve as the main definers of this group of colors.

Primitive marks have a connotation, due to their name, of occurring in primitive or local breeds, and they do indeed occur at a high frequency in most primitive breeds, such as Sorraia, Dülmen, and Konik. However, they also occur in many highly developed horse breeds that are far removed from any primitive ancestry, such as the Mulassier draft horse of France and the Norwegian Fjord horse. **Primitive marks** are, by themselves, no indication of more primitive breeding in a horse. The marks are indeed so variable, even in primitive breeds, that many **linebacked dun** horses of those breeds may lack some of the **primitive marks**. All **duns** do have the **backstripe**. The most common mark to be missing is the **wither stripe**, and sometimes the **zebra stripes** on the legs are also absent, especially if the legs are dark.

The most common group of **linebacked duns** are the **zebra duns**, and this is the group of colors most likely to be called simply "**dun**." **Zebra duns** have black points, **primitive marks** (which are usually black, but more rarely brown or red), and bodies some shade of tan. **Zebra duns** tend to be a distinctly tan shade rather than a lighter or clearer yellow, and it helps to think of **zebra dun** as dun dilution based on a **bay** color. The head of a **zebra dun** is usually a slightly darker shade than the body, but is still basically the same color as the body. This is in contrast to the **cream**-related colors, on which the head is usually the same shade of color as the body with the colors tending to be brighter and more yellow.

The terminology for the **zebra dun** group is somewhat variable. Some horse fanciers call these primitive-marked tan-based colors **buckskin**, but the general trend is to reserve that term for yellow horses that have black points but lack **primitive marks**. Similarly, many breeders refer to the **cream**-related varieties that lack the **dorsal stripe** as **dun**, especially in breeds of British extraction. The nomenclature is therefore somewhat hopelessly confusing because both of the terms, **dun** and **buckskin**, are used very specifically to designate different ones of these colors in different situations and different breeds.

In order to assure that each name goes with one color, this guide reserves **dun** for **linebacked** colors and reserves **buckskin** for black-pointed yellow horses lacking the full array of **primitive marks**. It is important to note that the use of the terms **buckskin** and **dun** are extremely variable throughout many breeds as well as many geographic regions. No system of nomenclature is inherently right or wrong, but it is important to note which system is being used for which breeds in order to avoid confusion and mis-identification of horses.

The middle shade of the **zebra dun** group tends to have tan body color. These are frequently the color of peanut butter and are sometimes called **peanut butter dun** (Figure 4.6). Some **zebra duns** are more of a yellow shade and are called **golden duns** (Figure 4.7), and a few are very pale and are called **silvery duns**. These last two are called **dunskin** by some observers, to convey the unique genetic combination that causes most of these. At the darkest extreme **zebra dun** could be confused with **bay**, except that the stripes are usually very prominent and the body color usually lacks the characteristic red tint of **bay** and is instead more of a dark tan. Those **zebra duns** with black counter-shading over the dorsal areas are called **coyote duns**, because they resemble the color of the coyote (Figure 4.8). A rare shade of **zebra dun** is **dusty dun**. **Dusty duns** have a flat beige body color, nearly like a **grullo** (GREW yo: in Spanish the double "l" is pronounced like "y" in English), but lack the black or dark head of the **grullo** classification. All of the variants of the **zebra dun** group have black points, although on some of these the black legs fade slightly at the coronary band above the hoof.

The **grullo** group of colors is generally darker than are the **zebra duns** and is also less frequent in most breeds. Relating **grullo** to a **dun** dilution on a base coat of **black** or

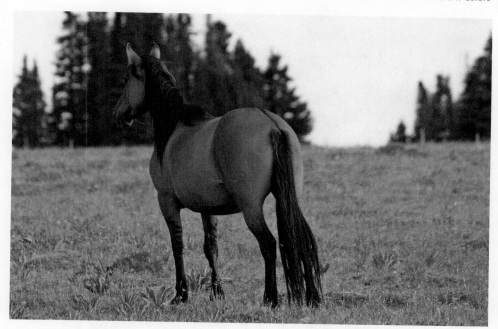

Figure 4.6 The usual shade of **dun** is a rich medium tan, sometimes called **peanut butter dun**. *Source: courtesy of* Dan Elkins.

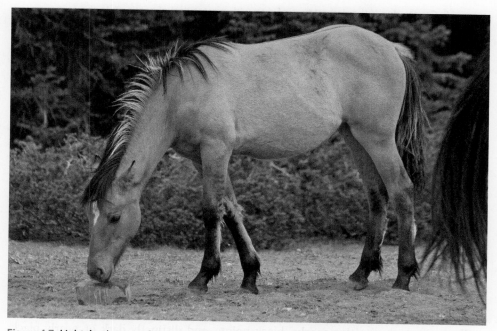

Figure 4.7 Light **dun** horses, often referred to as **golden duns**, can be mistaken for **buckskin**, except they have the **primitive marks** and nearly always have a head that is darker than the body. *Source:* courtesy of Dan Elkins.

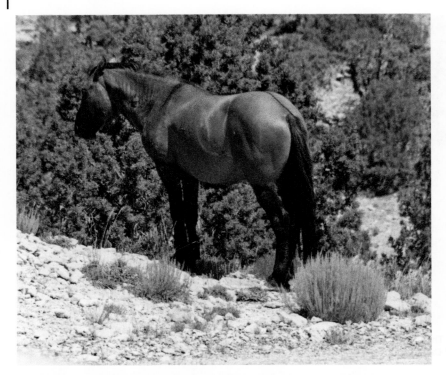

Figure 4.8 **Coyote dun** is the darkest type of dun, with a great deal of sootiness in the coat.

seal brown can be helpful in understanding this color. **Grullo** is the Spanish name for the crane bird, and these horses are similar to the bluish color of the sand hill crane. **Grullo** (on males, **grulla** on females) is the western term for this color and is more commonly used than the eastern terms, which are **blue dun** or **mouse dun**. A very few people refer to **grullos** as **smoky**, which can lead to confusion with the **smoky** that is related to the *cremello* allele. **Grullos** consistently have black points and also usually have dark or black heads that contrast dramatically with the body color. The **primitive marks** on **grullos** are characteristically black.

The body color of **grullos** varies among shades of flat beige (with little or no hint of tan or red tones) or, more commonly, slate. The middle shade is a clear bluish grey and is called **slate grullo** (Figure 4.9). The lightest shade is **silvery grullo**, and some of these have blue eyes (Figure 4.10). Those with **sooty** black countershading on the dorsal areas are called **lobo duns** (*lobo* is Spanish for "wolf") and can be quite dark (Figure 4.11). The dark color of some **lobo duns** results from an overall darkness of body color (from the **shade** effect). This type of **lobo dun** lacks **sooty** countershading and is more rare than the **sooty** type. Many lighter **grullos** tend to have a yellowish cast to the body color and are called **olive duns**, but they still retain the nearly black head that is one of the unifying characteristics of the **grullo** group (Figure 4.12). The essential hallmarks of the whole **grullo** group are **primitive marks**, black points, and distinctly dark or nearly black heads. As with **zebra dun** horses, the black legs on some **grullos** will fade slightly at the coronary band above the hoof.

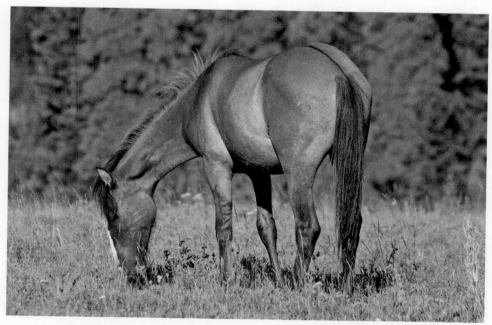

Figure 4.9 **Slate grullo** is a clear shade of greyish beige, with a dark head. *Source:* courtesy of Dan Elkins.

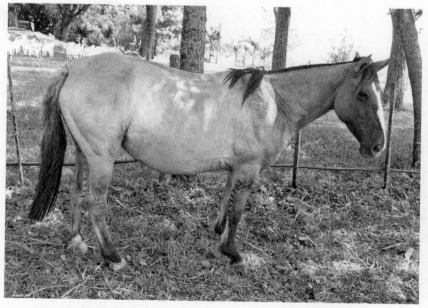

Figure 4.10 Light **grulla** color is rare, and retains the distinctly bluish grey tone of the entire group.

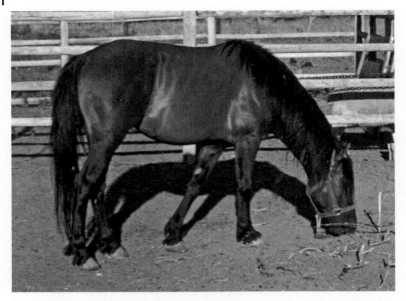

Figure 4.11 **Lobo dun** is the darkest of the **grullo** colors. Some of these horses have the **sooty countershading** as illustrated here.

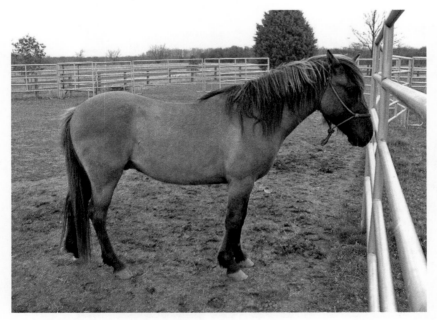

Figure 4.12 **Olive dun** is a **grullo** with a distinct tan tint to the body color, but with the black head typical of **grullos**.

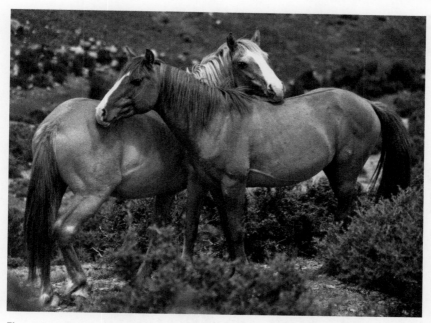

Figure 4.13 **Red dun** and **apricot dun** are similar colors, and the darker shades are nearly the same color as **sorrel** or light **chestnut** horses.

Linebacked duns with nonblack points are an extremely variable group, and when grouping them together it can help to think of them as **dun** dilution on a base color of **chestnut**. These colors tend to be less common than **zebra duns** but are more common than **grullos**. These colors are usually lumped together rather than split finely into different shades of color. When lumped together these colors are all referred to either as **red dun** or **claybank dun**. Similar to the case with **zebra duns**, the terms **red dun** and **claybank dun** are also used in a stricter sense for specific shades within the broader **red dun** group (Figures 4.13, 4.14, and 4.15).

The darkest **red duns** have brownish points and a paler brown body color. The mane, tail, and head are usually dark (Figure 4.14). This color is **muddy dun**. **Muddy duns** are quite rare. The next three shades are more common. **Red dun** is a reddish body color with darker red points. **Red duns** can be nearly the color of a **light chestnut** or **sorrel**, but have the very distinct **primitive marks** (in a darker red color) that distinguish them from **sorrels** or **light chestnuts** (Figure 4.13). **Orange dun** is a lighter body color, and generally the mane and tail are lighter as well, although they can be the same shade as the body or darker. **Apricot duns** are the lightest of this group, and most are distinguished by a very pale body color (Figure 4.15). Most, but not all, **apricot duns** have **mealy** shading and are lighter on the belly and between the legs. Most **apricot duns** have lighter manes and tails, but some do have darker manes and tails. Black countershading on any of the **red duns** is rare and is simply designated by adding **sooty** to the color name, as in **sooty red dun**, for example.

The final group of varieties of **linebacked dun** without black points includes those that fit nowhere else. Some of these horses are pale, yellow to reddish, and have brown or red points. These colors are usually simply called **claybank dun** (Figure 4.16).

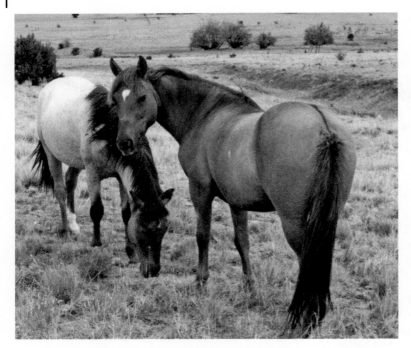

Figure 4.14 **Muddy dun** is the darkest of the **red dun** shades, and is rare.

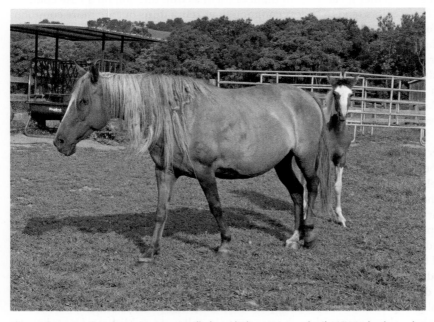

Figure 4.15 **Apricot dun** horses generally have light manes and tails. Most also have the **mealy** effect, which this horse lacks.

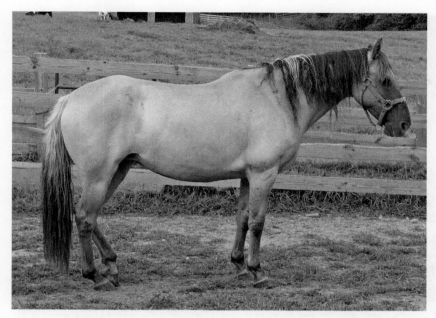

Figure 4.16 **Claybank dun** horses are pale and fit no other neat classification of **dun**.

Claybank duns can be similar enough to **palomino** to be confused with that color. The usual distinction is that the manes and tails of **claybank duns** are browner or redder than those of **palominos**, and the lower legs are also redder or browner. Red or brown points do not occur on **palominos**. An occasional **palomino**-colored horse will have **primitive marks**, in which case it is called **linebacked palomino** (Figure 4.17). Some **cream** horses have **primitive marks** and are then **cream duns** or (less accurately) **white duns**. These can also be called **dunalino**, which conveys their likely genotype.

The whole group of **linebacked dun** colors is characteristic of (but not limited to) primitive or rugged breeds. They are a consistent feature of the Tarpan (usually **grullo**), Sorraia, Dülmen, and Przewalski's horse (these last three are usually **zebra dun**, although the Sorraia is also commonly **grullo**). The Przewalski's horse (*Equus przewalski*) is unfortunately the only remaining species of wild horse; all of the others are domesticated breeds (*Equus caballus*) that are changed in several ways from the wild ancestor.

Linebacked dun colors also occur in some highly developed and specialized breeds. Therefore, their presence alone is no indication of primitive type. In some breeds, most notably the Fjord, these colors are a consistent feature. **Linebacked dun** colors are also common in Spanish breeds from North and South America, although this class of colors is now rare in Spain, where the ancestors of these breeds originated. Breeds such as the American Quarter Horse are likely to get the **dun** colors from the Spanish foundation stock that contributed to the breed. **Linebacked duns** are common in northern European pony breeds and are present in a few draft breeds, such as the Mulassier. **Linebacked duns** are rare, but persistent, in some saddle horse

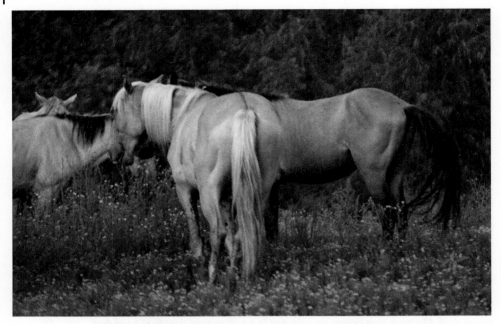

Figure 4.17 **Linebacked palomino** horses have the gold color of **palominos** but also the **primitive marks** typical of **duns**.

breeds from Europe. **Linebacked duns** are notably lacking in the Arabian and Thoroughbred breeds.

The naming of **linebacked dun** colors in the Fjord breed varies from the approach taken by most other breed registries. Part of the reason for this is that the color names used in the Fjord breed by breeders in the USA tend to be direct translations from the original Norwegian for these colors (Figures 4.18, 4.19, and 4.20). **Zebra dun** is generally called **yellow dun** or **brown dun**, depending on the depth of the background shade (*bruunblakk* in Norwegian, with *lys* for light and *mørk* for dark). The lightest colors are called *ulsblakk* or *borket* and are silvery. **Grullo** is referred to as **grey** (*grå*), which could lead to confusion if used in a different breed because **grey** in most breeds refers to a pattern of white hairs and definitely does not refer to **grullos**. **Red dun** is conveniently referred to as **red dun** (*rødblakk*). Yellower horses with light points are called *gul*. Occasionally, very pale Fjord animals are born, and these are called **white** (*kvit*) or **white dun**, and they do retain some hint of **primitive marks**. The Fjord breeders' approach to the **linebacked dun** group of colors is obviously not consistent with usual North American usage, but this is of little consequence because this breed displays only **linebacked dun** colors and no others. The result is that their color names cannot lead to confusion within that one breed, but they certainly would lead to confusion if used outside the Fjord breed.

Folk wisdom holds that **linebacked duns** are very tough and durable and are good horses for extreme situations. They generally have a reputation for being very dependable and standing up very well to hard use. Some variation in acceptance of the shades within the group is present. The Argentines, for example, praise **grullos**, while some

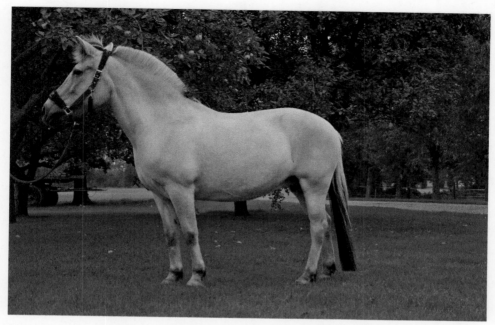

Figure 4.18 Fjord horse **duns** are generally lighter than those of other breeds. The light overlay of the central black mane is dramatically emphasized by the trimming of the mane undertaken by most breeders and owners. *Source:* courtesy of Anouk Schurink.

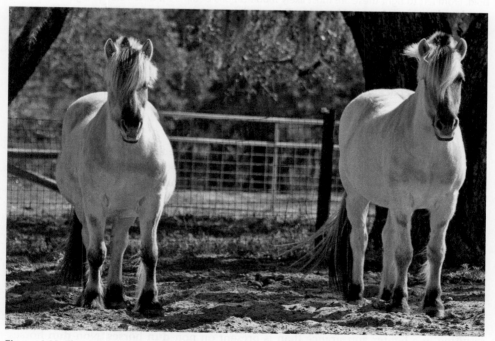

Figure 4.19 The color called **grullo** in most breeds is called **grå** for "grey" in the Fjord breed. It is characteristically pale, as are all the Fjord variants of **dun**. This pair shows the limited extent of the black region on the head, typical for this color in this breed. *Source:* courtesy of JoAnn Bellone.

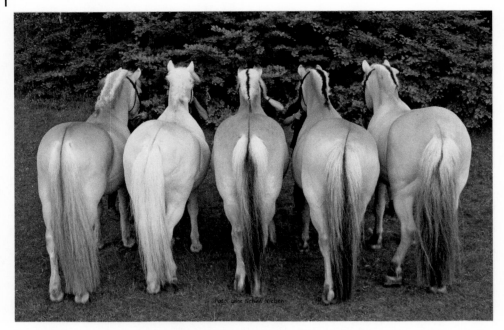

Figure 4.20 These are the main variations of **dun** in the Fjord breed. All of them are paler than similar colors based on the same basic genotypes in other breeds. This is most likely due to selection for pale shades. The dorsal stripes on these colors in this breed also tend to be delicate rather than bold. From left to right these are most likely modifications of different base color backgrounds: **sorrel**, **perlino**, **black**, **bay**, and **buckskin**. The overall paleness can make fine distinctions of base color difficult to assess in this breed. *Source:* courtesy of Line Shøn Nielsen.

Mexican horse traditions disparage these. Cowboys from the western USA generally favored all **linebacked** shades.

4.1.2 Genetic Control

The dominant allele, Dn^+, at the *Dun* locus is responsible for **linebacked duns**, and is sometimes abbreviated Dn^D. This allele is considered to be the wild-type allele because all of the current related wild species exhibit some variation of **dun** color. These include Przewalski's horse, the only remaining species of wild horse, and the various wild asses. This nomenclature may be confusing, but only because this group of colors is now relatively rare in most breeds of domesticated horses, while the non-dun colors have become the general rule. The effects of the Dn^+ allele are summarized in Table 4.1. The *dun* allele causes black on the body to be lightened to a slate blue grey or beige, and red on the body to be lightened to tan (on **bays**) or light red (on **chestnut**). It tends to leave points unaffected, as well as leaving the head darker than the body.

The dun phenotype is caused by asymmetrical deposition of pigment in the hair, resulting in a lighter appearance than is present on non-**dun** horses. Non-**dun** horses have pigment that is deposited symmetrically around the hair shaft. The differences in

Table 4.1 *Dn+* modifications of base color, **sooty**, and **shade**.

| Base color | Linebacked **dun** derivative | | | |
	Sooty variant	Dark shade	Medium shade	Light shade
Black	Lobo dun	Lobo dun Dark grullo	Slate grullo	Silvery grullo Olive dun
Seal brown	Shaded lobo dun	Shaded lobo dun Shaded dark Grullo	Shaded mealy Grullo	Dusty dun
Bay	Coyote dun	Dark dun	Zebra dun	Golden dun Silvery dun
Chestnut	Sooty red dun	Red dun Muddy dun	Red dun Orange dun	Clayblank dun Apricot dun
Sorrel	Sooty Apricot dun	Apricot dun	Apricot dun	Apricot dun

the colors are controlled by three alleles that regulate *T-box 3* (*TBX3*) on horse chromosome 8 (Figure 4.21). The *wild-type Dn⁺* allele is specific for the **dun** phenotype, and the other two alleles are associated with non-**dun** phenotypes. These two alleles are *non-dun 1* (*Dn^{d1}*) and *non-dun 2* (*Dn^{d2}*).

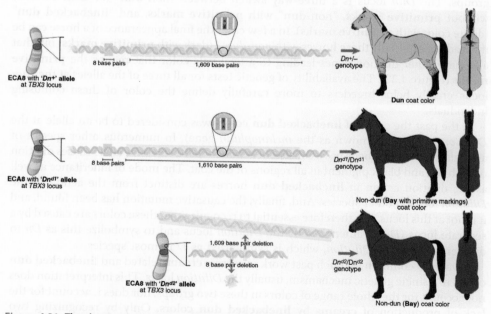

Figure 4.21 The **dun** coat color is controlled by three alleles at the *TBX3* locus. Horses that have at least one copy of the *wild-type* allele have the **dun** phenotype. Non-**dun** horses can be homozygous for the *non-dun 2* allele and are then dark with no **primitive marks**. Horses that are homozygous for the *non-dun 1* allele, or heterozygous for *non-dun 1* and *non-dun 2*, are dark but also have **primitive marks**, at least a **dorsal stripe**. *Source:* courtesy of Francesca Gianino.

Horses that are heterozygous or homozygous for the Dn^+ allele are a **dun** color with **primitive marks**. The *non-dun 1* (Dn^{d1}) allele has a single base pair change, with G changing to T in the genetic code. This allele allows for the presence of a **dorsal stripe** but does not dilute the body color (Figure 4.21). This allele has been found in pre-domestication horse samples, indicating that it is an old variant. The third allele, *non-dun 2* (Dn^{d2}), results from two deletions of portions of the DNA code of the *TBX3* gene. The two deletions are close to one another. One of them is 1609 base pairs long, and the other is only 8 base pairs long. These deletions affect the expression of the gene and cause an even distribution of pigment in the hair, and therefore a dark coat color. The *non-dun 2* (Dn^{d2}) homozygotes usually have no expression of **primitive marks**, and have dark coats. Horses that are heterozygous for *non-dun 1* and *non-dun 2* ($Dn^{d1}Dn^{d2}$) have non-**dun** coat colors but may show **primitive marks**. A genetic test is available for all three alleles.

Primitive marks are characteristic of horses with Dn^+. **Primitive marks** are associated with these colors as an integral part of the action of Dn^+. The **primitive marks** are generally lacking in horses having only *non-dun 2* (Dn^{d2}) but are expressed in horses homozygous for *non-dun 1*. The three-allele system explains the **dun** coat color, and also explains the presence of the dorsal stripe in some dark colored horses.

The result of Dn^+ is that **black** is changed to **grullo**, **seal brown** to a subtly shaded **grullo** that is usually only slightly different than **grullo**, **bay** to **zebra dun**, and **chestnut** to one of the **red dun** colors. The Dn^+ allele generally leaves **sooty** areas fully expressed. The shade of body color can vary on **linebacked duns**, just as it does in other color groups. The *Dun* locus is a three-way switch between "non-**dun**" (or dark colored) without **primitive marks**, "non-**dun**" with **primitive marks**, and "**linebacked dun**" (dilute color with **primitive marks**). In a few cases the final appearance of a horse can be misleading, especially those horses with *non-dun 1* (dark with **primitive marks**) but that also have other dilution genes leading to a final pale color that retains the **primitive marks** (Figure 4.22). The availability of genetic tests for all three of the alleles at the *Dun* locus greatly helps breeders to more carefully define the color of these confusing individuals.

In the past the cause of **linebacked dun** colors was considered to be an allele at the *Dilution* locus (also known as the *melanophilin* gene). In numerous other species of animals the *Dilution* locus has a consistent action in that a recessive allele causes dilution of both red and black pigment in all regions of the coat. The mode of inheritance as well as the dilution action in **linebacked dun** horses are distinct from the action of the *Dilution* locus in other species. And, finally, the causative mutation has been found, and it is not at this locus. It is therefore essential to recognize that these colors are caused by a separate locus (*Dun*) rather than by the *Dilution* locus and to symbolize this as *Dn* to differentiate it from *Dilution*, which is symbolized as *D* in most species.

It was also common in much past work to ascribe **cream**-related and **linebacked dun** colors to a single genetic mechanism, usually the *Dilution* locus. This interpretation does not account for the whole range of colors in these two groups, nor does it account for the lack of production of **creams** by **linebacked dun** colors. Only by recognizing two separate loci as responsible for these colors is it possible to account for all of the various colors in the **dun** group and to understand the genetic mechanisms producing them. Fortunately, the mutations responsible for these color variations have now all been documented and described.

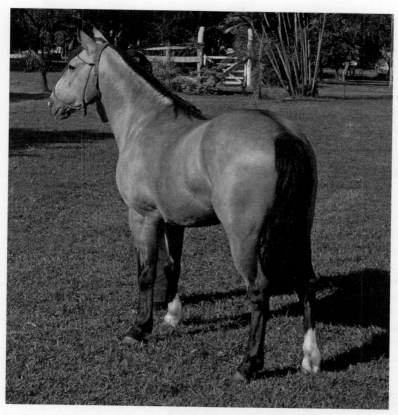

Figure 4.22 Some dark horses have **primitive marks**, although on most dark base colors this can be subtle and often is missed. When those colors are combined with the *cremello* allele, the results are more obvious. This horse is homozygous for the *non-dun 1* allele, leading to the backstripe, but is also a **golden buckskin** as betrayed by the uniformity of the gold yellow color that lacks the dark head of **zebra dun**. On most *non-dun 1* horses the dorsal stripe is weaker than on **duns**, and rarely extends completely to the withers.

4.2 Cream-related and Pearl Colors

4.2.1 Definition and Classification

The **cream**-related colors derive mainly from dilute red and yellow pigment, and include many different horse colors. This is an important group of colors for many horse breeders. The accurate classification of these colors is essential for breeding programs interested in producing **buckskin** and **palomino** colored horses. The **pearl** colors are recently documented as part of this group. The **pearl** colors are rare, but their genetic relationship with **cream**-related colors makes it best to discuss them in the same section.

Accurate classification of these horses is especially important if the production of extreme dilute horses is to be avoided. Avoiding the so-called **creams** with blue eyes and pink skin is a fairly common goal in breeding programs working with these colors, although some few breeders have been using **cream** horses to their advantage in the production of both **buckskin** and **palomino** foals.

Buckskin is the term commonly used for the horses that have a yellow body and black points, although this nomenclature is by no means universally accepted. These are basically **bay** horses with a dilute coat. In British or eastern usage this color is frequently referred to simply as **dun**, although that can lead to much confusion because western usage tends to reserve **dun** for **linebacked duns** (as described earlier). The color lacking the **dorsal stripe** is usually called **buckskin** in western usage, although **buckskin** is used by some horse fanciers to designate a similar **linebacked** variety. Various breed registries differ on the definition of **buckskin** and **dun**. The approach presented here is by no means universal; for example, **dun** is frequently used for the color designated here as **buckskin**. This is especially true for pony breeds of British origin. The approach in this guide is to reserve **dun** for the **linebacked** varieties and **buckskin** for the varieties lacking the **primitive marks** caused by $Dn^{+}+$.

Shade can vary on **buckskins**, just as on other color groups. The darker ones are sometimes brownish yellow and are called **dusty buckskins**, although more frequently the darker ones tend to be a gold color and are called **golden buckskins** (Figure 4.22). The medium shade is **buckskin** (or **yellow buckskin**), and the lightest is **silvery buckskin** (Figure 4.23). **Sooty buckskins** have dorsal countershading and are also called **dark buckskins** (Figure 4.24). Some of these can be very dark, and most of the dark ones are strongly dappled. Some of the darkest colors can be confusing because they are so dark as to be nearly black, but they have the characteristic yellow highlights

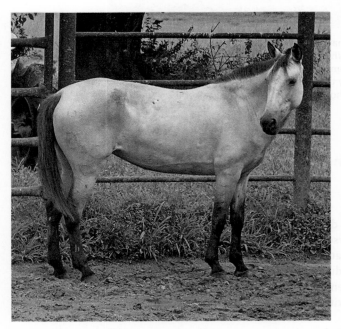

Figure 4.23 Lighter **buckskin** horses are sometimes called **silvery buckskin** to indicate the pale body color.

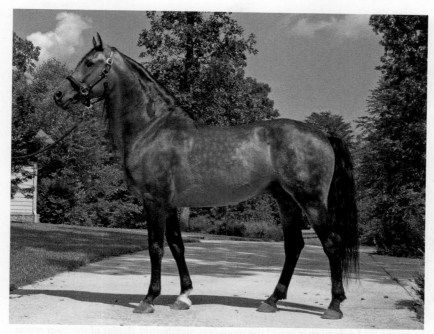

Figure 4.24 **Sooty buckskin** horses generally end up being a color that is difficult to describe or to classify. Many of them are strongly dappled, which shows off dramatically due to the contrast of the black countershading with the gold background color. *Source:* courtesy of Laura Hornick Behning.

of the **buckskin** group of colors. These highlights usually persist in the flank, behind the elbow, inside the legs, and from the ears to the jaw. These light areas remain on even the darkest of the **sooty buckskins**. The **mealy** effect is rarely noted on buckskins, although it can occur.

On a few **buckskin** horses the point color, especially on the legs, is not really black but instead is a very dark brown. This color can become lighter at the coronary band, but usually the lower leg is black enough to avoid confusion with other colors, and these horses are indeed genetically **buckskins**.

Palominos are yellow horses with nonblack points, and they generally have pale manes and tails. They are **cream**-dilute **chestnuts**. Head, body, and leg color are usually all the same on these. **Palominos** vary from a rich gold shade to a clear yellow shade. The classic definition of **palomino** is that they should be the color of a newly minted gold coin and have white manes and tails. In reality the **palomino** color is much more variable than this, and the desired **golden palomino** shade is one of the rare variants within this color group (Figure 4.25). **Sooty** (or **smutty**) **palominos** have black mixed in with the yellow body coat hairs (Figure 4.26). **Sooty palominos** can be quite dark and can be very difficult to distinguish from **chestnut**. Many **sooty palominos** are dramatically **dappled**. The very palest **palomino** shades have dark cream bodies and occasionally have amber eyes. These are called **isabelos** (Figure 4.27).

Some **palominos** have considerable amounts of dark hair mixed into their manes and tails. On **palominos** this mixture is especially likely to be called **silver** (although this

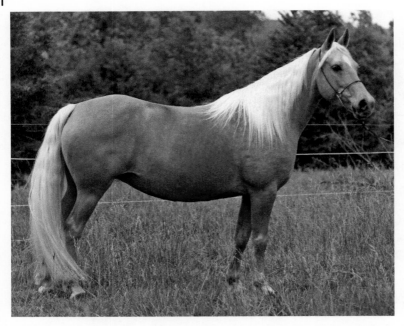

Figure 4.25 The bright gold **palomino** is one of the more rare, and desired, shades of the color group. *Source:* courtesy of Dyan Westvang.

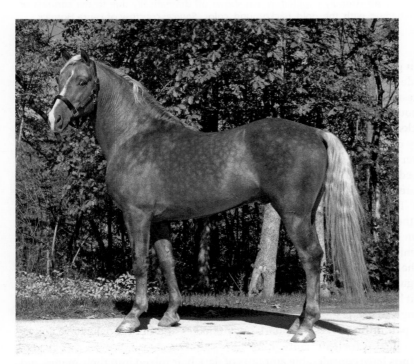

Figure 4.26 **Sooty palomino** is an unusual color, and is often mistaken for several other colors. Many of them have **silver** manes and tails, some of which are quite dark. They tend to be strongly **dappled**. *Source:* courtesy of Laura Hornick Behning.

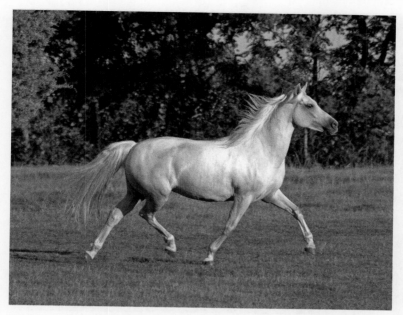

Figure 4.27 The lighter **isabelo** shade is more common among **palominos** than the darker, golder shades. The skin and eye color of this horse clearly indicate its **palomino** color rather than confusing it with a **cremello**, which would have pink skin and blue eyes. *Source:* courtesy of Laura Hornick Behning.

should not be confused with the **silver dapple** colors discussed later). **Bend Or spots** are fairly common on **palomino** horses, much as they are on **chestnuts**. The contrast of the darker **Bend Or spots** against the yellow or gold color of **palominos** makes these spots much more noticeable than they are on **chestnut** horses.

One rare horse color, which is usually missed as being part of the **cream**-related group, is **smoky**. **Smoky** horses are best described as "off black" and are only included in the discussion of these colors because they have important genetic ties to the **cream**-related colors. **Smoky** horses are usually a flat color that is not quite **brown**, not quite **liver chestnut**, and not quite **black** (Figure 4.28). The points are black, but observers sometimes miss the subtle differences between the point and body colors. **Smoky** horses are frequently registered as either **brown** or **dark liver chestnut** despite the black points. They frequently have hazel eyes. **Smoky** horses occur rarely, and only in breeds in which **palomino** or **buckskin** horses also occur. Because **smoky** horses are likely to be misregistered as another dark color, they can often produce surprises when **buckskin** or **palomino** foals are born. A few horses are **smoky** with yellow highlights in the flanks, muzzle, and around the eyes. These are essentially light **seal brown** horses, and can be called **smoky seal** to distinguish them from ordinary **seal brown**.

The very palest horses (that are not **white**) are cream colored. In many instances the only way to determine that these horses are not white is to look for a slight color difference at the boundary of a white facial or leg marking. These cream-colored horses are often simply called **creams**. The term **cream** is often used for this entire group of very dilute colors, and often the lightest ones are called **cremellos** to provide for more accuracy (Figure 4.29).

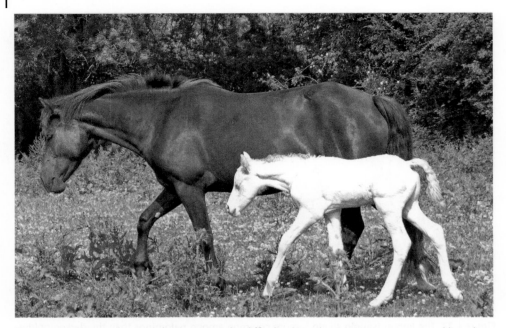

Figure 4.28 This **smoky** mare demonstrates the difficulty this color presents to owners and breeders. Many are registered either **chestnut** or **brown**, but can easily produce **perlino** foals, like this one, when mated to **buckskin** mates. *Source:* courtesy of Finola Mulholland.

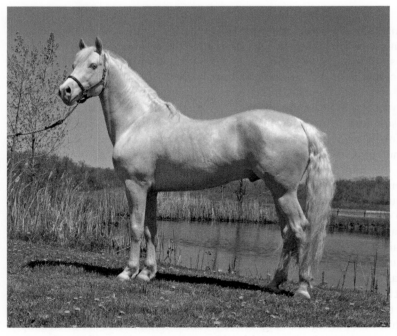

Figure 4.29 **Cream** horses have subtle differences that can correlate to the underlying color genotype. The lightest ones are nearly white, with light manes and tails. These are **cremellos**. *Source:* courtesy of Laura Hornick Behning.

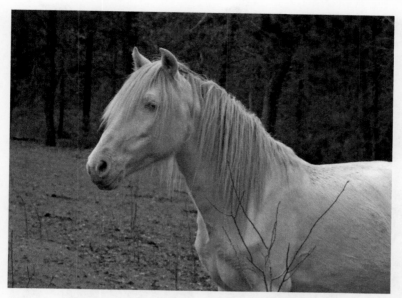

Figure 4.30 Most **perlino** horses retain manes and tails that are slightly darker than the body color. *Source:* courtesy of Jeannette Beranger.

Cremellos have pink skin and blue eyes. Their body color is off-white, and their manes and tails are white or nearly so. Two other subtypes of **cream** horses occur and are easily confused with **cremellos**. These are more important for genetic considerations than for identification purposes and include **perlino** and **smoky cream** colors. **Perlino** horses have similar body color to **cremello** horses, but the points are distinctly darker, usually a pale brown (Figure 4.30). **Smoky cream** horses are rare, and generally a pale brown color on both body and points (Figure 4.31). **Smoky cream** has also been called **silver smoky**, but this terminology can lead to confusion with other uses of the term **"silver"** in horse color terminology.

To some extent **cremello**, **perlino**, and **smoky cream** all can be confused with one another, because they are all cream-colored horses. The differences, when present, can be that most **perlinos** retain pale tan color in the mane, tail, and lower leg, while some **smoky creams** retain even more pigment in these areas and sometimes also on the body. Still, all three are cream-colored horses with pink skin and blue eyes, and they generally are lumped under **cream** or **cremello** for most identification purposes even though breeders find it useful to separate them due their different potential for base color production.

These three **cream** colors (**cremello**, **perlino**, and **smoky cream**) occur only in breeds in which **palomino** or **buckskin** occur. In many breeds none of the **cream** colors can be registered, even though **palomino** and **buckskin** horses are offered full registration by registries for these breeds. This trend is changing, though, and many registries that barred these in the past now accept them for registration.

The American Albino and Creme Horse Registry (they prefer the "creme" spelling to the more usual "cream") has four categories for cream-colored horses with pink skin and blue eyes. Their "A" classification is for cream-colored horses with lighter manes

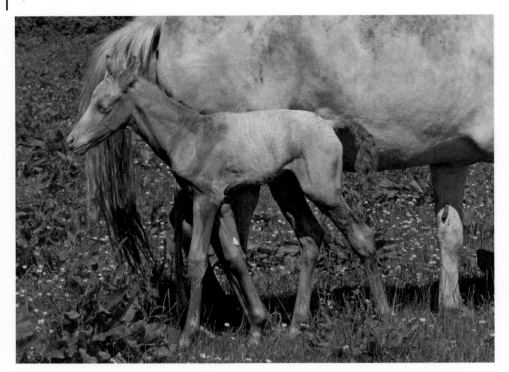

Figure 4.31 **Silver smoky** horses usually have a pale brown color on mane, tail, and body.
Source: courtesy of Finola Mulholland.

and tails, which essentially denotes **cremellos**, although some **perlinos** and **smoky creams** probably end up fitting this description as well. The "B" classification is for cream horses with darker manes and tails, and usually this includes **perlinos** and **smoky creams**. The "C" classification is for darker creams that usually have manes and tails the same shade as the body. This is sometimes fulfilled by darker **perlinos** and especially by **smoky creams**. The "D" classification is for creams with some sootiness, which is rare, and may be **sooty** countershaded **cremellos**, **perlinos**, and **smoky creams**. "Albino" in the registry name is confusing, because complete albinism (in its strictest sense) has not been reported in horses. **Creams** closely approach being albinos, but they lack the essentially white coat color and pink eye characteristics that are typical of albinos in other species. These colors in horses are due to a different genetic mechanism than the albinos of most other species.

Cream-related colors occur in a fairly wide distribution of breeds, especially British ponies, as well as in New World Spanish breeds and their derivatives such as the American Quarter Horse. They occur as a rare variant in many others, including the Thoroughbred, other saddle breeds, some Warmblood breeds, and in the Mulassier draft horse from France. These colors are not present in the Arabian horse.

The **palomino** color is the basis of a registry for horses of the appropriate color and specific saddle horse backgrounds. **Palomino** is a color with an identity apart from the Palomino registry and does occur as a color in many breeds, so the color should not generally be confused with a specific breed. The **buckskin** term is also used for a few registries, although these registries are based on **linebacked duns**. The use of **buckskin** for the **linebacked dun** colors was once widespread but is decreasing, and it is important to note that **buckskin** as presented here refers to the **cream**-based color rather than a **linebacked dun** color. The use of **buckskin** by the Buckskin registries is in keeping with a separate system that includes all **linebacked duns** as variants of **buckskin**.

Palomino and **buckskin** are considered by folk wisdom to be flashy but somewhat thin skinned. As a result they have generally not been favored for hard work under trying conditions. Part of the reason for the low regard for these colors is that it is difficult to keep these (and all other) light colors clean and looking good, especially in harness horses. In other situations, such as parade and saddle use, these colors are highly desired by many people because they are flashy and eye-catching.

Folk wisdom generally considers **cream** to be associated with weak horses. Part of the reason for this is that pink skin is considered weaker than black skin. Another disconcerting aspect of these colors, at least for some observers, is light-colored eyes. Many people consider amber or blue eyes to have reduced vision compared with the usual brown eyes of horses. Most light-eyed horses, however, see perfectly well and are at no disadvantage relative to their dark-eyed herd mates. A few do seem to be impaired, but anecdotal evidence is that most are visually sound. No evidence in the literature supports reduced vision for these colors.

Some breeders in the Connemara breed society surveyed owners of **cream** horses years ago, with the result that most breeders were satisfied that their horses had normal vision. A few had horses with obviously impaired vision, but no more than was considered about the same rate as dark horses. The conclusion was that the **cream** horses did not have any propensity for defective vision. In contrast, some breeders of Lusitano horses prefer **cream** horses to other colors for horses destined for high school dressage work, insisting that this color results in horses easier to train to higher levels. In this breed "**cream**" likely also includes another type of dilute color known as **pearl**.

Pearl horses are related to the **cream**-based colors. **Pearl** horses vary in color, but nearly all are either gold or light tan. They have pink or mottled skin, and **amber** eyes. The darkest ones have a pinkish cast to the color; the lightest ones are gold but usually lack the very light manes and tails of **palomino** horses. Dark ones are called **sable pearl**, or **classic pearl**. The middle range usually has darker manes, tails, and points and is called **amber pearl**. The lightest are distinctly gold throughout body, mane, and tail and are called **gold pearl**. The lighter end of the range is a light beige color, usually darker than **cream**, and with light eyes that are somewhat darker than the eyes of **cream** horses (Figures 4.32 and 4.33).

Pearl colors very closely resemble **champagne** horses, and cause substantial difficulties if the goal is a one-to-one correspondence of nomenclature with genotype. The difficulty arises because **pearl** horses and **champagne** horses are visually identical colors in many cases. The result is that a distinct nomenclature for **pearl** really demands that observers know the genotype, and does not allow observers to rely solely on the appearance of the horse in front of them. In cases where it is certain that the horses are **pearl** and not **champagne**, it is appropriate to use **pearl** nomenclature.

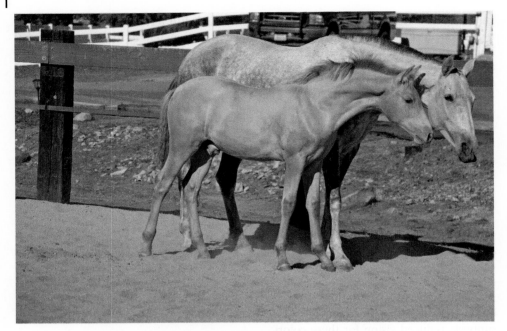

Figure 4.32 This colt is a **pearl** based on **bay**. *Source*: courtesy of Suzan Sommer.

4.2.2 Genetic Control

The genetic control of the **cream**-related and **pearl** colors is at a single locus, the *membrane-associated transporter protein* (*MATP*) locus. The *MATP* locus codes for a transporter protein involved in a biochemical pathway of pigmentation. This protein regulates the pH of the organelle that produces pigment (melanosome), and therefore influences the first step of pigment production. Three *MATP* alleles are known to contribute to pigmentation differences in horses. These are *wild-type* (C^+), *cremello* (C^{Cr}), and *pearl* (C^{pr}). Mutations at this locus can affect both eumelanin and pheomelanin. This is a situation where older nomenclature does not correspond well to current scientific knowledge. The old assignment of the $C^{Cr}Cr$ allele to the *Albino* locus was an error, though it is now difficult to change the well-recognized C^{Cr} nomenclature.

The *cremello* allele, C^{Cr}, is due to a single base-pair change in exon 2 at the *MATP* locus that results in a missense mutation. A genetic test is available for this allele. This allele is incompletely dominant and causes pigment to be lightened or diluted. Homozygotes have a more pronounced phenotype than do heterozygotes. The effects of the *cremello* allele are summarized in Table 4.2. Red is lightened to yellow in heterozygotes (C^+C^{Cr}), resulting in **bay** becoming **buckskin** and **chestnut** becoming **palomino**. Heterozygotes express **sooty** areas and can also be different **shades**. When results of testing for C^{Cr} are combined with the results of testing for E^e and A^a it is possible to more accurately classify **cream** horses and predict their color production potential in a breeding program.

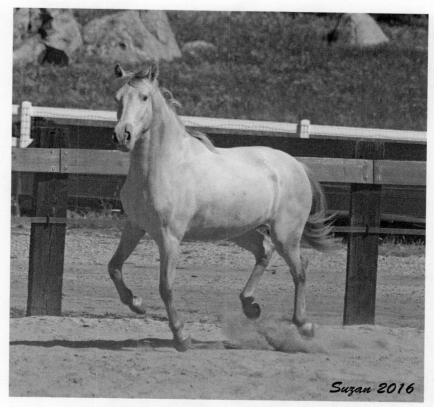

Figure 4.33 At maturity the combination of **pearl** and **smoky** remains light, and is one of the light colors favored for high school dressage in Portugal. *Source*: courtesy of Suzan Sommer.

A tricky detail of C^{Cr} is that it does not affect black in the heterozygous condition. Most **black** horses with one copy of C^{Cr} cannot be distinguished from **blacks** lacking it. Some **black** horses are subtly lightened to **smoky**, and some also have telltale amber eyes. **Smoky** horses can provide interesting surprises in a breeding program because many of them do not show visual signs of the *cremello* allele, but they can pass it along to offspring that have the more obvious **buckskin** or **palomino** colors associated with the allele.

Seal brown horses with one *cremello* allele have subtle differences from those that lack it. The black areas are minimally lightened, but the tan or red areas are lightened to a yellow color that is distinctive. These horses could easily be missed as having the *cremello* allele, but **smoky seal brown** can be used to distinguish those with yellow highlights from those with the more usual tan or red highlights.

Both red and black pigments are lightened to **cream** by the presence of two C^{Cr} alleles, and it is occasionally difficult to distinguish among **cream** horses with a **bay**, **chestnut**, or **black** base color. Even though homozygotes can be tough to distinguish as to original base color (**black**, **bay**, **chestnut**), long usage has favored the use of **cremello** for those **creams** on a **chestnut** background, **perlino** for those on a **bay** background, and **smoky cream** for those on a **black** background. Sometimes these three can be distinguished visually due to the fact that many **smoky cream** horses have darker points and bodies

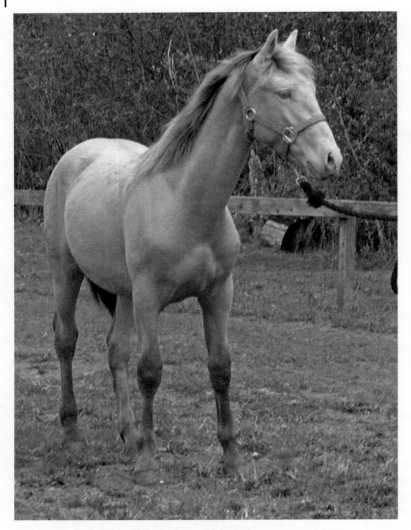

Figure 4.33 *(Continued)* *Source*: courtesy of Ginger.

than do **perlinos**, which in turn are darker than **cremellos**. However, most $C^{Cr}C^{Cr}$ horses are about the same shade of cream regardless of whether on a **black**, **bay**, or **chestnut** base and are usually lumped together as **creams** or **cremellos**. This inability to accurately distinguish base colors of cream-colored horses can produce some surprising results in a breeding program using **cream** horses. In situations where knowing the base coat color is important it is advisable to test for the genotype at the *Agouti* and *Extension* loci. Homozygote **creams** are generally uniformly cream colored with no expression of **sooty** and little, if any, of **shade**.

The combinations of the Dn^++- genotype with the C^+C^{Cr} genotype produce some interesting subtleties in color. On a **black** background the result is a pale **grullo**, although this can be difficult to appreciate as different from a normal **grullo** on most

Table 4.2   Effects of C^+C^{Cr} and $C^{Cr}C^{Cr}$ on dark base colors.

Base color (C^+C^+)	C^+C^{Cr}	$C^{Cr}C^{Cr}$
Jet black	Black	Smoky cream
Black	Smoky or black	Smoky cream
Grullo	Light grullo or olive dun	Cream dun
Seal brown	Smoky seal brown	Smoky cream
Brown	Sooty buckskin	Perlino
Blood bay	Golden buckskin	Perlino
Red bay	Yellow buckskin	Perlino
Sandy bay	Silvery buckskin	Perlino
Zebra dun	Golden dun, silvery dun, dunskin	Cream dun, dunalino
Liver chestnut, sooty type	Sooty palomino	Cremello
Liver chestnut, dark shade type	Golden palomino	Cremello
Chestnut	Palomino	Cremello
Light chestnut	Isabelo	Cremello
Red dun	Linebacked palomino	Cream dun, dunalino

horses. On a **bay** background the **primitive marks** usually remain but the ground color of the body is more yellow, like that of **buckskins**, rather than the more tan shade of the usual **zebra dun**. The resulting combination is usually a **golden dun** or a **silvery dun**. Many breeders call this combination **dunskin**, which is an allusion to the genetic combination rather than any visual appearance. Somewhat confusingly, Kiger Mustang breeders call the same combination **claybank**. On **chestnut** the result of the combination is **linebacked palomino**. Most of these horses have **primitive marks**, but a few do not and therefore cannot be distinguished visually from the more usual sort of **palomino** caused by C^+C^{Cr} alone.

The net effect of the combination of $C^+C^{Cr}, Dn^+ +-$ is the expression of whichever gene leads to more extreme dilution of the base color. For example, **chestnut** is lightened to **palomino**, which is more extreme than **red dun**. Bay is lightened to a **golden dun**, usually retaining the stripes but much lighter than the usual **zebra dun**. **Black** is lightened to **grullo**, which is lighter than **smoky**. **Creams** that have Dn^+ ($C^{Cr}C^{Cr}Cr$, $Dn^+ +-$) usually retain at least a hint of the **primitive marks** and are **cream duns** or **white duns**, although **dunalino** is increasingly used as a term that springs from the genetic basis of the combination.

Because the *cremello* allele is incompletely dominant, its action must be thought of as a three-way switch between "intense pigment" (C^+C^+, neither red nor black pigment diluted), or "dilution of red to yellow" (C^+C^{Cr}) or "dilution of red and black to cream" ($C^{Cr}C^{Cr}$).

Pearl is due to a separate recessive mutation at the *MATP* locus. In keeping with traditional nomenclature, this is symbolized C^{pr}. The mutation for **pearl** has been identified, and a DNA test is available. In the homozygous condition *pearl* changes **chestnut** to **gold pearl**, **bay** to **amber pearl**, **seal brown** and **brown** to **sable pearl**, and **black** to **classic pearl**. These names are adopted from the nomenclature for **champagne**

colors discussed later, although time may change that to a more specific choice of names. Owing to the rarity of these colors, most observers simply call them **pearl** and do not subdivide the group.

This mutation is recessive, so heterozygous *pearl* animals, in the absence of other diluting alleles such as *cremello*, are usually dark and appear as the normal base coat color of whatever color is present. Despite the generally recessive character of the *pearl* allele, heterozygotes do have changes in the skin color consisting of a slightly lighter color and small pale spots.

In the event that a horse has both *cremello* and *pearl* alleles it is impossible for the horse to have the *wild-type* allele, and therefore the result is dilute rather than dark. This is because both copies of the gene have a mutation, even though the *pearl* allele by itself is recessive. Horses that are heterozygous with one each of the *pearl* and *cremello* alleles are dramatically changed to pale colors (Figure 4.33). These vary from nearly white in appearance on a **chestnut** background color, to light beige with brown points on a **bay** background, to a more uniform tan with dark tan points on a **black** background. These are all similar to the **pearl** colors resulting from homozygous *pearl* horses, but in each case are lightened further than the **pearl** colors. Eyes on these horses are usually blue or pale amber, but typically darker than the eyes of homozygous **cream** horses. These combinations are all rare and can be usually denoted by their visual appearance as **ivory pearl**, **light gold pearl**, **light amber pearl**, or **light classic pearl** depending on the actual color.

The combination of *pearl* with *cremello* ($C^{Cr}C^{pr}$) is the cause of most "**cream**" or lighter Lusitano and other Iberian-derived horses, although pale horses in these breeds could also be **cremello**, **perlino**, or **smoky cream**. Many of these "**creams**" occur as complete surprises when an obvious **buckskin** or **palomino** is mated to a **bay** or **chestnut** *pearl* heterozygote. This dramatic result is logical once it is realized that these two alleles are at the same locus.

Pearl horses are rare and occur in Lusitanos, Paints, Gypsy horses, and American Quarter Horses. They also occur rarely in New World breeds with an Iberian connection, such as Paso Fino and Peruvian Paso horses. Now that a DNA test is available, **pearl** horses are being detected in an increasing array of breeds. Table 4.3 outlines the result of *pearl* on several background colors.

Table 4.3 Effect of the *pearl* allele on various base colors.

Base color	Heterozygous *pearl*	Homozygous *pearl*
Black	Black with minor skin changes	Classic pearl
Seal brown	Seal brown with minor skin changes	Sable pearl
Brown	Brown with minor skin changes	Sable pearl
Bay	Bay with minor skin changes	Amber pearl
Chestnut	Chestnut with minor skin changes	Gold pearl
Smoky	Light classic pearl	—
Seal smoky	Light sable pearl	—
Buckskin	Light amber pearl	—
Palomino	Ivory pearl (common)	—
	Light gold pearl (rare)	

4.3 Champagne

4.3.1 Definition and Classification

The **champagne** dilute colors are a separate group of pale colors that can easily be confused with the **cream**-related colors caused by the *cremello* allele, and are especially similar to the **pearl** colors. In North America the **champagne** colors are generally more frequent than the **pearl** colors, although the frequency of these two is highly dependent on the breeds involved. The whole **champagne** group consists of pale colors, most of which have pinkish or light brown skin (often called **pumpkin** skin) and amber eyes. Most of these horses are born with blue eyes that darken to amber sometime after birth and sometimes continue to darken until they are nearly the familiar dark brown color of most horse eyes. The skin can also become dusky or mottled but always lacks the uniform darkness associated with the skin of most other horse colors. Amber eyes and light skin with darker mottling are the hallmarks of this group of dilute colors and are present in all but a few of these horses.

The colors in the **champagne** group vary from chocolate brown to various shades of yellow with varying point color. Some of these are a pale brownish color, nearly a dove or lilac color in many horses. **Lilac dun** has been used for some of these colors in the past (especially the darker ones), although they generally lack **primitive marks**. **Champagne** is currently accepted as the term for these colors, especially in the Tennessee Walking Horse breed. The **champagne** colors frequently exhibit a bright sheen, and reversed dappling is fairly common (darker dapples with pale peripheries). **Champagne** foals are frequently born a dark color and lighten to the **champagne** color after shedding the foal coat (Figure 3.40). This phenomenon is the reverse of most other horse colors and contributes to the confusion surrounding these colors. The **champagne** colors are frequently mistaken for other colors when the foal coat is noted for registration, and that confusion often leads to misidentification of the final color. This can be frustrating to breeders trying to trace the colors back through a pedigree.

The entire **champagne** group encompasses many different combinations of body and point color within the general framework of pale skin, pale eyes, and light, shiny colors. These colors have historically been very rare, but are currently increasing in popularity. Terminology has only recently been developed for them, and this varies from registry to registry. The names used in this section are not universally accepted, but do attempt to match the actual colors with appropriately descriptive names. A reasonably standard nomenclature helps to define these colors.

The darkest of these colors is called **champagne** or **classic champagne** (Figure 4.34), which is **champagne** dilution on a **black** base coat. These horses have a pinkish or beige body color and generally have medium to light brown points that are darker than the body color. The **champagne** color is very distinctive and difficult to confuse with any color other than **pearl**, although it has historically been registered as **buckskin** because breeders did not know exactly how to classify the lighter shades of this color.

The second main variant in the **champagne** group is called **amber champagne**, which is a light tan or yellow body color with points that are medium to light chocolate brown (Figure 4.35). This is **champagne** dilution on a **bay** base coat. This color could be confused with **claybank dun** except that **primitive marks** are missing. **Amber champagne** horses are frequently registered as **buckskin**, which can result in some confusing

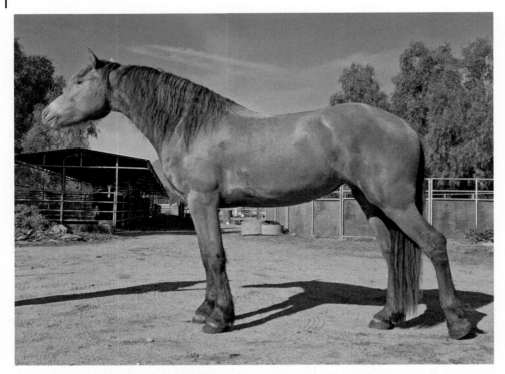

Figure 4.34 Classic champagne is a light beige with darker brown points as well as the typical skin changes of the color group. In addition, all **champagne** horses generally have bright shiny coats. *Source:* courtesy of Aimee Ziller.

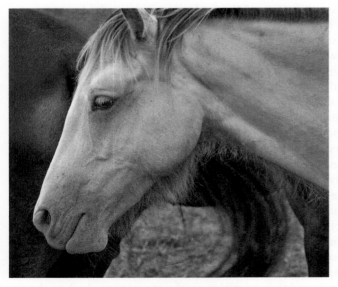

Figure 4.35 Amber champagne horses have tan bodies and light brown points. *Source:* courtesy of Neil Chapman.

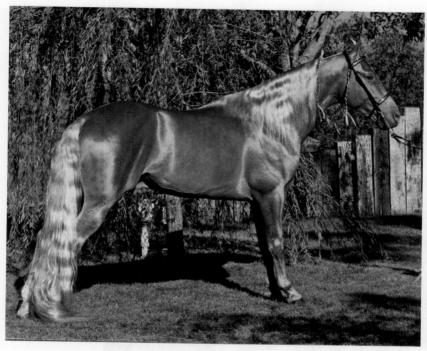

Figure 4.36 **Gold champagne** is often mistaken for **palomino**, but is more likely than **palomino** to be a rich gold color. *Source:* courtesy of Midge McGoldrick.

results in breeding programs. **Sable champagne** is between **classic champagne** and **amber champagne**, much as **brown** resides between **bay** and **black**.

The third major variant in this group of colors is **gold champagne**, which has a bright golden body color, usually coupled with a white mane and tail (Figures 4.36 and 4.37). These are the result of **champagne** dilution on a **chestnut** base coat. **Gold champagne** horses are usually registered as **palominos**, even though the pale skin is distinctive and the body color is usually much more gold and shiny than that of most **palominos**. In past work these were called **pink-skinned palominos**, but calling them **gold champagne** more adequately distinguishes the fact that these horses are indeed phenotypically and genetically different from **palominos**. **Gold champagne** horses tend to have very golden-yellow bodies. Mane and tail color is variable on **gold champagne** horses. Most of them have white manes and tails, but gold and even red manes and tails also can occur and can lead to confusion in naming this color.

Very light **champagne** horses are difficult to classify, and the nomenclature for these varies. Some are **ivory champagne**, and are the result of a combination of **champagne** and **cream** (Figure 4.38). These usually have light skin that is somewhat darker than **creams**, and dark blue or green eyes. Some are **silver champagne** with a very pale and very shiny body color and eye characteristics typical of **champagne** horses.

An alternate approach to these pale **champagne** colors is to simply add whatever other genes are present to the **classic, sable, amber,** or **gold** designation, so that *champagne* and heterozygous *cremello* on a chestnut background becomes **gold cream**

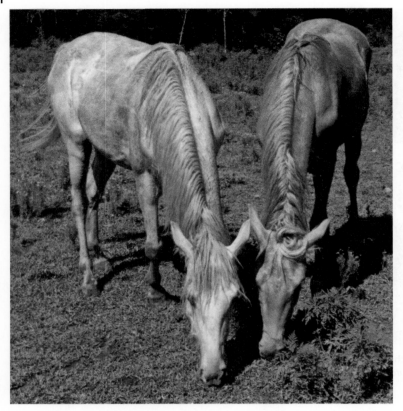

Figure 4.37 **Gold champagne** varies, as do all **champagne** colors, and in the darker versions is often misregistered as **sorrel**. This is especially when foals are registered early, because **champagne** foal coats are darker than are the mature final colors. *Source:* courtesy of Liz Nutter.

champagne. This has an advantage in clearly establishing the genes that are present, but works only poorly for quick field use, as all of the combinations of *champagne* and one copy of *cremello* are pale and most of them are relatively easily confused one with the other. In addition, most horses called **gold cream champagne** are a very light ivory color, and the use of "gold" implies a darker color so that the color name and the actual color of the horse correlate poorly.

Horses of the **champagne** group of colors occur in a variety of breeds. Historically these have been rare, but selection in favor of them has increased the frequency of these colors in several breeds. They are documented in the Spanish Mustang, Tennessee Walking Horse, American Quarter Horse, and various pony breeds. In Argentina, the paler members of this group are called *palomo*, or dove colored. The group of **palomo** colors in Argentina also includes **creams**, possibly **isabelos**, and also **pearls**.

A very pale **gold champagne** color is a breed characteristic of the American Cream Draft Horse. In this breed the color results from the *champagne* allele on a pale **sorrel** background color. The ideal color for this breed is a medium to pale cream, with all of the skin and eye characteristics of **champagne** horses. The breeders of American Cream

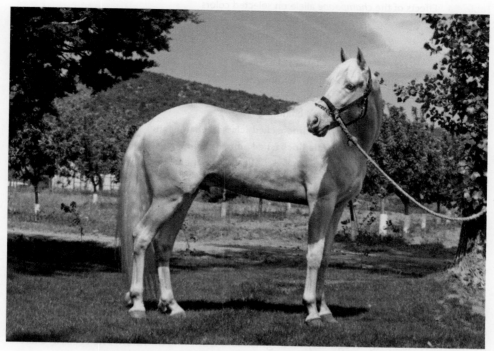

Figure 4.38 **Ivory champagne** is the result of combining **gold champagne** and **palomino**. This very light shiny color also has light skin and eyes. *Source:* courtesy of Midge McGoldrick.

Draft Horses refer to the color as **cream**, although it must be remembered that this is not the blue-eyed **cream** that is associated with the homozygous condition of the *cremello* allele. It is also important to note that the American Cream Draft Horse is not uniformly homozygous for the *champagne* allele. As a result, foals that lack this allele are produced and these are usually **sorrel**. To complicate the issue further, some horses that do have the *champagne* allele are dark enough to be classed as **sorrel** rather than the desired **cream** that the breed standard dictates.

4.3.2 Genetic Control

The genetic control for the **champagne** group of colors is a dominant allele, whose actions on various colors are summarized in Table 4.4. The allele is a consequence of a missense mutation in exon 2 of the *SLC36A1* gene. This is a transport protein, solute carrier 36 family A1. The missense substitution changes the amino acid threonine to an arginine in the protein produced from the gene. This changes the function of the protein and yields the dilute color.

The *champagne* allele (Ch^C) is dominant, and in the heterozygous state it dilutes black to brown and red to yellow. The result of the homozygous state is usually slightly paler than heterozygous horses, with paler skin and eyes. However, the colors of the palest heterozygotes and the darkest homozygotes do overlap, so it is not always possible to

Table 4.4 Effects of the *champagne* allele on selected colors.

Base color	Champagne variant
Black	(Classic) champagne
Seal brown and brown	Sable champagne
Bay	Amber champagne
Chestnut	Gold champagne
Grullo	Pale linebacked (classic) champagne
Zebra dun	Pale linebacked amber champagne
Red dun	Linebacked amber champagne
Smoky	Pale (classic) champagne or classic cream champagne
Buckskin	Pale amber champagne or amber cream champagne
Palomino	Ivory champagne or gold cream champagne

neatly separate the two different genotypes by appearance alone. In that regard, the *champagne* allele can be considered a true dominant allele in which heterozygotes and homozygotes are only irregularly distinguishable from one another. The recessive allele is the *wild type* (Ch^+) and allows for fully intense colors.

The locus can be considered to be a two-way switch between "non**champagne**" and "**champagne**." It is important to remember that the *champagne* allele is currently rare in most breeds. Selection favoring these colors in some breeds is rapidly resulting in the allele becoming more common. Breeders in many breeds are becoming increasingly familiar with these colors and their genetic control.

The **champagne** group of colors is highly variable. Each different base color, and the combinations of these with the other dilution genes, also has a **champagne** counterpart in which the skin is pale and the eyes amber. Any black is replaced by chocolate brown, and red is lightened to gold or yellow.

Black is changed by Ch^C to **champagne** or **classic champagne** (sometimes called **lilac dun**). The combination of **champagne** and **bay** results in **amber champagne**, which has a yellow body, brown points, and the skin and eye characteristics typical of this group. **Brown, seal brown,** or **brown-black** combined with **champagne** results in **sable champagne**, which is intermediate between **classic champagne** and **amber champagne**. In field situations it would be difficult to accurately distinguish it from those other colors.

The **champagne** effect on the E^eE^e genotypes (**chestnut** and its derivatives) usually results in a gold horse with either a gold or white mane and tail, which is **gold champagne**. In the past, most of these horses ended up being registered as **palomino** due to their very gold body color, although the intensity of the color as well as the skin and eye characteristics are distinct from those of true **palomino** horses. The pale skin of **gold champagnes** is a telltale feature that clearly distinguishes them from **palominos**. **Gold champagne** horses do not reproduce as if they were palominos, but rather as if they are in the **champagne** group of colors. Of the three main colors in this group (**champagne, amber,** and **gold**), **gold champagne** is the most likely to be missed as part of this group of colors because **gold champagnes** with white manes and tails are so likely to be misclassified as **palomino**.

The degree to which the color is lightened by the Ch^C allele is extremely variable, and minimally affected horses may be easily misidentified as not having this allele. The **champagne** colors, therefore, present something of a nomenclature nightmare, because the resulting color of any of the genotypes is so highly variable that color designations need to include more variability than is typical of those in most other color classes. Minimally affected horses are commonly misregistered. Very dark **champagne** horses can be misregistered as **black** or **brown**. Dark **amber champagne** horses can end up registered as **bay**, or occasionally as **buckskin**. The darker range of the **gold champagne** color is very orange and is frequently misregistered as **sorrel**. These misregistered horses can be very confusing in pedigrees and even more confusing in ongoing breeding programs unless their color is correctly identified.

Some of the past misregistrations can be attributed to the fact that these colors are darker in foals than they are in mature horses; and if horses are registered based on observations made when they are foals, many **champagne** horses will be misidentified as lacking the allele. The telltale skin characteristics are indeed noticeable in foals, and noting those would help to avoid this confusion. However, the darkness of **champagne** foal coats is unusual when compared with nearly every other horse color, and this contributes greatly to misunderstanding and misregistering the colors of this group. The availability of a DNA test for the *champagne* allele, in combination with the ones for *cremello* and *pearl*, makes classification and registration much more accurate.

Not all combinations of the Ch^C allele with other background colors are well documented. The combination of Ch^C— and C^+C^{Cr} heterozygotes usually results in cream or ivory-colored horses with pale greenish-blue eyes that have a tinge of amber. The eyes of foals are usually lighter and bluer. These could easily be confused with **cream**-colored horses, but they are heterozygotes at two loci instead of homozygous at the *C* locus. One strategy is to call these pale horses **ivory champagne** instead of **cream** to acknowledge their genetic distinctions from **creams** that are homozygous $C^{Cr}C^{Cr}$. **Ivory champagne** horses do have mottled or dusky skin instead of the pink skin typical of **creams**, so the distinction is usually easy to make if the horse is inspected closely.

The total range of colors resulting from other combinations of Ch^C with C^{Cr} and Dn^+ are difficult to predict and are rarely encountered. The International Champagne Horse Registry prefers to use **classic cream champagne, sable cream champagne, amber cream champagne,** and **gold cream champagne** for the combination of **champagne** colors with the *cremello* allele. This nomenclature does have the advantage of conveying the genotype very well. A disadvantage is that these names imply much darker colors than the very pale color of most of these combinations. Nearly all of these horses have a pale tan or light beige body color, with points that vary from nearly white to a light brown that is distinctly darker than the body color. These can all be reasonably difficult to separate one from the other without genetic testing, although the **classic cream champagne, sable cream champagne,** and **amber cream champagne** all tend to retain more pigment in the points than do the **gold cream champagne** horses.

The **champagne** dilute colors are unusual and can be confused with other more common colors. In some cases **smoky cream** could be dark enough to be confused with

champagne, but **smoky cream** is unlikely to reproduce itself with any regularity in most breeds, so that the color pedigree, as well as the blue eyes of the **smoky cream**, usually helps in distinguishing these two. **Smoky cream** is also likely to produce **buckskins** and **palominos** in most breeds, which is not the case with **champagne**. The most common confusion comes from combinations of **champagne** with red body colors (such as **bay** and **chestnut**). These combinations resemble **palominos** and **yellow silvers**. For many of these colors the skin and eye characteristics are the only reliable indicator that the horse is a variant of the **champagne** color. The result of Ch^C with colors other than the dark colors will continue to be better appreciated and documented as breeders increasingly develop these combinations.

4.4 Silver Dapple

4.4.1 Definition and Classification

The **silver dapple**, or simply **silver**, group of colors is extremely variable. In some countries (notably Australia) this whole group of colors is called **taffy** instead of **silver**. **Taffy** has its advantages because these colors frequently lack any silver character. A disadvantage is the lack of historic use of **taffy** for any horse color in the USA. Rocky Mountain Horse breeders tend to classify all of these colors as "**chocolate**," even though many of them lack the brown color associated with that name. Despite the limitations of "**silver**" for these colors, this guide will continue with it because it has been historically the more widely accepted term for these colors.

Some few manifestations of this group are light enough to be considered as part of the overall group of dilute colors. Many manifestations of this group are as dark as the darkest of the nondilute colors. **Silver** horses were uncommon in North America for decades, and the colors have historically been associated only with pony breeds. These colors have always occurred as a rarity in several breeds of all size classes. They are now becoming increasingly common as selection is favoring them in many breeds. All of the **silver dapple** colors are very easily misidentified due to a superficial similarity to colors based on **chestnut**.

The most distinctive group of **silver dapple** variants is called **blue silver**, **black silver**, **chocolate silver**, or **silver dapple** (Figures 4.39 and 4.40). These horses have a body color that varies from nearly black to a flat sepia brown body color that is frequently heavily dappled. The manes, tails, and lower legs vary from nearly black to nearly white. At the lighter extreme these points are easily confused with the **flaxen** points of some **chestnut** and **sorrel** horses, but are totally separate in terms of genetic control.

Eyelashes and coarse muzzle and facial hairs on most **silver dapples** are nearly white, which can be a useful tip-off to this group of colors when they are minimally expressed. Unfortunately, exceptions to this useful rule are common enough that this is not an absolutely foolproof test.

In breeds such as the Rocky Mountain Horse and Icelandic Horse, in which **silver dapple** colors are fairly common, the **silver dapple** group is split into subtypes. The **black silvers**, **chocolate silvers** (with many Rocky Mountain Horse breeders calling these **chocolates**), and **blue silvers** (Icelandic Horse terminology) vary from a nearly

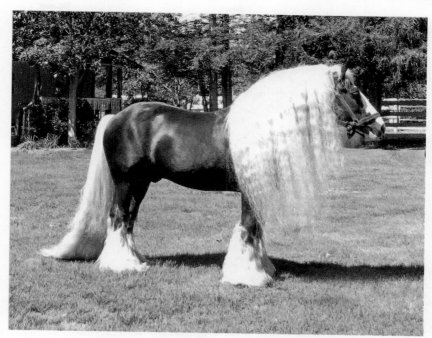

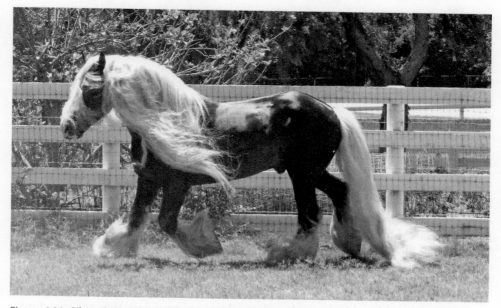

Figure 4.39 **Silver dapple** is easily mistaken for **flaxen liver chestnut**. *Source*: courtesy of Celeste Huston.

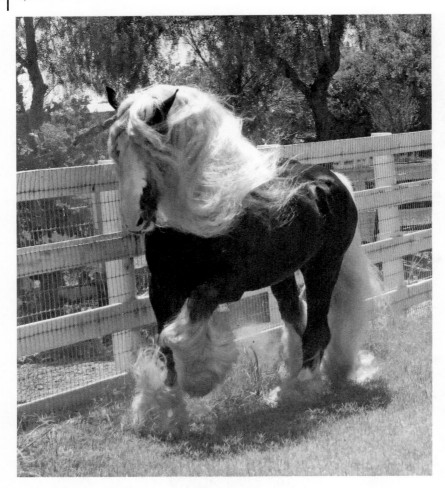

Figure 4.39 *(Continued)*

black body color with light points, through a dark chocolate body color, to a bluish body color, and then to the more classic **silver dapple** (or **light chocolate silver**) color that is a pale "dead grass" brown and is usually heavily dappled. The approach taken here is to include all of these as **blue silver** (**black** base coat with **silver** dilution) while acknowledging that the darkest and lightest extremes lack the blue tint that is usually present in the middle range of shades.

At the darker end of the range the **blue silvers** are easily confused with **flaxen liver chestnuts**. When **blue, black,** or **chocolate silvers** are very dark they are sometimes called **black chestnut** or **coal chestnut**, but the presence of light points and eyelashes is generally consistent. Some **silver dapple** horses do have darker points, but nearly all have some pale hairs among the dark ones, cleanly separating these from truly black-pointed horse colors. Many **silver dapple** horses have manes and tails that become darker with age. While it is possible to confuse **blue silvers** with **chestnuts**, a reliable

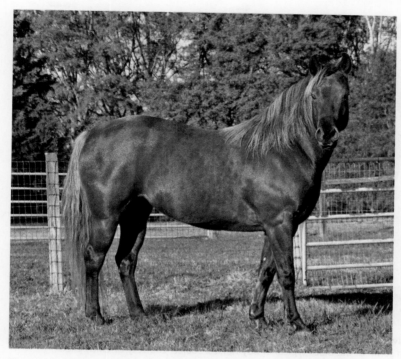

Figure 4.40 The most common shade of **silver dapple** is a medium brown, most often with a light mane and tail that become darker with age. After the mane and tail become dark the color can be especially confusing because it resembles dark **chestnut** shades. *Source*: courtesy of Laura Hornick Behning.

tip-off is the fact that **blue silvers** lack any red tint to the body color. Only an exceptional **chestnut** horse will lack the red cast to its color, and this is especially true of the lower portions of the legs.

Red silvers or bay silvers (**red chocolate**, curiously, to Rocky Mountain Horse breeders) generally have a clear **bay** body color but the points are **flaxen** with varying amounts of black in them (Figure 4.41). Nomenclature varies on these, but the approach here is to group them all as **red silvers** (**bay** base coat with **silver** dilution) while acknowledging that this does not always reflect the trend among all breeders or all breeds.

The points of **red silver** horses vary from almost entirely pale to nearly black, but most are combinations of black and pale hairs that are fairly easily distinguished from the colors of **chestnut** horses with **flaxen** points. When the points are extremely pale, **red silver** can be confused with **flaxen chestnut**. In general, the mane and tail are lighter than the lower leg, which retains some black areas. Usually, the lower leg nearest the hoof is lighter than portions closer to the body. The result is a pale color (**flaxen** or "dead grass" brown) near the hoof, with black above this region in the areas expected to be black on black-pointed horses, with the black area finally undergoing a transition to the body color as the upper leg is approached.

This orderly transition of colors along the lower leg is quite noticeable on **red silvers** because the red body color contrasts with the black point color on the upper leg, which

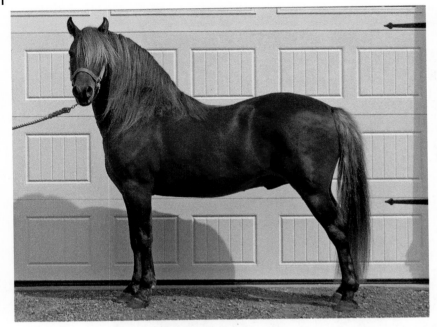

Figure 4.41 **Red silver** can be a confusing color, but usually the lower legs give hints of the true color because they retain some of the black typical of **bay** horses. *Source:* courtesy of Cindy Dietz.

then fades to the paler, more flaxen color toward the hoof. This same phenomenon is present, but not noticeable, on **chocolate silvers**. On these the point color resembles the body color, so the contrast between the body and point color is very subtle and missed by most observers.

Red silvers are sometimes very subtle, and when this is the case they are often misclassified as **bay**. The intensity of the body color of **bay silvers** is usually similar to **bays** or **chestnuts**, and they frequently combine characteristics of both **bays** and **chestnuts** to a casual observer. This causes confusion surrounding the classification of **red silver**. Once it is realized that **red silvers** are a separate category from **bay** and **chestnut** this color becomes much less confusing.

The **silver dapple** combination on a **brown** base color results in a color in which the dorsal parts of the body are a chocolate or blue shade and the ventral portions are red. This combination is called **brown silver** and occupies a position between **blue silver** and **bay silver**, much as **brown** horses are between **black** and **bay**.

The **silver dapple** counterpart of **zebra dun** and **buckskin** is yellowish, with typical changes in point color (Figure 4.42). These horses are called **yellow silvers** (**linebacked yellow silver** if appropriate) and are by far the rarest of **silver dapple** colors. **Yellow silvers** can be very confusing. If the points are very light it is easy to mistake them for **palominos**. If the points retain more of a brown or black color they can be confused with **buckskin, zebra dun, claybank dun,** or **amber champagne**. Detailed inspection can usually determine which specific components are present, although some of the final combinations are difficult to accurately classify (Figure 4.43).

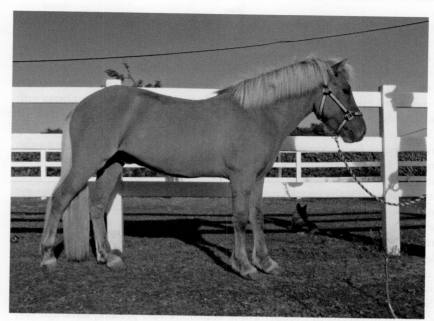

Figure 4.42 **Yellow silver** results from various combinations of **silver dapple**. Usually, these are with **buckskin**, or with **zebra dun** as is the case with this horse. *Source:* courtesy of Lucinda Nold.

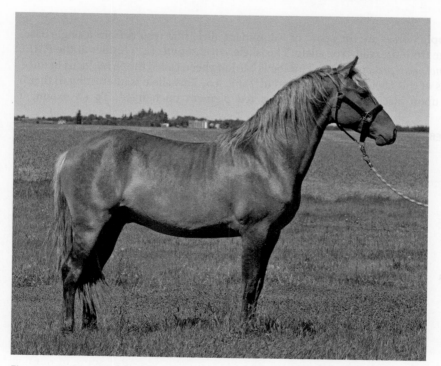

Figure 4.43 **Silver dapple** colors can be quite variable depending on which components are present. This Morgan horse is a combination of **silver, sooty, dun,** and **bay,** resulting in a fairly dark tan body color with distinct **primitive marks** and the characteristic mane and tail changes. *Source:* courtesy of Cindy Dietz.

Silver dapple horses are often very pale at birth, and then darken to the usual **silver** color. Many of them then continue to darken throughout life, so that mature horses that were easily recognized as **silver** when young can be more difficult to classify later in life. This is especially true of the mane and tail, which can darken dramatically with age.

Many horses with **silver dapple** colors have ocular abnormalities that include either fluid-filled sacs called cysts (usually denoted only as "cysts" on phenotype), or cysts with additional ocular abnormalities known as "multiple congenital ocular abnormalities" or MCOA as an abbreviation. The more severe expressions of these anomalies typically involve some improper formation of the iris (the pigmented part of the eye), but can also include abnormal formation of the cornea (the clear outer layer) or retina (back of the eye). In more severe cases vision is affected. Some horses can accommodate even relatively severe defects in the eye, so predicting a horse's visual function from an eye exam alone can sometimes be misleading. While these defects need not condemn the entire color group, breeders must be aware that they exist and take steps to minimize their occurrence in foals that are produced. More details are given in Section 4.4.2.

Silver dapple colors are becoming more popular in many breeds of gaited horses. These are common in the recently standardized gaited breeds from the Appalachian region, including the Rocky Mountain Horse, Mountain Pleasure Horse, and Kentucky Mountain Saddle Horse. **Silver dapple** colors also occur in a wide variety of pony, saddle, warmblood, and draft breeds in Europe. These colors are also present, although very rarely, in breeds such as the American Quarter Horse.

4.4.2 Genetic Control

Silver dapple horses are the result of a dominant allele that results from a single base-pair change from the wild-type allele. This allele, *silver dapple* (Z^Z) resides at the *PMEL* (*pre-melanosomal protein*) locus. This locus has long been called the *Silver* locus in mice. The effects of this allele are summarized in Table 4.5. This allele is interesting in that it acts only upon black pigment but leaves red pigment unchanged. To an extent, it

Table 4.5 Effect of the *silver dapple* allele on various base colors.

Base color	Silver variant
Black	Blue silver Black silver Coal chestnut Black chestnut Dark chocolate silver Light chocolate silver
Seal brown	As for **black** in most cases, **brown silver** in some
Brown	Brown silver
Bay	Red silver Bay silver
Zebra dun	Linebacked yellow silver
Buckskin	Yellow silver (can resemble some **pale champagne** colors)
Grullo	Linebacked chocolate silver

functions as a sort of opposite to the heterozygous state of the C^{Cr} allele at the $MATP$ locus in which the red pigment is affected but the black is unaffected. However, it differs from what is observed with *cremello* because the homozygous condition still does not affect red pigment.

The effect of the Z^Z allele varies from obvious to minimal, but it usually betrays its presence in some form or other on any color with black points: **black, seal brown, brown, bay, zebra dun, grullo,** or **buckskin.** One reasonably (but not absolutely) consistent and subtle action of this allele is the pale eyelashes. It changes **black** horses to **blue silvers,** including **chocolate silver, black chestnut** or **coal chestnut,** and **black silver.** The "chestnut" nomenclature is unfortunate here, because these colors are not related to **chestnut** genetically. Historic usage includes these two, though, so they must be indicated here for completeness.

Brown silvers are the result of Z^Z on a **brown** background, and these usually resemble **chocolate silvers** but have a distinct redness on the lower parts of the body, just as do **brown** horses. The effect on **seal brown** is usually subtle enough to be missed, so that these are usually classified the same as the combination of Z^Z on **black.** The *silver dapple* allele changes **bay** to **red silver,** which is essentially a red body with light points. These colors could be confused with **flaxen chestnuts** or **sorrels,** but usually the presence of Z^Z betrays its presence by irregular changes of color where leg color normally changes from black to red. This is due to the persistence of some black pigment, especially at the junction of the body color with the point color, which would be very uncharacteristic of **chestnut** or **sorrel.** Manes of **silver dapple** horses likewise usually have some indication that they were black before being lightened to brown or flaxen by the Z^Z allele. Eyelashes are usually pale or white, which is a reasonably consistent betrayal of the presence of the *silver dapple* allele.

Silver dapple combinations with **zebra dun** or **buckskin** are more subtle than those with **black** or **bay.** On these paler colors **silver dapple** can give little indication of its presence. It can happen that **silver dapple buckskin (yellow silver** or **buckskin silver),** for example, could be easily confused with **palomino** due to the gold body color and pale points. Such horses are rare, but do account for some very unusual results in color prediction of foals. **Yellow silvers** usually do retain some black or brown pigment in the points and are therefore usually not confused with **palomino. Yellow silvers** with C^{Cr} are likely to have light skin, and some are therefore superficially similar to various **champagne** colors.

Because **chestnut** and **chestnut**-based colors lack black areas (except for **sootiness**), the *silver dapple* allele does not affect them, and it is carried without any outward evidence. This can be the cause of surprising colors when **chestnut** carriers of the *silver dapple* allele are mated to **bay, brown,** or **black** horses. The *silver dapple* allele does, interestingly, affect **Bend Or spots** on some **chestnut** horses that have both the spots and the *silver dapple* allele. The *silver dapple* allele causes these spots to be paler than they are on **chestnut** horses that lack the allele. This effect is probably most obvious on those horses with nearly black **Bend Or spots** and a very light-colored manifestation of the **silver dapple** modification.

Several genetic mapping and sequencing studies have shown that the associated ocular defects are most likely the result of the *silver dapple* allele itself. The ocular changes that are usually associated with colors of this group occur in all breeds in which this allele occurs, so breeders should be aware of the potential of ocular defects and should assure that horses with **silver** colors have their eyes tested for presence or absence of any abnormalities. Available studies support that heterozygotes have the "cysts only" phenotype, whereas homozygotes have the more severe "MCOA" disorder, which includes cysts and additional abnormalities. Therefore, heterozygotes have normal vision (or nearly so), while homozygotes with the more profoundly affected eyes can have impaired vision.

A simple breeding strategy to avoid producing the severely affected horses is to not produce homozygous horses. Fortunately, a genetic test for the *silver dapple* allele is now available, so it is possible for breeders interested in these colors to identify horses with the allele. These can then be mated to horses lacking the allele in order to avoid the production of horses that are visually impaired. By this strategy it is possible to reduce or eliminate the production of horses with the more severe ocular defects while retaining this attractive group of colors.

4.5 Mushroom: Definition, Classification, and Genetic Control

Mushroom horses are a color very similar to **silver dapple**. The body color is usually a flat beige or sepia color, and the manes and tails are usually paler than the body (Figures 4.44 and 4.45). On most **mushroom** horses **dapples** are subtle or nonexistent. Eyelashes are usually darker than those of silver dapple horses; and of course, **mushroom** horses test negative for the *silver dapple* allele.

Mushroom is a recessive mutation, tentatively called *mushroom* at the *Mushroom* locus (Mu^{mu}) until investigations can establish its exact location in the equine genome. That is distinct from *silver dapple*. Confusingly, most **mushroom** horses are $E^e E^e$, and therefore lack black pigment. The close mimic to **silver dapple** is perplexing, because

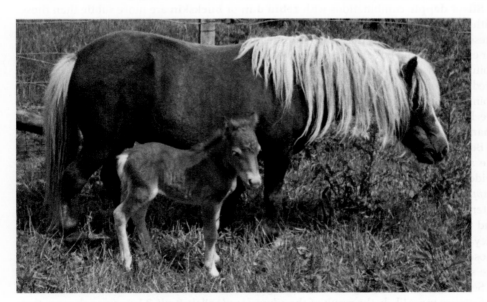

Figure 4.44 **Mushroom** is a rare color, based on **chestnut**, but nearly identical to **silver dapple** phenotypically. The contrast between the **mushroom** dam and the **chestnut** foal is striking. *Source*: courtesy of Elisabeth Mead.

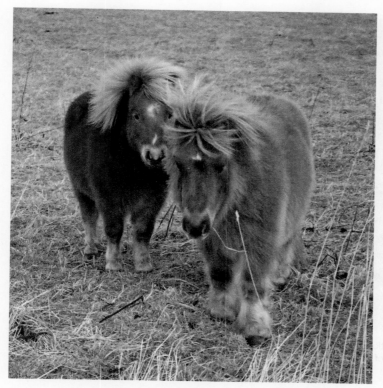

Figure 4.45 **Mushroom** and **chestnut** are quite distinct, although the one is simply a single-gene modification of the other. The final shade of **mushroom** is quite variable. *Source:* courtesy of Elisabeth Mead.

mushroom is a modification of **chestnut**, while *silver dapple* has no effect on a **chestnut** background color. The few **mushroom** horses that have been tested have lacked the *silver dapple* allele and have had a **chestnut** base color.

Mushroom has only been documented in a few breeds, such as the Shetland pony, Haflinger, and perhaps the American Quarter Horse. It is very rare wherever it is found, so details such as the color resulting on a bay or black background have not been determined, but early observations indicate some dilution of these black-pointed colors.

4.6 Lavender

Lavender foals are a specific dilute color in Egyptian Arabian horses. The foals are born with a pale color variously described as pale grey, pewter, or light chestnut. Along with the distinctive color are neurologic abnormalities, including seizures, and other abnormalities that prevent the foal from nursing and lead to its death.

The defective allele is recessive, and is at the *MYO5A* locus. The mutation is a deletion in exon 30 of the gene, leading to a frame shift that causes an abnormal protein.

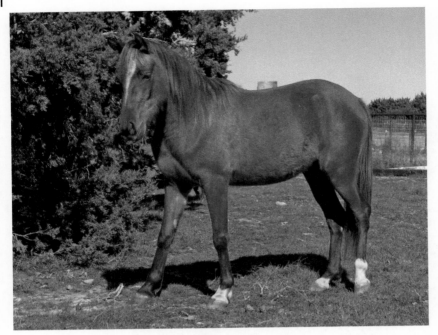

Figure 4.46 Some dilutions, such as on this Arabian horse, have yet to be characterized at the molecular level. *Source:* courtesy of Dan Stanfield.

4.7 Other Dilutions

A few horses that are obviously lighter than the usual dark colors occur in breeds in which dilution is otherwise rare or nonexistent. These rare horses point to the possibility that other mechanisms for dilution do occur in horses.

One of these dilutions has occurred in a few Arabian horses (Figure 4.46). These horses have a color lighter than **black** but darker than **classic champagne**. While their skin is subtly lighter than normal, it is not as light as the skin of most **champagne** horses. The eyes are amber rather than dark brown. The results of testing for color genes indicate that these horses are genetically **black** at *Agouti* and are negative for *pearl*. Related horses have a similar light color, suggesting that these light colors might be due to a recessive allele. No other dilution allele has been documented in Arabians other than a few tantalizing **silver dapple** look-alikes. The only known recessive dilutions in horses are *pearl* and *mushroom*. The *pearl* allele has been eliminated as a candidate cause for these colors by the results of the DNA tests, and the mutation for **mushroom** is unknown.

A few other candidates for dilution occur in other breeds. Some Friesian horses, for example, are distinctly lighter than black. It is likely that further mechanisms for dilution occur in other breeds if only as very rare mechanisms. Occasional horses that are similar to **silver dapple** occur in a number of breeds, but lack the allele and are black based, so are neither **silver dapple** nor **mushroom**.

Other potential dilutes are more subtle, and some are difficult to classify. Within Missouri Fox Trotters some foals are born with pinkish skin that darkens to freckled, and

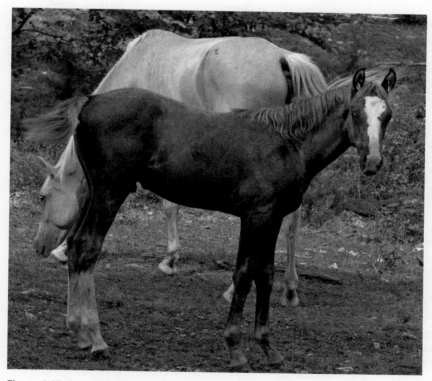

Figure 4.47 Some dilutions can have unusual final results. This colt has a genotype $E^+E^e,C^+C^{Cr},Sb^+Sb^1$ and has no *silver dapple*, *champagne*, or *pearl* alleles. He appeared to be **sooty palomino** as a foal. *Source:* courtesy of Dyan Westvang.

blue eyes that darken to amber. The color is lightened a bit, so that **chestnut** horses have a distinct gold sheen. These are negative for *pearl* and *champagne*. Others are dark, but with distinct yellow undertones, and test negative for known dilutions. Sorting through all of these rare variants is challenging.

The more common dilutions, **dun** and **cream**, can sometimes have unusual final results, and can be confusing to breeders. This is especially so when horses are classed by color as foals (Figures 4.47 and 4.48). At maturity, most of these more closely reflect their underlying genotype, although some remain confusing at maturity.

4.8 Compound Dilute Colors

Each of the diluting alleles (*dun, cremello, champagne, pearl, silver dapple,* and *mushroom*) has a very distinctive interaction with the background colors of **bay, brown, seal brown, chestnut**, and **black**. In many breeds (especially the gaited breeds) these colors are all enjoying increasing popularity, and with that popularity come increasing instances of horses having multiples of these diluting alleles. Some of the resulting combinations are difficult to identify accurately. Combinations involving several of these are outlined in Table 4.6.

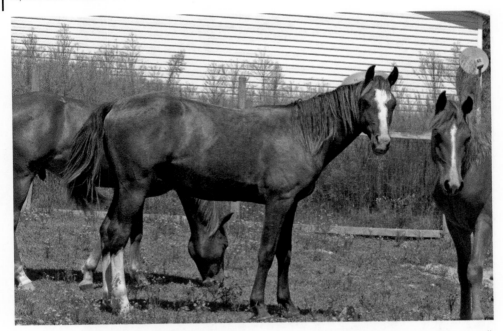

Figure 4.48 The foal in Figure 4.47 matured into a more usual **smoky** color, but still retained the overall "non**black**" appearance that leads to **smoky** horses being misregistered as **brown** or even as **chestnut** in some cases. *Source:* courtesy of Dyan Westvang.

The classification of compound dilute colors is especially problematic because the effects of both *silver dapple* and *champagne* are so highly variable. The notation and discussions of distinct and different colors of the different combinations can give the false impression to readers that these colors are, in fact, easily distinguishable. In truth, however, many combinations involving either or both of these two alleles have pale beige bodies and pale brownish manes and tails (Figure 4.49). Such horses can be very difficult to accurately classify, especially in breeds such as the Rocky Mountain Horse and Mountain Pleasure Horse, which have all of these alleles segregating at relatively high frequencies.

In compound dilute horses, even the usually diagnostic skin features can be confusing and misleading because *cremello* (C^{Cr}) and *silver dapple* (Z^Z) both can lighten skin, especially when combined with each other or one of the other diluting alleles. The resulting phenotype can easily resemble *champagne* (Ch^C) or *pearl* (C^{pr}). Many of these horses are best described as "pale" because they are darker than **cream** and yet have few distinctive features other than pale yellow body color and washed out, pale brown point color. Attempts at detailed nomenclature that is based on the genotypes of these combinations of dilutions can easily mislead people into thinking that they are easily distinguished colors, when the truth is that they often are close mimics one of another.

Table 4.6 Various combinations of Dn^+, C^{Cr}, C^{pr}, Ch^C, and Z^Z on dark background colors.

Base color	Black	Seal brown	Brown	Bay	Chestnut
Dn^+, C^+C^{Cr}	Light grullo	Light grullo	Gold coyote dun Coyote dunskin	Gold dun Dunskin	Linebacked Palomino
$Dn^+, C^{Cr}C^{Cr}, -,-$	Linebacked smoky Cream	Linebacked smoky Cream	Linebacked perlino Dunalino	Linebacked perlino Dunalino	Linebacked cremello
$Dn^+, C^{Cr}C^{pr}$	Linebacked pale Pearl	Linebacked pale Pearl	Linebacked pale pearl	Linebacked pale Amber pearl	Linebacked Ivory pearl
$Dn^+, C^{pr}C^{pr}$	Linebacked classic Pearl	Linebacked sable pearl	Linebacked sable pearl	Linebacked amber Pearl	Linebacked gold pearl
Dn^+, Ch^C	Linebacked champagne	Linebacked Champagne	Linebacked sable Champagne	Linebacked amber Champagne	Linebacked gold Champagne
Dn^+, Z^Z	Linebacked blue silver	Linebacked blue silver	Linebacked yellow Silver	Linebacked yellow Silver	Red dun
Dn^+, Ch^C, Z^Z	Linebacked pale Champagne/silver	Linebacked pale Champagne/silver	Linebacked pale Champagne/silver	Linebacked pale Champagne/silver	Linebacked gold Champagne
Dn^+, C^+C^{Cr}, Ch^C	Linebacked pale Champagne	Linebacked pale Champagne	Linebacked pale Champagne	Linebacked pale Champagne	Linebacked ivory Champagne
Dn^+, C^+C^{Cr}, Z^Z	Linebacked pale Blue silver	Linebacked pale Blue silver	Linebacked pale Yellow silver	Linebacked pale Yellow silver	Linebacked Palomino
$Dn^+, C^+C^{Cr}, Ch^C, Z^Z$	Linebacked pale Champagne/silver	Linebacked pale Champagne/silver	Linebacked pale Champagne/silver	Linebacked pale Champagne/silver	Linebacked ivory Champagne
$Dn^+, C^{Cr}C^{pr}, Ch^C$	Linebacked pale Champagne/pearl	Linebacked pale Champagne/pearl	Linebacked pale Champagne/pearl	Linebacked pale Champagne/pearl	Linebacked ivory Champagne/pearl
$Dn^+, C^{Cr}C^{pr}, Z^Z$	Linebacked pale Pearl/silver	Linebacked pale Pearl/silver	Linebacked pale Pearl/silver	Linebacked pale Pearl/silver	Linebacked Ivory pearl
$Dn^+, C^{Cr}C^{pr}, Ch^C, Z^Z$	Linebacked Pearl/silver/champagne	Linebacked Pearl/silver/champagne	Linebacked Pearl/silver/champagne	Linebacked Pearl/silver/champagne	Linebacked ivory Champagne/pearl
$Dn^+, C^{pr}C^{pr}, -,-$	Linebacked pearl	Linebacked sable Pearl	Linebacked sable Pearl	Linebacked amber Pearl	gold Pearl

(continued)

Table 4.6 (Continued)

Base color	Black	Seal brown	Brown	Bay	Chestnut
C^+C^{cr}, Ch^C	Pale champagne/classic cream champagne	Pale champagne/sable cream champagne	Pale champagne/amber cream champagne	Pale champagne/amber cream champagne	Ivory Champagne/gold cream champagne
C^+C^{Cr}, Z^Z	Pale blue Silver	Pale blue Silver	Shaded yellow Silver	Yellow silver	Palomino
C^+C^{Cr}, Ch^C, Z^Z	Pale champagne Silver	Pale champagne Silver	Pale champagne Silver	Pale champagne Silver	Ivory Champagne
$C^{Cr}C^{Cr}, \_, \_$	Cream/smoky cream	Cream/smoky cream	Cream/perlino	Cream/perlino	Cream/cremello
$C^{Cr}C^{pr}, \_, \_$	Pale pearl	Pale pearl	Pale pearl	Pale pearl	Ivory pearl
$C^{pr}C^{pr}, \_, \_$	Classic pearl	Sable pearl	Sable pearl	Amber pearl	Gold pearl
Ch^C, Z^Z	Champagne Silver	Sable Champagne/silver	Shaded sable Champagne/silver	Amber champagne Silver	Gold champagne

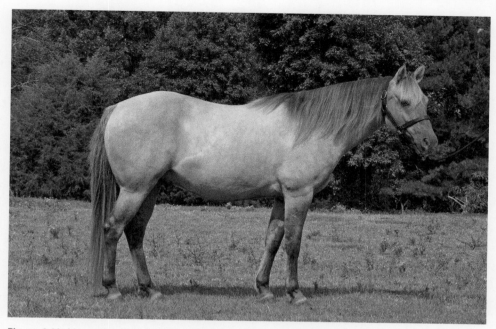

Figure 4.49 Many of the combinations of different dilutions result in fairly similar pale colors with pale brown points. This horse is a **silver smoky grullo**, so a genotype of $A^aA^a,E^+-,C^+C^{Cr},Dn^+Dn^{d2},Z+Z^Z$. *Source: courtesy of Jennifer R. Kuipers.*

5

Overview of the Genetic Control of Horse Color

Several genetic loci interact to build the various colors of most horses. The coat color loci and their alleles are summarized in Table 13.3. Each of these loci and its alleles control some basic aspect of pigmentation, and therefore influences the visible color of a horse. The final color is the result of a cascade of choices at each of several loci. The consequences of these interactions, without considering dilutions or white patterns, are summarized in Figure 5.1. The combinations that follow addition of the dilutions multiply these choices even further.

To summarize briefly, the *Extension* (also known as *MC1R*) locus controls the switch that determines if a horse will have black points or be **chestnut** (non**black** points). The *Agouti* (or ASIP) locus controls the switch on non**chestnut** horses to determine whether the body is black (**black**), red (**bay**), or **seal brown**. These two loci determine the basic color of the horse, which can be modified by the other factors. Other proposed alleles (*dominant black, extension brown, wild bay*) either have somewhat subtle effects or are rare, but their presence could serve to complicate the situation in some breeds.

Some of the remaining factors affect the character of the colors within a general color grouping. Shade is likely polygenic and controls the relative lightness or darkness of pigmentation, and is relevant for all base coat colors. Shade can arbitrarily be split into **dark**, **middle**, or **light**.

Sooty is important as a source of the black countershading that can be superimposed on any basic color. The genetic control of **sooty** is not straightforward, and the control is likely to be different in **chestnut**-based colors than it is in colors with black points. It is convenient and accurate for identification purposes to consider **sooty** as a single switch between present or absent, regardless of the specific locus involved.

The **mealy** characteristic, controlled by the *Pangaré* locus, controls the distinctive pattern of pale red to yellow areas on the muzzle, over the eyes, and on the flanks of some horses. The switch for **mealy** controls whether it is present or absent. **Mealy** only changes the color designation when it is present on **black** and **chestnut** horses. **Black** horses with the *mealy* allele are nearly identical to **seal brown**, despite arriving at that color from a different genetic mechanism than the *black and tan* allele at the *Agouti* locus. **Chestnut** horses with the *mealy* allele are **sorrel**.

Flaxen is complicated genetically, but determines the relative lightness or darkness of manes and tails (and lower legs, on at least some horses) within the group of colors based on **chestnut**. Any division of these point colors into groups is arbitrary because all intermediates occur. Still, the colors of manes and tails on **chestnuts** can usually be divided into four groups: **dark**, **red**, **light**, and **flaxen**.

Equine Color Genetics, Fourth Edition. D. Phillip Sponenberg and Rebecca Bellone.
© 2017 John Wiley & Sons, Inc. Published 2017 by John Wiley & Sons, Inc.

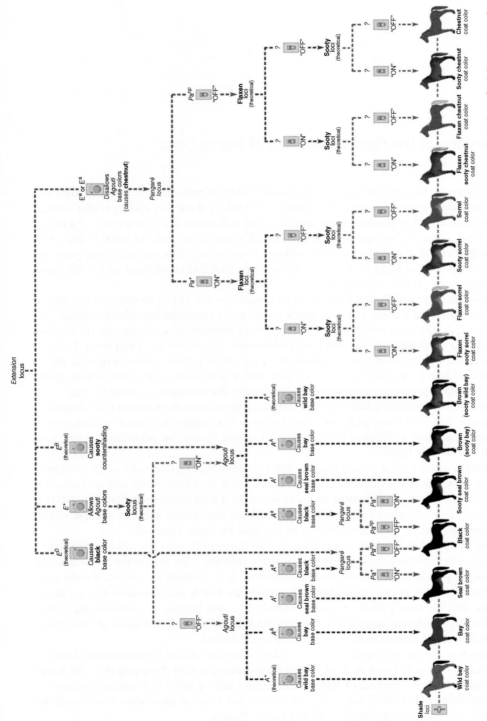

Figure 5.1 Control of the basic coat colors is the result of choices at a few key loci. These choices cascade down and interact to yield the final distinctive colors. *Source:* courtesy of Francesca Gianino.

Brindle refers to a horse that has stripes of one color on a different background color. It is a rare factor, and is therefore usually ignored has having much importance in the determination of horse color. Multiple mechanisms can result in **brindle**. Two that have been documented are X-linked alleles: one at the *MTFPS2* locus (this one is *BRI*) and the other at the *IKBK* locus (this one is associated with a skin disorder). Another source of **brindle** is the chimeras resulting from fusion of embryos. Other mechanisms may be discovered in the future.

Several independent factors are responsible for causing dilute (light) colors. The dilute colors are modifications of the darker, intense, colors. These are independent of the base coat colors, and can be added together for a host of subtly different pale colors, and are too numerous to illustrate in a single figure.

The *Dun* locus (*T-box 3* or *TBX3*) is responsible for controlling the expression of **linebacked dun**, in which both black pigment and red pigment are changed to lighter colors, with the points largely unaffected. Three alleles reside at the *Dun* locus: *wild type* (**linebacked dun**), *non-dun 1* (**linebacked dark**), or *non-dun 2* (dark, not **linebacked**). The last allele is very common, and is the cause of all fully intense dark colors that lack the **dorsal stripe**, which are the most common colors in most breeds.

The *membrane-associated transporter protein (MATP)* locus determines whether or not pigment will be lightened to the pale, **cream**-related group of colors, or to the **pearl** colors. The presence of three alleles with different modes of action complicates the idea of a switch. The most common three choices are phenotypes and genotypes associated with *cremello*, and these are "no copy," "one copy," or "two copies." With one copy of the *cremello* allele at the *MATP* locus, red pigment is lightened to yellow, and black pigment is unaffected. With two copies of the *cremello* allele, both red and black pigments are lightened to a cream color. The visual consequences are therefore (1) "red and black unchanged," (2) "red becomes yellow, and black is unchanged," and (3) "red and black changed to cream." The *pearl* allele is at the same locus, but is a recessive allele that mimics *champagne* in appearance. The array becomes five final choices for the locus: (1) dark color, (2) one *cremello* allele (red changed to yellow), (3) two *cremello* alleles (red and black both changed to cream), (4) two *pearl* alleles (mimicking **champagne**), or (5) one *cremello* and one *pearl* (dark **cream**).

The *Champagne* locus, *solute carrier 36 family A1 (SLC36A1)*, controls the expression of the **champagne** colors in which black pigment is lightened to a pale chocolate brown color and red is lightened to yellow. The choices at this locus are "**champagne**" and "non**champagne**." The mutant allele is dominant, with homozygotes variably paler than heterozygotes.

The choices for the switch at the *premelanosomal protein PMEL* locus are "**silver**" or "not **silver**." This locus controls the colors in which red pigment is unaffected, but black pigment is lightened in varying degrees. At the lightest extreme the black areas become cream colored, or **flaxen**.

The switch at *Mushroom* appears to be a straightforward recessive that changes **chestnut** to **mushroom**, which is very similar to **silver dapple** in appearance when viewed from a distance. Its effect on other background colors is undocumented. The locus involved in this effect is undetermined, and the genotypes' interactions with different base coat colors has not been fully explored.

The "Arabian dilution" and other dilutions are rare, and may have a limited breed distribution. The choices for these are "dark color" or "dilute." The final phenotype

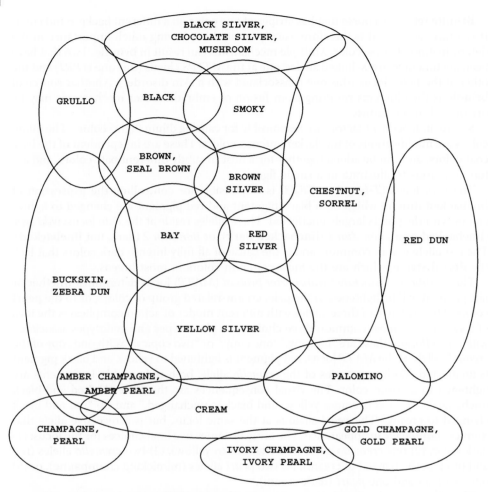

Figure 5.2 Relationships of the various color groups of horses. Each group abuts or even overlaps other groups, and specific examples of colors that occur in the overlapping areas between groups can be confusing. **Bay**, for example, shares overlapping areas with **buckskin** and **zebra dun**, **brown** and **seal brown**, **brown silver**, **red silver**, and **yellow silver**. This indicates that, within the overall **bay** color group, individual horses occur that could be confused with each of these other colors. For example, a very dark **bay** might easily be confused with a **brown** horse. This figure demonstrates the difficulty of assessing the genotype from the phenotype in some horses. The Argentines have a useful designation of "a seven-colored horse." This does not indicate a horse with seven colors, but rather a horse whose color would be designated seven different ways by seven different observers. Fortunately, such horses are rare. They usually occur in one of the overlapping areas at the margins of several of these ovals.

depends upon which specific mechanism is in play, but most moderately lighten both black and red pigments, and most are likely to be recessive alleles.

The original color of wild horses before their domestication was probably a type of **zebra dun** based on a **wild bay** background color, with the distinct light areas caused by **mealy**. The resulting genotype was probably $A^+A^+, C^+C^+, Ch^+Ch^+, Dn^+Dn^+, E^+E^+,$

Mu^+Mu^+,Pa^+Pa^+,Z^+Z^+. This is a pale shade of tan characterized by a lighter belly that is typical of wild mammals. From this color all of the other colors were developed by mutation and selection over the millennia during which horses have been domesticated.

The genetically based approach to horse colors does leave a few holes. Some colors, such as **muddy dun** and **claybank dun**, remain poorly explained. Some colors with a single designation, such as **liver chestnut**, and **brown** (if this includes several options such as countershaded **brown, seal brown**, and **brown-black**), also complicate the overall picture because they can result from multiple distinct interactions of the factors. This contrasts with the situation for most colors, each of which results from a single combination of various alleles. Even some of the more common colors, such as **bay**, may be more complicated than previously recognized, especially if the possible genetic mechanisms for **shade** are included. These may have one mechanism that is common, as well as a handful of more rare mechanisms that lead to close mimics. The development of additional genetic tests for several alleles will eventually help to explain these unusual cases.

The genetically based approach to horse color identification and classification also disregards the fact that each of the colors is observed as occurring over a range and not as an isolated point. It is possible for an observer to create several lists where colors can subtly vary, but just exactly where a line can be drawn between them is uncertain. Very pale **blond sorrels**, for example, are lighter than the darkest **palominos**. Usually, subtle aspects of the body and point color reveal the true genetic makeup of colors, even those that are difficult to discern or those which occur only rarely. Figure 5.2 illustrates various color groups and the areas along their borders that are shared by other color groups. Colors in these overlapping border areas can be difficult to classify accurately, although in many cases DNA tests can help. Currently, tests are available for: *black* at *ASIP* (*Agouti*); *chestnut* at *MC1R* (*Extension*); *dun, non-dun 1*, and *non-dun 2* at *T-Box 3*; *cremello* and *pearl* at *MATP* (*C* in the older nomenclature); *champagne* at SLC36A1; and *silver* at *PMEL* (*Silver Dapple*).

6

Patterns with Individually Distributed White Hairs

6.1 General Considerations

Many variations in what is loosely termed "horse color" are caused by patterns of white hairs that are superimposed over the base coat colors. These white patterns interact with the base coats to give a wide range of variation in the overall appearance of horses. The patterns of white hairs occur in two major groups, although some overlap does occur between the two groups. In one pattern group the white hairs occur as individual white hairs mixed in with colored hairs, which is referred to here as "patterns of individually distributed white hairs." The other group consists of patterns that have discrete patches in which all hairs are white, with little intermixture of white and pigmented hairs. These are "patterns with white patches."

Genetic control of the patterns of white is conceptually different from that of the basic horse colors that were discussed in the previous chapters. Each basic horse color is unique, and each arises from specific combinations of several different but interacting genetic factors. The result of these interactions is one and only one basic color designation for each horse. For example, a **linebacked yellow silver** horse has just that one description, but is the result of the interaction of *bay (Agouti)*, *wild type (Extension)*, *wild type (Dun)*, and *silver dapple (Silver dapple)*.

In contrast, each of the white patterns can be thought of as an independent addition to the genetic recipes that are described in the chapters dealing with color. Each pattern is the result of a separate factor acting independently of the equally independent factors causing other white patterns. Each individual pattern is essentially controlled by a separate switch that chooses between "present" or "absent." These unique patterns of white can occur in several different combinations, and can be added on to any base color. So while each horse can only be described by one final color name, it is easily possible that a single horse can sport multiple different patterns of white.

The final appearance of the patterns boils down to two questions: "Is the pattern present?" and "If present, how extensive is the pattern?" The answer to the first question is determined by the presence or absence of the main controlling gene for each pattern. The answer to the second question is that usually control is by modifying genes at loci other than the main determining gene. Very little is known about the specific genetic mechanisms involved in these modifying genes that control the range of expression of most of these patterns. Experience with most patterns suggests that some modifiers contribute to enhanced expression, while others contribute to suppression. In addition

Equine Color Genetics, Fourth Edition. D. Phillip Sponenberg and Rebecca Bellone.
© 2017 John Wiley & Sons, Inc. Published 2017 by John Wiley & Sons, Inc.

to the modifying genes, it is also likely that variation in the extent of the patterns is influenced by nongenetic influences, such as uterine environment or chance.

The range of each of the patterns can vary from minimal to maximal. When minimal, horses can be mistakenly classified as lacking the pattern even though they have the genetic recipe to produce the pattern. While most horses that have the genetic machinery for a pattern are indeed obviously patterned, a few patterns are notorious for occasionally being masked so completely that horses are misidentified. This happens with **leopard** complex patterns most frequently, but also occurs frequently enough with **frame overo**, **sabino**, and **splashed white** that the phenomenon of suppression is an important one. Very little is known about this phenomenon at the molecular level. However, horses on which the patterns are masked can provide surprises in foal production, because patterned foals can appear where they are not expected. Other patterns, like **roan**, **grey**, and **tobiano**, are masked only in very rare instances.

The variable expression of patterns occurs even with clones, which are basically genetically identical. In nearly all cases the white marks on a group of clones vary from individual to individual. This can be unsettling to some observers, because the thinking is that genetically identical horses should appear completely identical. One way to tease out the details is to consider that the underlying genetic question for most of these patterns is essentially "Is the pattern present or absent?" Clones are almost invariably identical when viewed from this angle, because they tend to all have the same basic pattern. The second question, "Which specific marks or degrees of expression are present?" is a different question, and obviously has both environmental and genetic input on the final outcome. Differences in uterine environment and chance events during the development of clones almost invariably lead to differences in the exact extent of any white pattern, despite their identical genomes. Studying the genetic component that controls the variability in the amount of white pattern has proven to be difficult because the final extent is controlled by both genetics and environment, and the environmental aspect is nearly impossible to quantify.

It is easiest to understand the various white patterns by considering them to be superimposed over whatever background color the horse exhibits. In most situations this background color can still be identified, although on horses that are largely white the color is impossible to see and therefore to recognize. For horses on which the background color can be detected it is always most accurate to first state the color of the horse and then to note any patterns of white that are present. For example, "**bay tobiano**" is more accurate than simply "**paint**," and "**liver chestnut with a blanket and leopard spots**" is a much better description than simply "**appaloosa**."

6.2 Patterns of White with Individually Distributed White Hairs: Grey and Roan

Patterns with individually distributed white hair are often lumped together and called **roan**. **Roan** is the general term used for the intermixture of white hairs and colored hairs in all animals. In this general sense, all of the patterns on horses that arise from such an intermixture could be called **roan**, and in some instances they are. However, it is important to note that the term **roan** also refers to a very specific pattern of distributed white hairs in horses, more specifically called **classic roan** for clarity, and discussed more thoroughly in Section 6.2.3. The use of **roan** in its general sense can be very misleading when describing horses, because when used loosely it encompasses an entire group of different patterns characterized by individually distributed white hairs, rather than a single one. Unfortunately, in some instances the use of **roan** in its general sense is unavoidable because no other word really captures the intermixture of white and colored hairs that is common to these many genetically different patterns. Whenever possible it is best to use the specific pattern.

6.2.1 Definition and Classification

Grey (also referred to as **gray** in some places) occurs very frequently and is considered to be a base color by many horse breeders and owners. **Grey** horses are generally born colored and progressively acquire individual white hairs throughout the coat as they age (Figures 6.1, 6.2, and 6.3). The base color of **grey** horses is usually betrayed by the color of the foal before it turns **grey**. This process usually starts in foals as white rings in the hair coat around the eyes, and this aspect is sometimes called "eye glasses." Greying usually involves the head and the legs very early in the process (Figure 6.2). **Greys** are frequently **dappled** at some point during the greying process. The speed of the greying process varies from horse to horse and also varies somewhat by breed. For example, Arabians and Welsh Ponies usually grey very rapidly, while Percherons tend to grey more slowly. Individuals vary greatly: one Welsh Pony mare did not begin greying until the age

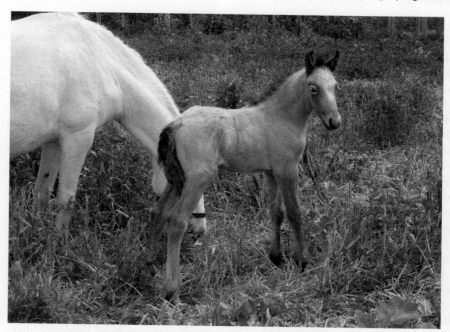

Figure 6.1 **Grey** horses with a light base color, such as **dun** or **buckskin**, rarely look truly grey, and instead are more yellow. This foal shows the yellow base color, and also the distinctive white "eye glasses" that many **grey** foals have. These "eye glasses" are often the first indication that a foal will turn **grey**. *Source: courtesy of Return to Freedom Sanctuary.*

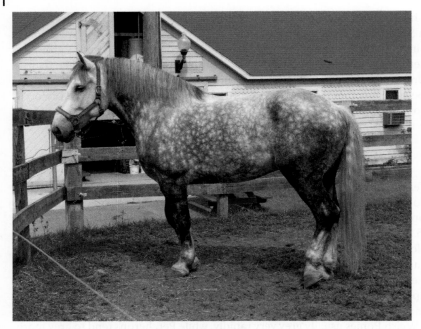

Figure 6.2 About halfway along the **greying** process, many **grey** horses are dappled. *Source:* courtesy of Jeannette Beranger.

of 8 years old, at which point she developed a very typical **grey** pattern. She also produced grey foals that were more typical in their rate of greying than was she, proving that she was genetically **grey**.

A few subtypes of **grey** horses occur. One of these loses pigment in the mane and tail hairs so that these become white (Figure 6.3). This type of horse can become completely white with age, although it usually does maintain pigmented skin. The pigmented skin underlying white hair is useful in distinguishing these aged **grey** horses from truly **white** horses, which have unpigmented skin. The other type of **grey** tends to maintain pigment (usually black or nearly so) in the mane and tail and also tends to keep some dark areas on the body or legs (Figure 6.4). In this type of greying the process tends to stabilize at some point, and some of these horses never become totally white.

In both types of **greys** the skin typically remains pigmented in most horses, although some horses can undergo a progressive depigmentation in the skin, called vitiligo (Figure 6.5). This is especially common in the Lipizzaner breed. Most **grey** horses develop melanomas (tumors of the pigment-producing cells in the skin) as they age. Unlike the case of deadly melanomas in humans, in horses these are generally more of a nuisance and in only a few cases do they become life threatening.

An interaction between **grey** and base colors occurs in such a way that many foals destined to become **grey** as adults will first undergo a darkening of the foal coat to become **black** or nearly so (Figure 6.6). This is such a pronounced tendency that Percheron breeders have a saying that "**greys** are born **black** while **blacks** are born **grey**" (referring to the ashy grey foal coat of **black** horses due to the recessive *Agouti* allele). Owing to this darkening phenomenon it is sometimes impossible to determine what base

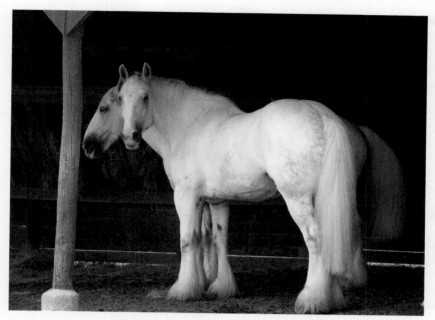

Figure 6.3 Many **grey** horses end up being white or nearly so, with pigmented skin underneath any areas that lack white markings. *Source:* courtesy of Jeannette Beranger.

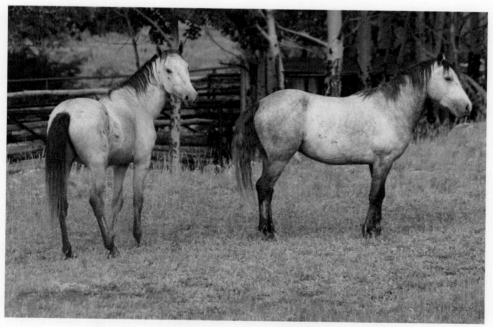

Figure 6.4 Some **grey** horses retain the dark pigment in manes and tails. This variant only rarely becomes completely **white** with age. *Source:* courtesy of Dan Elkins.

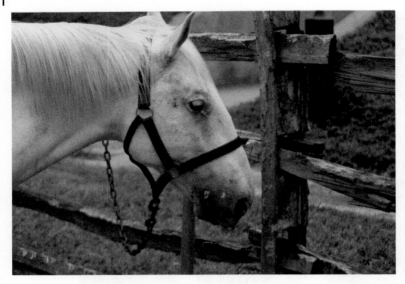

Figure 6.5 Some **grey** horses lose the pigment in their skin along with that in the hair, a condition called vitiligo. This horse has the pink skin typical of the condition, both around the eye and on the muzzle.

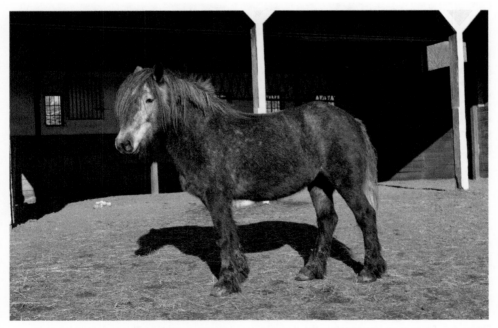

Figure 6.6 The process of producing a **grey** horse usually starts on the head and lower legs, and in most cases the base coat darkens to appear **black** or nearly so. *Source:* courtesy of Jeannette Beranger.

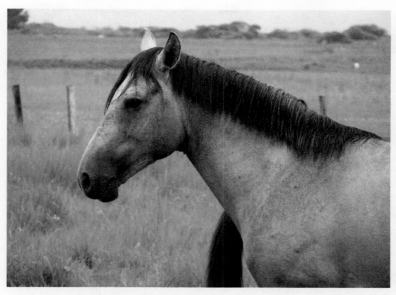

Figure 6.7 Horses that go **grey** from a **chestnut** or **bay** background sometimes retain a reddish color, and are called **rose grey**. The process is the usual one that eventually leads to a nearly white horse.

color a **grey** horse would have had. This is especially true of the dark colors **bay**, **brown**, **chestnut**, or **black**. It is sometimes easier to determine the original base color of a foal soon after birth than it is later, although in some cases even this approach can lead to wrong conclusions. Fortunately, the advent of DNA testing for many color genes can sort out the confusion.

Some horses, most notably in the Arabian breed, stay a **red chestnut** and then grey from this base to give a reddish color, which in this breed is termed **rose grey** (Figure 6.7). Horses with light base colors that are **greying** are sometimes referred to as **roan** instead of **grey**, because the overall color of these horses is never truly grey in appearance. This is especially the practice in the Thoroughbred breed. Referring to these red-based **greys** as **roan** leads to confusion, because **roan** in horse color nomenclature usually indicates a specific pattern (**classic roan**), which is genetically distinct from **grey** and is discussed in detail in Section 6.2.3.

When light colors (**dun**, **cream**-related colors, **champagne**, **pearl**, **silver dapple**, or **mushroom**) are destined to become **grey**, they usually do not darken, but instead they remain one of several light colors (Figure 6.1). This results in unusual intermediate stages as the greying process proceeds. Even the **greys** that do not truly look grey are undergoing the same process as those with a darker base color, and they will eventually end up just as white as the more usual **greys**. Very light colors, such as **cream**, that become **grey** can have such minimal evidence of greying that the process remains undetected.

Occasional **grey** horses have a very pronounced expression of **primitive marks**, especially while they are young. This includes the **dorsal stripe** as well as the **zebra stripes** on the legs. Such horses occur in breeds, including the Arabian, in which **duns** do not occur, and the significance of the striping is therefore uncertain. It may be that at

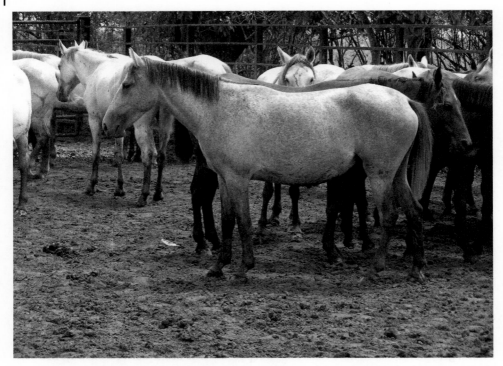

Figure 6.8 **Fleabitten grey** horses most often have a reddish appearance due to the presence of small red flecks in the otherwise white coat overlying pigmented skin.

least some such stripes are the result of the *non-dun 1* allele discussed in Chapter 4. The expression of the stripes on **greys** is transitory in nearly all cases, although those few horses that are **grey** on a **dun** background will retain at least some minimal evidence of striping for a longer time than will other, usually nonstriped, base colors.

It is common for **grey** horses to maintain small flecks of color throughout the coat. These **greys** are called **fleabitten greys**, and the flecks of color are usually red (Figure 6.8), although sometimes they are black (Figure 6.9). The differences in color in **fleabitten** areas can give a clue to the underlying base color. Some **greys** develop distinct large patches of color as they age. These patches are usually red and tend to enlarge as the horse ages. These are called **blood marks** and very rarely will enlarge and coalesce to result in a mostly red horse if the horse survives to great age (Figure 6.10). Some people refer to the body area covered by the **blood marks** when designating color, for example a **bloody shouldered grey**. These peculiarities are all somewhat independent of both the background color and the stage of greying.

Specific names have been used to denote peculiarities of **greys** at specific stages, so that **dappled greys** have **dapples** (Figure 6.2), **iron greys** lack **dapples**, and **porcelain grey** is sometimes used to describe those older **grey** horses that have white hair over pigmented skin. These names describe the stages of greying and can be useful as a temporary identification of a horse, but they are useless for a permanent identification because most **greys** ultimately lighten to nearly white.

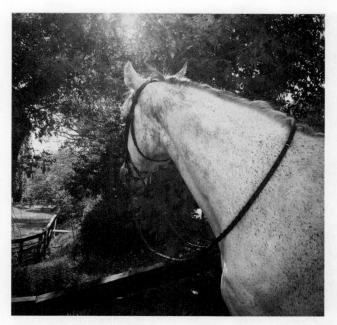

Figure 6.9 **Fleabitten grey** horses have small flecks of color that grow back into the areas left white by the usual **grey** process. Rarely are they black, as on this horse. *Source:* courtesy of Lyndsey Marsh.

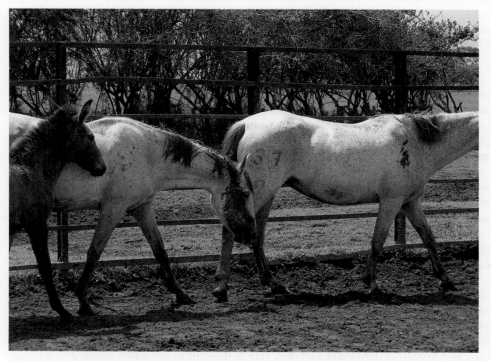

Figure 6.10 **"Blood marked greys"** have distinct patches of red pigment, and these can grow larger and larger with age. Especially among Arabian breeders, and when on the shoulders, this is called a **"bloody shoulder."** These two Criollo Venezolano mares are **fleabitten grey** as well as **blood marked**.

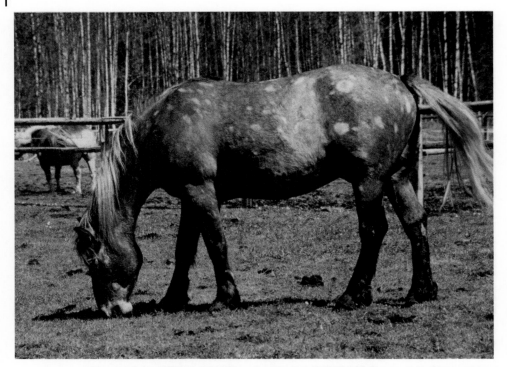

Figure 6.11 Some **grey** horses, especially when young, have odd lighter patches. The color usually becomes a more even, less unusual, and more obviously **grey**, over time. *Source:* courtesy of Evelyn Simak.

Some **grey** horses go through temporary stages during which they have irregular patches of white or dark hair scattered in the coat, and in some individuals these can almost look like the white patches typical of other patterns (Figure 6.11). These horses usually become more uniformly **grey** within months after displaying these irregular patchy areas. Scars or brands in **grey** horses tend to grow white hairs, although some **greys** will grow dark hairs in these injured areas.

Grey is a common pattern and is very widespread among most horse breeds worldwide. Most of the breeds in which it does not occur are those breeds that have a narrow and specific color range, such as Fjord, Suffolk, Friesian, Cleveland Bay, and Haflinger. In some breeds, such as the Andalusian and Lipizzaner, **grey** is so common that other colors of any sort are a minority in these breeds. In these breeds the action of **grey** serves to cover up a great deal of variation in background color, with the result that occasional foals of colors unusual for these breeds are still produced.

Folk wisdom holds that **grey** horses are phlegmatic. They are generally considered to have a quiet, biddable temperament, and have been highly valued for this. **Grey** is an eye-catching color, especially when it is a highly dappled medium shade, and this is partly the reason for favoring grey in breeds used for official state use (Windsor Greys) or draft use (Percheron). **Grey** horses are highly regarded in the tropical *llanos* of Venezuela where the combination of light color and dark skin is thought to provide resistance to intense sun as well as seasonally flooded environments.

6.2.2 Grey: Genetic Control

Grey is due to a dominant allele, G^G. This allele is due to a 4.6 kilobase duplication into intron 6 of the *STYX17* (*syntaxin-17*) locus. It is located on chromosome 25. The mutation appears to first cause an increase in the numbers of melanocytes associated with hair follicles, which is consistent with the relative darkening of the birth coat of **grey** foals. This initial increase in melanocytes is thought to slowly deplete the pool of cells that are needed to produce pigment in the hair in subsequent hair growth cycles, resulting in the progressive whitening of the hair color as the horse ages. The **grey** pattern, along with its genetic basis, is clearly more than just a color, but is related instead to a more general disruption of pigment cell biology and function. This same mutation is believed to also increase the number of melanocytes in the skin, which likely explains the high incidence of melanomas in **grey** horses.

The rate at which horses turn **grey** seems to be at least partially under genetic control. Some of this variation is the result of independent modifiers, but a large portion is due to homozygotes turning **grey** faster than heterozygotes. In some breeds, such as the Percheron, selection in the past for a very slow greying process has resulted in some **greys** achieving the medium, nicely dappled stage at about 9 years of age. These are likely heterozygous, but have other modifiers for a slow rate of greying. In other breeds, such as most Arabians, Welsh Ponies, and many Iberian-derived breeds, greying is very rapid, and 3-year-olds (especially if homozygous) are essentially white. Studies suggest that, in addition to homozygosity for *grey*, horses homozygous for *black* at *Agouti* may also turn **grey** at a faster rate.

Evidence from several breeds, including Percherons in Australia, suggests that heterozygotes are more prone to develop the **fleabitten** appearance than are homozygotes. The small spots of **fleabitten greys** and the **blood marks** of some may well be somatic reversions to the normal *wild-type* allele of this locus, although this has never been tested.

Homozygotes are more likely to have melanomas, and are also more likely to have vitiligo (progressive loss of pigment from the skin). Horses that are homozygous for the *grey* allele have four copies of the 4.6 kilobase region that is duplicated. A non**grey** horse would have only two copies, one on each chromosome. It is theorized that these extra copies cause the initial rapid increase in the number of pigment cells in the skin, leading to melanoma (a neoplastic tumor of pigment cells). It is therefore logical that homozygous horses would go **grey** faster than heterozgyotes, and would also have a higher incidence of melanomas. Studies of DNA isolated from the melanomas of **grey** horses have identified even more copies of this sequence in the more aggressive tumors, which is a possible reason why melanomas are life threatening in some **grey** horses, while others have less aggressive growths. It has also been suggested that horses that go **grey** from an A^aA^a background color are more likely than others to develop melanomas. Other studies have shown that additional modifying loci may be involved in both the progression of melanomas and the extent and rate of the loss of pigment.

The differences between **greys** that keep dark points and those that have white points are not known to be genetic. The peculiarities of **dappled** versus **iron greys** have likewise not been shown to have a genetic basis.

6.2.3   Classic Roan

6.2.3.1   Definition and Classification

Other patterns that are characterized by white hairs mixed into a base coat color are all much more rare than is **grey**, at least in most breeds of horses.

Roan is among several horse color terms that are subject to confusing and variable definitions. In the loose sense, **roan** is used to denote any mixture of white and colored hairs in which the white hairs are individually scattered rather than occurring as white patches. This loose definition is applied to many **grey** horses, especially of the Thoroughbred breed, and in that breed is used to denote horses of lighter base color that are undergoing the greying process. This is somewhat logical, because these horses never truly look **grey**, as they would if the base color were **black** or another very dark color.

In a narrower sense, **roan** is used to identify a specific pattern in which white hairs are intermixed into the base coat color of a horse. This pattern is also called **true roan** or **classic roan** to avoid confusion with the other patterns that cause roaning. On **classic roan** horses the intermixture of white hairs occurs on the body, but generally spares the head, mane, tail, and lower leg (Figure 6.12). **Roans** are rarely **dappled**, and the few that are usually have **reversed dapples**, on which the borders of the dapples are darker than the surrounding areas rather than lighter. Most importantly, **classic roan** is not progressive as is **grey**. **Classic roan** horses are born **roan** or shed to **roan** after the foal coat. On some foals the **roan** pattern is uneven and is usually paler on the

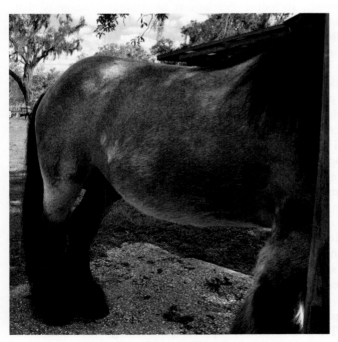

Figure 6.12 **Classic roan** is a mixture of white and pigmented hairs on the body of the horse. *Source:* courtesy of JoAnn Bellone.

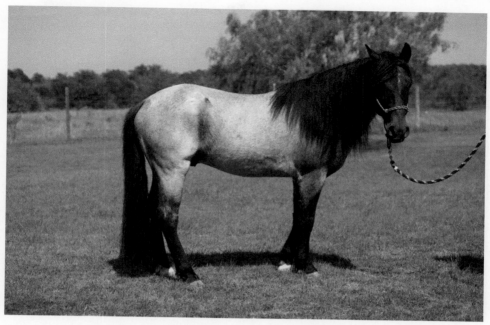

Figure 6.13 Seasonal color changes on **classic roan** horses can be dramatic. This **purple roan** mustang is lightest when first shedding in spring, but retains the dark points and head typical of **classic roan** horses. *Source:* courtesy of Joan Smith.

rump. This stage in the pattern can be confused with the **leopard** complex patterns, especially the **blanket** pattern (discussed in detail in Chapter 8). This confusing stage is temporary, and when the foal coat is shed the **classic roan** pattern is usually unmistakable. On most **classic roan** horses the pattern is consistently present after the shedding of the foal coat.

Classic roan is subject to changes related to season of year and age of horse (Figures 6.13, 6.14, and 6.15). **Classic roans** are lightest in spring when first shedding winter hair, then are medium shades throughout summer, and become dark enough to be confused with non**roans** in winter. These seasonal changes are fairly consistent across most **classic roan** horses. Some **classic roans** also become progressively darker with age, the opposite of what is seen in **grey** horses or in the **varnish roaning** associated with the **leopard complex** (Chapter 8). This can be extreme enough that some **classic roans** can be mistaken to be non**roan** late in life. This seems to be related to different lines of breeding and also seems to affect more mares than it does stallions or geldings. Seasonal changes in the shade of roaning lead to the Icelandic term for **roan** (*litförótt*), which is translated as "always changing color." The shade of **roan** is dependent on the relative amount of white and colored hairs and is subject to individual variation. Some individual **classic roan** horses are dark (fewer white hairs), whereas others are very light (many white hairs) even in the same season of the year and at the same age.

A variety of specific terms are used for **classic roan** horses, depending on the background color of the horse. These are summarized in Table 6.1 and illustrated in

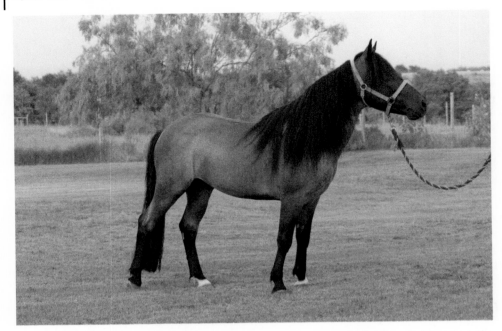

Figure 6.14 The same mustang stallion as in Figure 6.13 is a more even shade of **purple roan** later in the summer. *Source:* courtesy of Joan Smith.

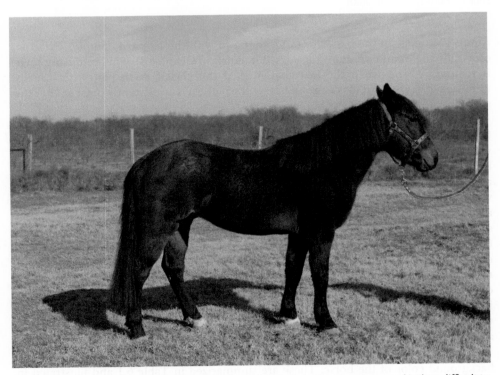

Figure 6.15 The same stallion as in Figures 6.13 and 6.14 is darkest in the winter, and is then difficult to identify as the **seal brown roan** that he truly is. *Source:* courtesy of Joan Smith.

Table 6.1 Specific names often used for **roan** horses with various background colors.

Background color	Roan variant
Black	**Blue roan**
Brown or **seal brown**	**Purple roan**
Bay	**Red roan**
Liver chestnut	**Lilac roan**
Chestnut or **sorrel**	**Strawberry roan**
Light chestnut or **light sorrel**	**Honey roan**

Figures 6.16, 6.17, and 6.18. **Classic roan** on **black** is generally called **blue roan**, although some people call these **black roans**. When **classic roan** combines with **brown**, **seal brown**, and **mahogany bay**, the slight redness shows through and the result is called **purple roan**, although many people tend to lump all of these with **blue roan**. On **bay** the result is **bay roan** or **red roan**. On darker **chestnuts** the combination is called **lilac roan**, while **strawberry roan** describes **classic roan** on the medium shades of **chestnut** and **sorrel**. Confusingly, some observers also use **red roan** for **chestnut roans**, so it has become difficult to be sure of the base coat color intended by people using **red roan** as a description. To avoid this confusion some registries are resorting to **bay roan** and **chestnut roan** as the official designation for these colors.

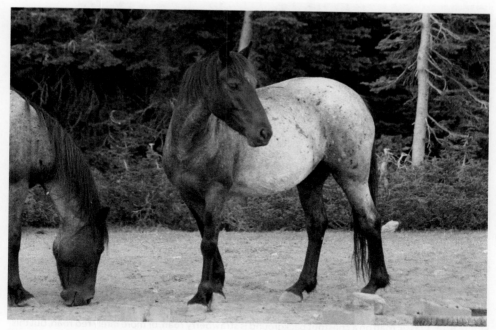

Figure 6.16 **Roan** on a **black** background is usually called **blue roan**. *Source:* courtesy of Dan Elkins.

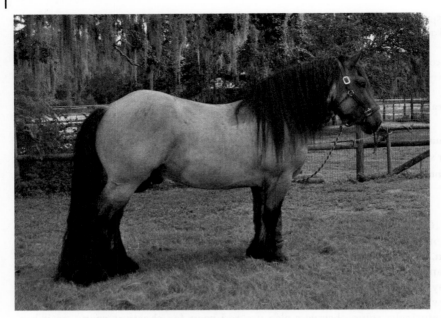

Figure 6.17 **Classic roan** on a **bay** background is usually called **red roan**, but **bay roan** has advantages to avoid confusion with **roan** on a **chestnut** background. *Source:* courtesy of JoAnn Bellone.

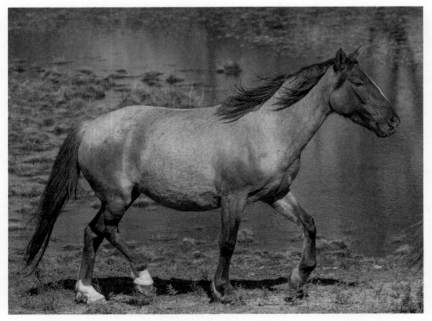

Figure 6.18 **Classic roan** on a **chestnut** background is **strawberry roan**, or more rarely **red roan**, but this last term can be confused with the pattern on a **bay** background. *Source:* courtesy of Neil Chapman.

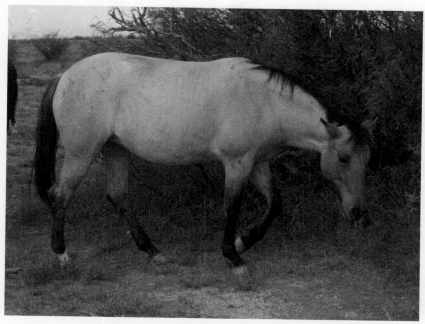

Figure 6.19 **Classic roan** can be superimposed over any background color. Many combinations, such as this **zebra dun roan**, have no specific colloquial name.

On **blond sorrel** the result is pale and is sometimes called **honey roan**. On any other base color **roans** are named by combining the base coat color and **roan** (**palomino roan**, **zebra dun roan**, etc.) (Figure 6.19). This approach of combining the base coat color name with **roan** is also sometimes used with the darker colors instead of using the specific combinations outlined earlier, so **bay roan** could be used instead of **red roan**, for example. This approach is less poetic, but does generate more accuracy for official identification purposes.

Dark spots grow into the coats of some **classic roan** horses (Figure 6.20). These are usually related to scars or brands, in which hair consistently grows back with the base color instead of **roan**. Some **classic roan** horses have dark spots that occur independently of scarring. Both the scarred and nonscarred dark spots are sometimes called **corn spots**, because they give an appearance similar to multicolored Indian corn. The term **corn** is used mostly in connection with the combination on **black** (**blue corn**), but the same spots can occur on **classic roan** horses of any background color. These are especially prominent in feral horses or those managed on extensive ranges. In these situations dominance battles are common, and along with them the nicks and cuts that can lead to the **corn spots**.

The **roan** pattern occurs at a low frequency in a wide variety of breeds. It is especially common in Brabant and Ardennes horses from Belgium, but does occur in nearly all breeds except a few, such as Arabian, or in those breeds highly selected for color, such as the Fjord, Cleveland Bay, Suffolk, Haflinger, and Friesian. **Classic roan** is especially common in British pony breeds, draft breeds, and several breeds with Spanish ancestry.

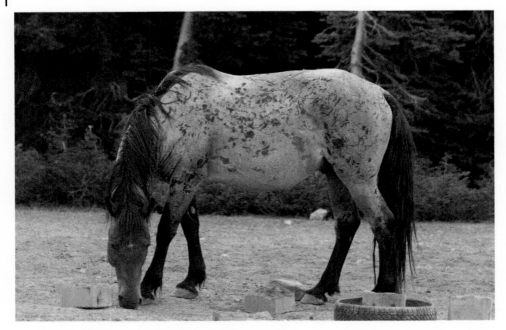

Figure 6.20 This **purple corn** stallion shows the consequences of scarring on **roan** horses. This is a Pryor Mountain Mustang and has weathered many dominance battles, which have left the numerous **corn spots** in his **classic roan** coat. *Source:* courtesy of Dan Elkins.

Folk wisdom holds that **classic roans** are durable and wear well under hard work. They are generally good, solid citizens that can work hard for long lives. They are especially valued in Europe as draft horses because they are reputed to hold up well under hard use. In German-speaking and many Spanish-speaking traditions **blue roans** are separated out as different from other **classic roans** and are more highly regarded. In a few breeds, such as the Peruvian Paso, the **classic roan** pattern is not favored, although this and all other fashions in color popularity are subject to change.

6.2.3.2 Genetic Control

The **classic roan** pattern is inherited as a dominant allele, so the *roan* allele is symbolized Rn^{Rn}. The genetic control for this pattern has been mapped to equine chromosome 3, and is reported to be close to the *KIT* locus. Mutations at the *KIT* locus cause several other white patterns described in Chapter 7. The exact genetic change causing **classic roan** at this locus is undocumented. However, assuming that the *KIT* gene is the culprit makes sense, because this locus has a major role in embryologic development and encodes a protein for mast/stem cell growth factor receptor. This receptor is involved in increasing the number of melanocytes early in embryogenesis and is also involved in maintaining melanocytes with each hair growth cycle. It is likely that the mutation causing **classic roan** reduces melanocyte numbers during embryogenesis, leading to some unpigmented (white) hairs. This knowledge is somewhat trivial to most horse breeders, but may eventually help explain the exact action of this allele and the pattern it produces.

The *roan* allele combines with any base coat color to produce the various shades of **classic roan**. For many years it was held that homozygotes for Rn^{Rn} were unknown, or at least very, very rare. In the data that showed this trend, crossing **classic roans** to one another resulted in two **classic roans** for every one non**roan** foal. This phenomenon is attributed to the death and subsequent loss of the homozygotes during early embryonic development. Such alleles are called embryonic lethal, but it is important to note that this loss is of early embryos and most breeders are unaware of the fact that a loss has occurred. These data were mainly from Belgian horses and generally were from early in the 1900s.

Since those data were published, several horses have been identified that reproduce as if they are homozygous **classic roan**. Such horses have been documented in the Quarter Horse, Spanish Mustang, and also in the Hokkaido Native Horse. The presence of homozygotes in widely divergent breeds suggests that *roan* is unlikely to be lethal to homozygotes as was once thought. Homozygous **classic roan** horses exhibit no phenotypic difference from heterozygous **classic roans**, so no visible hint is available to distinguish between the two genetic constitutions.

Classic roan, being a dominant trait, should never skip a generation. It does sometimes seem to do so, at least in the Welsh Pony breed. In most such cases a close inspection of the horses in the intervening non**roan** generations reveals that these are very minimally **roaned**. This complicates the picture somewhat, because many lightly **roaned** horses, identical to these dark **classic roans**, reproduce as if they are genetically nonroan. Despite the fact that the causative mutation is not known, mapping of this trait has led to the successful development of a DNA test that is often used to determine zygosity for *roan*, as well as detecting those minimally affected horses that carry the mutation.

The *KIT* locus is part of a linkage group that includes *Extension, Roan, Tobiano*, and some loci coding for specific proteins that were once used in blood-typing (including *Esterase, Vitamin D binding protein*, and *Albumin*). Linked genes are located close together on a chromosome, and the closer together they are physically the more likely they are to be passed as a unit rather than recombining in different combinations. The distance between *roan* and *Extension* is considered to be close and expresses itself as rather unusual segregations for some of the combinations.

In one case of a **bay roan** being mated to **chestnut** mares the result was 14 **bay roan** foals, 15 **chestnut** foals, and only 1 each of **chestnut roan** and **bay** foals. This demonstrates that the nonchestnut (*wild*) and *roan* alleles were the linked ones in this case (E^+, Rn^{Rn}) but that occasionally it is possible for the linkage to cross over, as in the **bay** ($E^+, Rn^+/E^e, Rn^+$) and **chestnut roan** ($E^e, Rn^{Rn}/E^e, Rn^+$) foals. In the absence of linkage the foals should have been produced at about eight foals each of **bay roan, bay, chestnut roan**, and **chestnut**, so it is easy to see that linkage changes the relative proportion of colors in the foal crop.

Linkage upsets the usual predictions of genes segregating independently from one another to pass on to the next generation (reviewed in Chapter 1). Consequently, some combinations are common and others are rare, depending on the specific linked combinations in the parents. These linkage relationships can be important in the color production of certain individual families, but they can be disrupted by crossover events frequently enough that they do not dramatically change the frequency of the different possible combinations when considered across a large population.

6.2.4 Frosty

One unusual and distinctive pattern of roaning results in a more uneven mixture of white than the **classic roan**, and such horses are called **frosty** instead of **classic roan**. **Frosty** horses tend to have roan areas mostly over the bony prominences, such as hip, down the spine, and over the shoulder. The mane and tail also tend to be roan, and the head can have roan areas on it as well (Figures 6.21 and 6.22). When present in extreme degrees this pattern is easily confused with **classic roan**, but the head, mane, and tail are roan, and the body pattern is usually less uniform than that of **classic roan** horses. Some breeders in the western USA refer to these roan manes and tails as **squaw tails** and **squaw manes**. **Frosty** horses are rare, and the occurrence of this pattern does not entirely seem to follow breed lines, with the exception that markedly **frosty** horses occur in the same breeds in which **classic roan** occurs.

Because **frosty**, at least in a high grade of expression, usually does occur in breeds in which **classic roan** also occurs it may simply be that **frosty** is a modification of **classic roan** that results in white hairs on the face as well as in the mane and tail in addition to those on the body. In the Spanish Mustang breed, horses that are **frosty** tend to develop heavily roaned manes and tails later in life. These horses have dark manes and tails of the more usual **classic roan** pattern early in life. The genetics of the **frosty** pattern are undetermined, and the pattern might be nothing more than a variant of the more usual **classic roan** pattern that is modified to give roaning in the points. Using the DNA test for the specific allele causing **classic roan** would quickly solve this mystery.

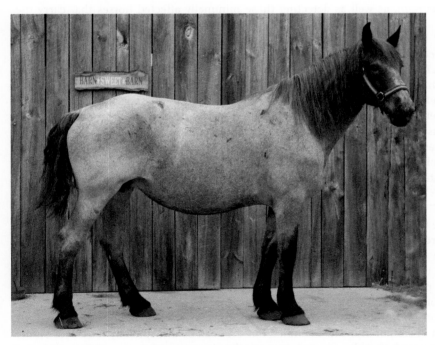

Figure 6.21 This **blue roan** Percheron mare is also **frosty**, including the distinctively roan areas on the head. *Source:* courtesy of Diane Blanzy.

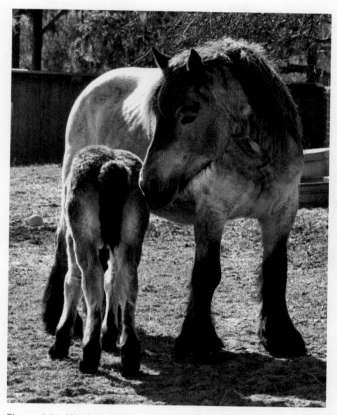

Figure 6.22 This Ardennes mare has the **frosty** pattern, barely detectable in her mane but more obvious on the face, which is more extensively **roan** than are most **classic roan** horses. *Source:* courtesy of JoAnn Bellone.

6.2.5 White Ticking

Other patterns of roaning are less common and are usually overlooked when identifying horses. One of these patterns, **white ticking**, is very specific and involves the base of the tail and the flank (Figures 6.23 and 6.24). The extent of this pattern is variable. Usually, however, the pattern is limited to a few white hairs at the base of the tail and in the flank. On horses with extreme manifestations the pattern is lightest in the flanks and can blend into vertical roan stripes over the ribcage area. This pattern is rarely extensive enough to be confused with **classic roan**.

White ticking does occur in most breeds, but usually the effect is minimal and it is therefore not noted in descriptions of horses. **White ticking** is the usual pattern described as **roan** in the Arabian breed in which the classic **roan** pattern does not occur. **White ticking** has never been the subject of formal genetic studies in horses. It seems to be passed along as a dominant trait in at least some families of horses. It is a subtle pattern, and is frequently mimicked by some **sabino** horses (discussed in

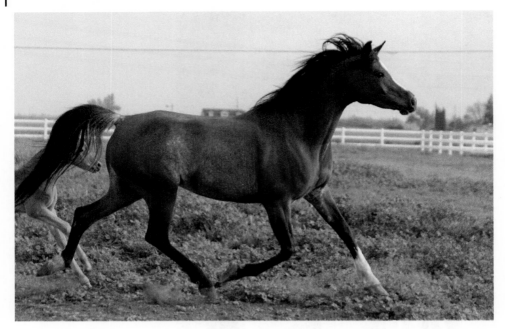

Figure 6.23 **Ticking** is a small amount of **roaning** in the flanks, and usually also at the top of the tail. When minimally expressed it is easy to miss when describing a horse. *Source:* courtesy of Alyssa Vieira.

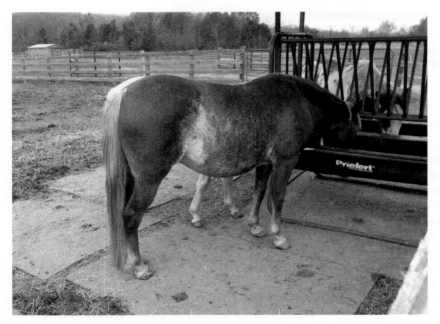

Figure 6.24 Higher grades of expression of **ticking** are distinctive, and usually feather out to stripes on the barrel.

Chapter 7), although many **ticked** horses lack the extensive white marks of **sabino** and therefore have a distinct and unique pattern unrelated to it.

The usual term for this pattern in English is **white ticking** or **highlights**, although it is sometimes called **skunk tail**, in reference to the whiteness in the tail hairs, or **coon tail**, when the roaning is somewhat striped over the base of the tail. In Spanish this pattern is called **rabicano**. It occurs on any background color and does not change over time.

6.2.6 Patterns of White Striping

Very rarely do horses exhibit patterns of very prominent **white striping** (Figure 6.25). Some horse fanciers classify this pattern separate from the others. Most such white striped horses are based on one of the patterns of white hairs, with the striping only occasionally being distinct enough to warrant notice. Prominent **white striping** especially occurs on some horses with the **white ticking** pattern, but is also seen with occasional **leopard complex** and **sabino** horses, as well as being seen rarely on **roan** or **grey** horses. These striped horses can resemble **brindle** horses in appearance (described in Chapter 3), but the striping is white instead of black. Occasionally, **white striping** shows no relationship to any of these other patterns, and in these cases it may be the result of an accident of gestation that simply leaves the pigment-producing cells out of the hair follicles in a striped pattern.

Horses with **white striping** are very distinctive, and it is unlikely that they are all due to a single mechanism. **White striped** horses are rare, and the genetic transmission is undetermined. A relationship of some **white striping** patterns to **brindle** has been

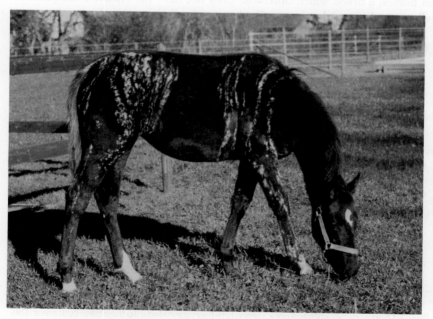

Figure 6.25 Coarse **white striping** is very unusual in horses, and can reflect underlying genetic mechanisms that are not fully expressed, such as **roan** or others. *Source:* courtesy of Evelyn Simak.

observed in some families. That both of these rare phenomena occur in the same horse families implies a genetic relationship between the two in at least some cases.

At least one **white striped** Thoroughbred in Australia, "Catch a Bird," has proven to have been a **classic roan** horse, based on genetic testing as well as foal production. This horse is an oddly marked animal with vertical white stripes on the body and has produced **classic roan** foals in a ratio consistent with his being a **classic roan** himself. This is all the more interesting because the *roan* phenotype was considered to be extinct in the Thoroughbred for a long period of time and has now reappeared through this horse.

6.2.7 Roaned

Some horses have a very light sprinkling of white hairs over the body (Figure 6.26). These are sometimes lumped in with **classic roan**, but if this is a very light sprinkling they are probably not genetically **classic roan**. In some instances these are termed **roaned**, as in **roaned bay** or **roaned chestnut**, for example. The **roaned** variant has never been shown to be genetic, which is not surprising because it is usually not noted in descriptions of horses and is therefore not tracked in records.

6.2.8 Other Roan Patterns

Occasional horses have patterns of white hairs that do not fit well within any of the recognized patterns (Figures 6.27 and 6.28). In a few cases these may be new variants, in other cases they are probably nothing more than unusual variants with relatively less or more white hairs than usual of more familiar patterns. One specific pattern occurs on rare Arabian horses, a breed which otherwise does not have the **classic roan** pattern. This is usually on a **chestnut** base coat. The horses usually have a uniform mixture of

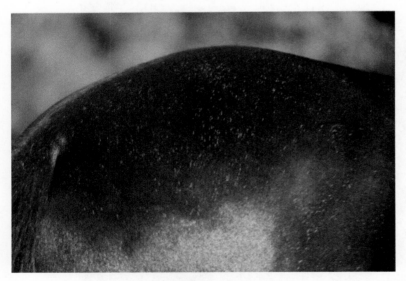

Figure 6.26 **Roaned** horses generally have only a few white hairs sprinkled into their base coat color. This is an example of a **roaned** horse that does not have the **classic roan** mutation, as shown by his foal production record.

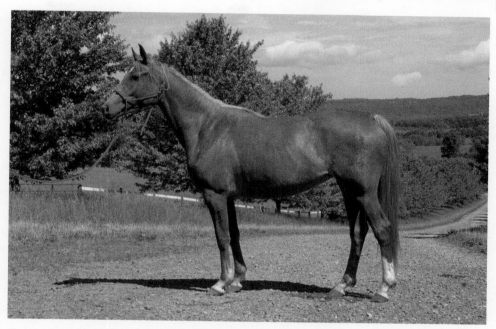

Figure 6.27 Arabian horses rarely have a type of **roan** pattern that mimics **classic roan** but usually also involves the head to an extent. It is nearly always on a **chestnut** background, and the horses also nearly always have some degree of **white marks**, but only rarely as extensively as would a **sabino** horse. *Source: courtesy of Tom Sayvetz.*

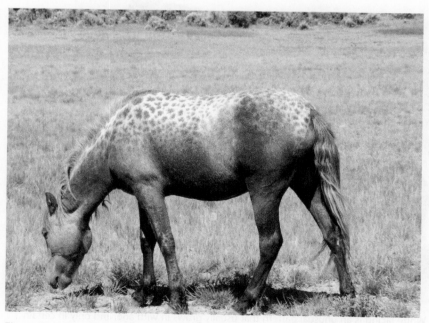

Figure 6.28 This is a distinctly **roan** phenotype that is also heavily **dappled**. The uneven distribution of the pattern suggests that it is distinct from **classic roan**. However, the fact that the **dapples** are reversed (dark centers) is typical of **classic roan** when it is dappled, and so this may be an odd variant of that pattern. *Source: courtesy of Sandi Claypool.*

white and colored hairs, including portions of the head. Most also have white markings on the face. Other examples that fit poorly with **classic roan** include highly dappled **roans**. These are unusual because the dapples are usually darker than the surrounding coat rather than lighter as is true of most colors and patterns.

6.2.9 White Lacing

A rare pattern of **white lacing** over the back of horses is known in the veterinary literature as *reticulated leukotrichia* (Figure 6.29). This pattern usually develops at about 1 year of age. It is limited to certain bloodlines, which suggests that heredity plays a role. Its development in some horses appears to be linked to use of certain vaccines or to a bout of the rare skin disease called *erythema multiforme*. In most cases the first change is development of linear crusts in the hair coat in the same pattern as the **white lacing** will ultimately take. The hair in the crusted areas then falls out, to be replaced by the typical **white lacing** pattern. At that point the skin abnormalities subside and the hair coat color is the only residual change.

Some owners indicate that horses with the typical pattern have not gone through any stage of skin changes, but that the typical pattern does grow into the coat unheralded by skin changes noted in other animals. In addition, some few horses are born with the marking, and it is present throughout life as a nonvarying pattern. In at least one

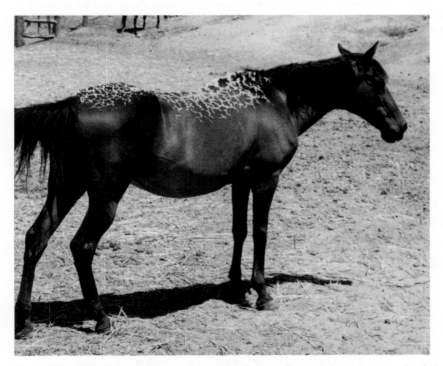

Figure 6.29 **White lacing** is an unusual pattern that usually grows in with age, and only in certain bloodlines. Minimal levels of expression are usually confused with saddle abrasions. *Source:* courtesy of Dr Deb Bennett.

instance, a stallion produced seven offspring all of which developed the **white lacing** at a few years of age, and none of which had any underlying skin changes. The stallion himself never developed the marking. While his plain color suggests a recessive mode of inheritance, the production of so many patterned foals is inconsistent with that interpretation.

White lacing is variable in extent, but usually covers portions of the horse's back from tail to withers. The lacy network of white lines is very distinctive. This pattern has been seen in Quarter Horses, Peruvian Pasos, Paso Finos, and in American Miniature Horses. Its distribution is probably wide throughout many breeds, but only as a rare condition. Rumors of "giraffe spotted" Akhal Teke or Turkoman horses in Iran may be referring to this pattern, which can resemble the pattern on a giraffe when the white lacing is extensive. Synonyms for this pattern include "**giraffe**" and "**marble.**"

6.2.10 Birdcatcher Spots

The **birdcatcher spots** are a white pattern that is rare and consists of small, random white patches scattered over the body (Figures 6.30 and 6.31). **Birdcatcher spots** are usually not numerous and usually not progressive. The name comes from a Thoroughbred horse named "Irish Birdcatcher," who sported these small white patches. They are unrelated to the **leopard complex** of colors, although if they are numerous they can resemble the **snowflake** pattern. In some cases they do increase in number with age, and on occasional horses they change locations from year to year.

Birdcatcher spots occur on horses of a wide number of breeds, but only in a very few individuals. Hairs in scarred or injured areas of any base color can grow in white, but

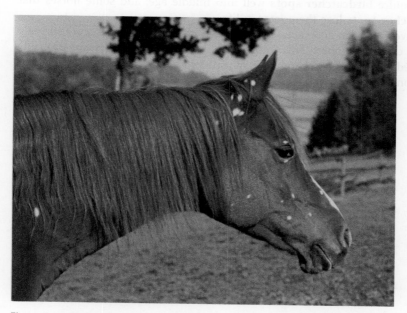

Figure 6.30 **Birdcatcher spots** are distinctive small white patches that often appear early in a horse's life. *Source:* courtesy of Evelyn Simak.

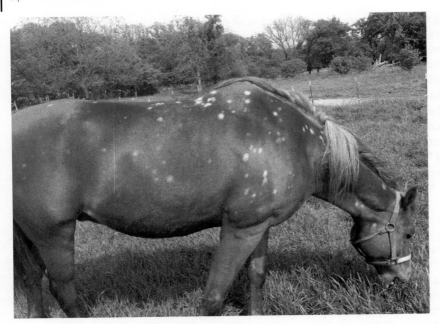

Figure 6.31 When **birdcatcher spots** are numerous they are a unique part of a horse's appearance. *Source:* courtesy of Mary Collins.

these blemishes are distinct from **birdcatcher spots**, which are unrelated to injuries. Some horses acquire **birdcatcher spots** well into middle age, and some horses that develop **birdcatcher spots** lose them later in life.

No studies have ever been done concerning **birdcatcher spots**, but they are strongly associated with certain families. This implies that such white patches are probably genetically caused, but details of the mode of transmission are unknown. Nor is it known if they result from action of a single allele.

7

Nonsymmetric Patches of White: White Marks, Paints, and Pintos

Many different patterns of white areas have been documented in horses. These are generally called "white spotting patterns" in animals because each adds white to the base coat color. Confusion on nomenclature creeps in with the terminology of "spots" because sometimes the pigmented areas are called "spots," and sometimes the white areas are called "spots." Using "spots" for both white and pigmented areas can be confusing, so this guide generally reserves "spots" for the pigmented areas in white regions, and "patches" for the areas of white. Also, to avoid confusion, "white pattern" refers to the individual patterns involved in producing the white patches.

White patterns fit into three major groups. The most common group consists of white marks on the heads and legs of horses, and these are commonly referred to as white face and leg marks. These marks occur on at least some horses of most breeds, although breeds vary in their approach to the specific names given to these white marks.

The other two main types of white patterns have white areas on the body. These patterns are not limited to the legs and head, and are generally are much less common than the usual white marks. The patterns with body patches have a much more limited range of occurrence in various breeds. This is usually due to past selection against them in many breeds, although in a few breeds the breeders actively select in favor of several of these patterns because they are associated with breed identity.

One group of white patterns with body patches consists of those with nonsymmetric white patterns. This group generally goes by the name **paint** or **pinto**. Within this group are several distinct patterns, each under separate genetic control.

The other group of white patterns with body patches consists of those that have reasonably symmetric areas of white on the body. These are typical of **leopard complex** patterns. This group is characteristic of the Appaloosa breed in the USA, and these patterns frequently go by that name even though they are also found in many other breeds both in the USA and worldwide. This type of white pattern is discussed in detail in Chapter 8.

All of the white patterns are generally accompanied by pink, unpigmented skin underlying the white areas. This is a consequence of the melanocytes being responsible for pigmentation of both hair and skin, so in areas where these pigment cells are absent both skin and hair are unpigmented.

Equine Color Genetics, Fourth Edition. D. Phillip Sponenberg and Rebecca Bellone.
© 2017 John Wiley & Sons, Inc. Published 2017 by John Wiley & Sons, Inc.

7.1 Face and Leg Markings

7.1.1 Definition and Classification

White marks on the heads and legs of horses are very common. They occur on horses of nearly all breeds, and usually their presence is barely noted except when used for identification of individual horses on registration or health papers. White marks are more likely to be noticed if they are extensive or otherwise distinctive. Some breeders actively select against them, leading to minimal expression and generally unmarked horses. Other breeders actively favor them. The white marks in those breeds in which they are favored are common and obvious. In most breeds they tend to be ignored, with individual breeders left to follow their own preference as to the presence and extent of the markings.

White marks on the head are subdivided into different classifications according to the area of the head that bears the white mark (Figure 7.1). Those between the eyes are called **stars**, those on top of the nasal bones are called **strips**, those above the upper lip are called **snips**, while **chin spots** reside on the lower lip. Each of these white marks can vary in size. They are also commonly connected in various ways, and some of the combinations have specific names. A **stripe** is a narrow connected **star**, **strip**, and **snip**. A **race** is a **stripe** that goes off to one side. A **blaze** is a wide **stripe**. **Baldfaced** describes horses with wide **blazes** that cover the nostrils or muzzle. **White muzzles** are white marks on the upper and lower lip and are usually associated with a **baldface** pattern or one of the patterns whiter than **baldfaced**. **Apronfaced** horses exhibit extensive white that extends down the bottom of the jaw to the throat, generally leaving color only over the eyes and ears. **Paperfaced** horses have entirely white heads, generally with colored ears. **Paperfaced** horses are sometimes called **bonneted**, due to the colored ears. It is unusual, even in very extensively marked horses, for the ears to be white.

White leg marks vary in extent, much as do facial markings (Figure 7.2). They nearly always begin at the hoof and extend up the leg a variable distance. **White coronets** involve only that portion of the leg immediately above the hoof and frequently are incomplete, only involving some of this area but not all of it. When **white coronet** marks are very small they are called **white spots**, and when they only involve the heel they are called **white heels**. **Half pasterns**, logically, involve only the lower half of the pastern. **White pasterns** are more extensive but extend up to the bottom of fetlock joint, while **white fetlocks** include that joint. **Socks** extend up to halfway up the cannon bone, with **stockings** extending further than **socks**. Some observers refer to **socks** as **boots**. **Stockings** can be subdivided into **three-quarter stockings** and **full stockings**, depending on how close to the knee or hock they extend. **Ermine spots** refer to small dark spots in white leg marks. These are usually right at the junction of the hoof and skin. **Ermine spots** are common and frequently lead to stripes in the hoof wall, growing from them when they involve the coronary band.

Most horses with white leg markings have white hooves on the marked legs. Many horse fanciers consider that white hooves on horses do not wear as well as black or striped hooves, although individual horses vary greatly and many horses have white hooves that are very durable. The general reputation for white hooves being weak is the reason that some breeders favor horses that do not have white leg markings. This bias is very pronounced in breeds such as the Friesian, Fjord, and Cleveland Bay, where such

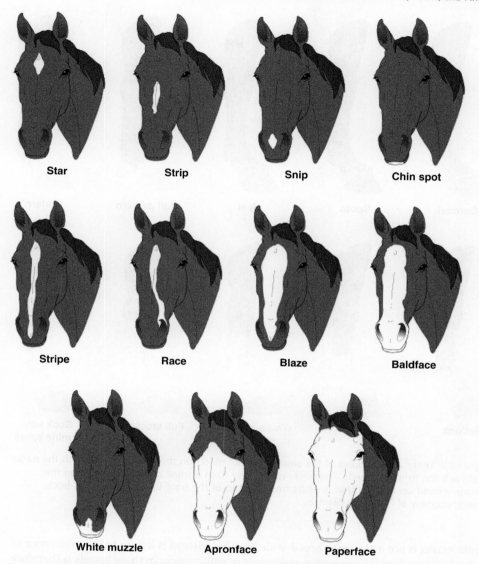

Figure 7.1 These are examples of the common white marks on the heads of horses, with the name that each has in most breeds. The white marks vary in extent from a small **star** located between the eyes to a face that is almost entirely white, usually called **paperfaced**. *Source:* courtesy of Francesca Gianino.

marks are penalized, but it is also present in breeds such as the Percheron and Suffolk, whose breeders simply prefer unmarked horses.

It cannot be denied that white marks on the head and legs do give a horse a flashy appearance. As a consequence, such marks are favored in some breeds, such as the Hackney and Clydesdale. The marks highlight the high leg action of those breeds. In the Welsh Pony and some other riding breeds the white marks are desired because they are attractive on a saddle mount. In many breeds the desirability or undesirability of

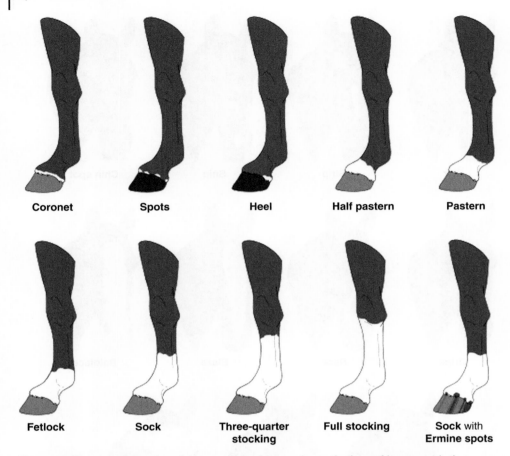

| Coronet | Spots | Heel | Half pastern | Pastern |

| Fetlock | Sock | Three-quarter stocking | Full stocking | Sock with Ermine spots |

Figure 7.2 These are examples of the common white marks on the legs of horses, with the name that each has in most breeds. The white marks vary from a small amount of white on the coronary band up to a leg that is white from the top of the hoof up to the knee or hock. *Source:* courtesy of Francesca Gianino.

white marks is not a matter of breed-wide bias, but instead is left up to the preference of individual breeders. The presence and extent of white marks in those breeds is therefore understandably quite variable.

Face and leg markings vary in extent, with a strong tendency to vary in tandem. Horses with extensive facial markings also usually have extensive leg markings, and vice versa. White leg markings are generally more extensive on rear legs than on front legs and also loosely tend to be more extensive on left feet than on right ones. Curiously, they are more extensive in male Arabian horses than in females, but more extensive in female Haflinger horses than in males.

All white markings are usually more extensive in **sorrels** (lighter or **mealy chestnuts**) than in darker **chestnut** horses, and both these colors are likely to be more extensively marked than are **bays**. **Black** horses usually have minimal white marks. This interaction of base color with white markings is consistent across breeds, although the general extent of white markings in a breed results from past selection either for or against (or ignoring!) these markings.

Early researchers postulated separate single alleles for each type of white mark, which turns out to have been too simplistic an explanation. This interpretation still surfaces from time to time, despite having been disproven by more recent studies. The usual white marks on legs and faces of horses have been documented as a quantitative trait in the Arabian, Thoroughbred, and other breeds. This means that more than one gene plays a role to produce the white marks.

As already noted, the genetic control of **chestnut** versus not-**chestnut** at the *MC1R* locus also influences the extent of white marks. This interaction between the base coat color and the extent of white marks is genetically influenced, so that **chestnut** horses tend to have more extensive white marks than do **bays**, which in turn are more extensively marked than **black** horses. This effect is interesting, in that **bays** carrying *chestnut* (A^A—E^+E^e) are more extensively marked than those not carrying *chestnut* (A^A—E^+E^+). This is evidence, for at least this one interaction, that the *Extension* locus allele for *chestnut* is incompletely recessive rather than completely recessive.

Recent research suggests that accumulations of mutations at both the *KIT* and *MITF* loci contribute to increasing the extent of white marks in the Franches-Montagne breed, a Swiss breed in which a great deal of molecular genetics work on pigmentation has been accomplished. In this breed, seven loci are thought to contribute to variation in the phenotype of face and leg markings. These loci include *MITF*, *KIT*, and *MC1R* along with other unspecified loci. The extent to which *MITF* and *KIT* contribute to the amount of white is dependent on the genotype for *MC1R*. On **chestnut** horses, *KIT* appears to modify the amount of white face markings more than does *MITF*. On bay horses, *MITF* seems to be the more important modifying locus.

Information about the genetic cause of these marks allows breeders to select for or against them more adequately, although the quantitative nature of these will make complete accuracy of selection nearly impossible. Several genes at separate loci control the marks, and the overall balance between the genes determines the extent of the white marks. In spite of a good start in understanding the genetic interactions important for the expression of these white marks, at this point no commercial test is available for the underlying genes.

To further complicate the issue, variation of white marks in the Franches-Montagne horses could not be fully explained by genetics alone, even when considering the seven loci that have been documented to be associated with their expression. This suggests that other factors in addition to genetic ones are also playing a role in the expression of white marks, which makes it difficult for breeders to succeed consistently in either increasing or decreasing their expression by selection of breeding stock.

Important issues for breeders interested in controlling these white marks can be somewhat separated into two major issues. One of these is whether or not the marks are present or absent. The second, only relevant if the marks are present, is the relative extent of the marks. Genetic factors are the most important influence on whether the horse has white marks or not. In contrast, the nongenetic influences are likely to be more important in determining the extent of the white marks on horses that have the marks.

The result is that breeding for face and leg markings is possible, but to some degree the exact extent of those marks is left to chance. For example, genetically identical cloned horses usually have different white marks. This can be perplexing to observers that think that genetically identical clones should be identically marked. If the genetic question is thought of as "Are white marks present?" then usually the two clones are indeed similar if not identical. It is just that the exact extent of those marks seems to be influenced by nongenetic factors that occur during development, with the end result that each clone ends up with a different extent of individual marks.

In some breeds other white patterns make important and large contributions to white marks. The most common of these is the **sabino** pattern. Minimally marked **sabinos** frequently have extensive white marks. The control of the **sabino** pattern is itself complicated, and its relationship to all white marks is unclear. Other candidates for a single gene effect on some horses are the *frame* (**bald faces**), *tobiano* (**white stockings**), and *splashed white* (both face and leg markings together). The presence of any of these patterns could easily confuse the issue when considering the inheritance of white marks, because the presence of these patterns puts marks on the horses regardless of the presence or absence of the usual genes for these marks.

The expression of white marks can also be complicated by mechanisms to suppress these. In addition to the usual genetic mechanism of various genes favoring their expression, it is also likely that a few genetic mechanisms actively suppress or impede the expression even in horses with a genetic propensity to have the marks. While the underlying genetic mechanisms are undocumented, some horses have marks (especially on the head) where the usual shape is altered by colored areas that seem to be superimposed over the white mark. This is visual evidence that mechanisms do exist that can mask the **white marks**, essentially by covering them up with pigment.

Miniature Horses consistently have less extensive expression of white marks than do horses of other breeds. This tendency for minimal expression extends to other white patterns, even in the presence of the genetic machinery for causing the patterns. This is further evidence for genetic influences that can suppress markings and other white patterns.

7.2 Nonsymmetric White Body Patches: Paint or Pinto Patterns

Patterns consisting of white patches on the body (whether symmetric or nonsymmetric) are important in some breeds and essential in a few. All of these patterns tend to occur in a more restricted array of breeds than do **grey** or **classic roan**. They also exist in a much narrower range of breeds because several breed registries specifically disallow them. In contrast, some North American breeds are built around these patterns, such as the Paint, Pinto, Appaloosa, and Pony of the Americas breeds. In other breeds, such as the Spanish Mustang and Miniature Horse, these patterns are allowed along with many other patterns and colors. In still other breeds, notably Trakehner, Dutch Warmblood, and some other Warmbloods, these patterns still persist in a minority of individuals, but are by no means common. As a result of selection that either favors or penalizes these patterns they usually become either very common in a breed or are eliminated nearly completely. Some few breeds, including the Icelandic, Arabian, and Thoroughbred, neither favor nor penalize these patterns on a breed-wide bias. In these few breeds some of the patterns persist at a low to moderate level of occurrence.

One distinct group of patterns consists of those with irregular, nonsymmetric patches of white on the body. This group of patterns usually goes by the name **paint** or **pinto**. The names Paint and Pinto are also used as breed names in addition to their less specific use for a group of white patterns. These names are therefore sometimes confusing, and at least in the Arabian breed the term **particolored** is used in an effort to avoid confusing breed and pattern when referring to patterned horses. When used to designate pattern, the terms **paint** and **pinto** generally mean any of the nonsymmetric white patterns.

The older English terms "piebald" and "skewbald" further confuse the terminology of paint and pinto patterns. **Piebald** refers to any black and white horse. This term derives from "magpie," a black-and-white bird. **Skewbald** refers to white patches on any color other than **black**. **Skewbald** derives from the Scandinavian *skjöt*, which also refers to the magpie. Neither **piebald** nor **skewbald** indicates which specific pattern of white is present, and the trend among horse fanciers is to no longer use these terms. Breeders of horses within the Gypsy group of breeds are an exception, where these terms are still commonly used.

An increasingly frequent practice is to indicate the base color of a horse, and then to designate the specific pattern of white that is superimposed on it. This approach yields the greatest accuracy in horse identification and is also important for horse breeders interested in only one of the several specific single patterns. With this approach the final name reveals a great deal about the alleles present in the horse.

The confusion of terminology in this group of patterns goes beyond the general terms **paint** and **pinto** and extends to the terminology of the individual patterns within this group. The resulting ambiguity has caused problems in the identification of these patterns, and accurate identification is a critical first step toward understanding the genetic control of these patterns, because genetic studies require accurate phenotypic identification of the animals involved. The genetic control behind most of these patterns is fortunately now well understood, which can help breeders to control the expression of specific patterns.

The whole group of **paint** and **pinto** patterns contains at least five distinct patterns, and maybe as many as seven. North American usage usually distinguishes **tobiano** as a distinct pattern, and lumps the others together as **overo**. It is important to understand that this **overo** group actually contains multiple patterns, including **frame, splashed white, manchado**, and **sabino**. **Sabino** likewise includes **sabino 1, white, dominant white**, and polygenic **sabino**. Each one of these patterns is genetically distinct from the others, and appreciating this detail is the key to understanding the entire group.

Each pattern within the group has a reasonably consistent placement and character of white patches, and this phenomenon helps observers to accurately classify the majority of nonsymmetric patterns on horses. Horses with minimal expression of white for each pattern usually have the white in locations that are very consistent and that involve only specific body regions. Likewise, horses with the maximal amount of white for each pattern usually have color remaining on a specific combination of body regions. It is generally the case that the white increases from the minimal to the maximal expression in an orderly fashion. Regions that are white in the minimally white horses tend to be white in all horses with the same pattern. Likewise, regions that are colored in the maximally white horses are generally colored in all horses with the pattern. This detail can help in accurately classifying horses. The progression of each of these patterns from least white to most white is illustrated in Figure 7.3.

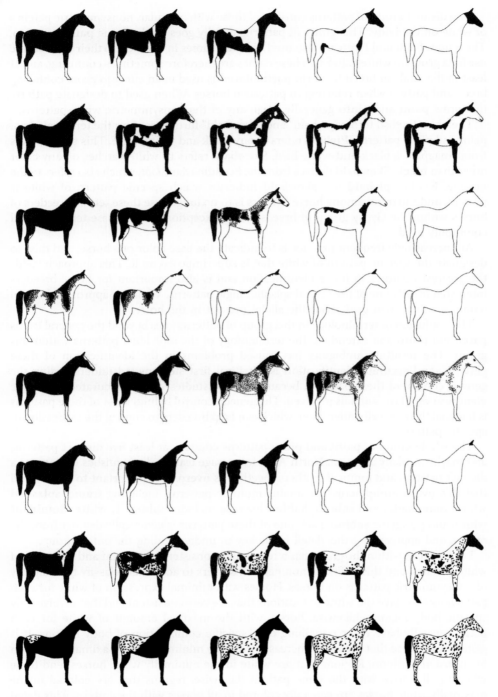

Figure 7.3 The progression of the extent of white in each of the **paint** patterns is generally orderly. Despite this trend, some individual horses can still be confused if classed solely by their own external appearance. The presence of common white marks can contribute to the confusion. The top rank in this figure is the **tobiano** pattern, second is **frame**, third is **sabino 1**, fourth is **dominant white**, fifth is polygenic **sabino**, sixth is **splashed white**, seventh is **overo manchado**, and the eighth is **leopard** complex.

7.2.1 Tobiano

7.2.1.1 Definition and Classification

The **tobiano** (toe bee AH no) pattern is fairly common in North America. The name **tobiano** comes from South America and originated when General Tobías came to Argentina from Brazil in the mid-1800s with a contingent of soldiers mounted on horses with this pattern. Prior to Tobías's arrival in Argentina, the **tobiano** pattern did occur, but was very rare. As a result, **tobiano** was originally lumped in with all other patterns and called **overo**. Following the arrival of Tobías, and with him so many horses of this previously rare pattern, the pattern acquired his name and was no longer lumped with all other types of white patterns under the general term **overo** (see Section 7.2.3).

The expected progression of the **tobiano** pattern is illustrated in Figure 7.4. **Tobiano** horses generally have white hooves and lower legs, and the white on the body usually crosses the topline somewhere between the ears and tail (Figures 7.5, 7.6, 7.7, and 7.8). The white areas tend to have sharp, definite edges and usually have a vertical character. As a rule the heads on **tobiano** horses are very conservatively marked, and those with white marks on the head nearly always have other genetic mechanisms in addition to **tobiano**. Most **tobianos** have dark eyes, although a few do have blue eyes. Some of these blue-eyed **tobianos** lack any of the other patterns that usually cause blue eyes, leading to the conclusion that the **tobiano** pattern itself is causing the blue eyes in a consistent but small minority of **tobiano** horses. Most **tobianos** have regions of white as well as regions of color in the mane and tail, and this has become a defining characteristic for this pattern in some registries even though this detail is not invariably present. The long mane and tail hairs can obscure the fact that these mixed manes and tails are growing from very crisp and distinct patches.

The minimal **tobiano** pattern is four white lower legs, usually from the knees and hocks down. Most minimally marked **tobianos** also have a small patch of white somewhere along the topline, and this is frequently in the mane or tail (Figure 7.4). The heads on minimally marked **tobianos** are usually solid with small or no white marks. **Tobianos** with a great deal of facial white, as is typical of the Gypsy family of breeds, have other genetic mechanisms at work to provide for those markings. Maximally marked **tobianos** often have completely white bodies and colored heads. Some retain colored patches in the flanks or on the chest. The variant with color only on the head is sometimes called the Moroccan pattern, although it has no direct connection with Morocco or with horses from that country (Figure 7.8). To further confuse the issue, the Moroccan Spotted Horse breed includes horses exhibiting each of the different **paint** patterns, not just the one manifestation of the **tobiano** pattern alluded to in the breed name.

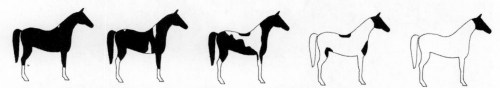

Figure 7.4 The progression of **tobiano** from minimal to maximal is difficult to confuse with any other white pattern. The white legs and colored heads are very distinctive, though common white marks can confound this by affecting the head.

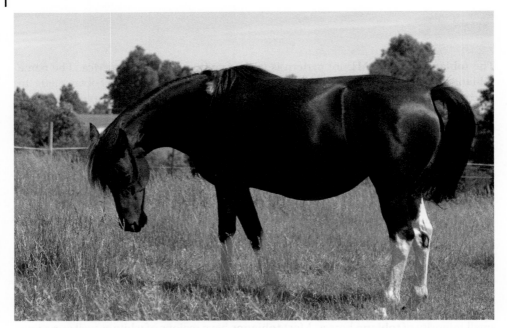

Figure 7.5 Minimally marked **tobiano** horses usually have dark heads, white lower legs, and a small white patch somewhere along or close to the topline. This horse has a white patch that is partially covered by the mane. *Source:* courtesy of Dyan Westvang.

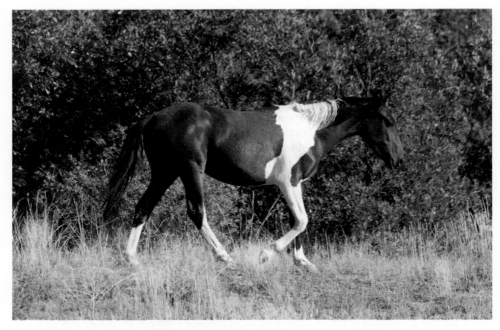

Figure 7.6 The mid-range of **tobiano** expression is usually easy to recognize, with white lower legs, vertical white patches that cross the topline, and a conservatively marked head. *Source:* courtesy of Dan Elkins.

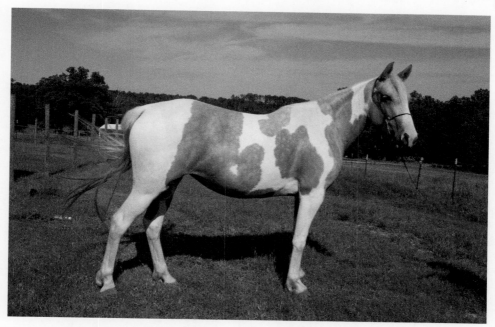

Figure 7.7 **Tobiano** horses with white facial markings usually have other white pattern genes at work, besides the obvious *tobiano* allele. *Source:* courtesy of Dyan Westvang.

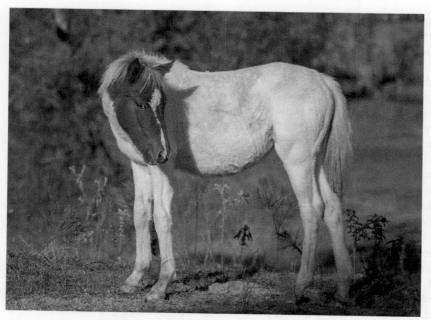

Figure 7.8 At the whitest extreme, **tobiano** horses usually have colored heads and are otherwise white. *Source:* courtesy of Neil Chapman.

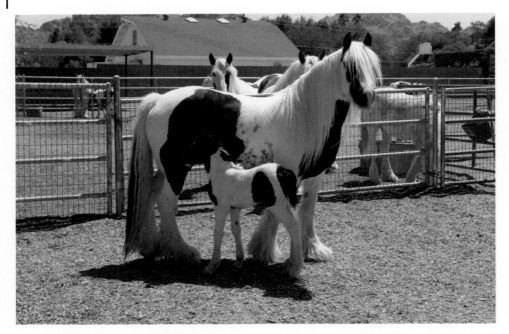

Figure 7.9 **Ink spots** are small dark or roan spots in the white areas of **tobiano** horses, like the ones on this mare. They are a useful tip to identify horses likely to be homozygous for the *tobiano* allele. *Source:* courtesy of Jennifer Gilson.

Ink spots are another peculiarity of some **tobiano** and other patterned horses. **Ink spots** are small spots of solid color or roan that occur in the white patches (Figure 7.9). They are usually small and round, can occur in groups, and are therefore distinct from the other colored spots on most **paint**-type horses. **Ink spots** are the expected background body color of the horse on which they occur. On some **tobianos** the white areas have smudgy roan patches in them, and the colored areas might also have smudgy roan patches as well. These are called **paw prints**, **cat tracks**, or **bear paws**.

On the **tobiano** pattern of some horses, pigmented skin extends a short distance into the white areas. The result is a shadow or halo between the colored and white areas on the horse (Figure 7.10). This effect sometimes causes the horses to be called **shadow paints**, **ghost paints**, **ribbon paints**, or **halo paints**. This peculiarity occurs on horses of other white patterns as well.

The **tobiano** pattern is very common in the Paint and Pinto breeds, for which it is one of the major defining patterns. **Tobiano** has a very wide geographic distribution, occurring in several northern European pony breeds, Mongolian Ponies, Asian breeds, several breeds of gaited horses, and also in various Warmblood breeds. **Tobiano** occurs, although rarely, in breeds derived from a Spanish influence 500 years ago and is still seen in some of them today. **Tobiano** is very common in the Gypsy family of breeds.

Many registries disallow the **tobiano** pattern, even though it was originally present in several of the breeds that now frown upon it. In some horse-breeding traditions any sort of white pattern was penalized because prevailing logic held that the white patches would become progressively larger through the generations, leading to whiter and whiter

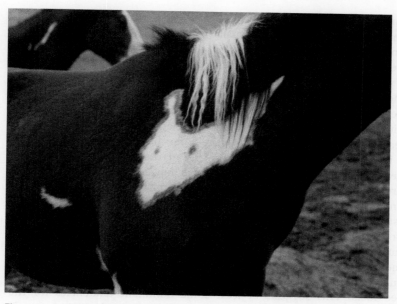

Figure 7.10 Ribbon paints have a border of dark skin under white hair adjacent to their white patches, creating a distinctive border between the white and colored areas.

horses. This assumption is erroneous, and the production of well-marked **tobianos** is easily possible through many generations.

Some anecdotal evidence from the Paint breed suggests that **tobianos** are superior performance horses, even though many of them apparently lack some subtle conformational edge that tends to put horses at the top of halter classes.

7.2.1.2 Genetic Control

The **tobiano** pattern is caused by the *tobiano* allele (To^T), which is dominant to its absence. This gene maps to equine chromosome 3, just downstream from *KIT* (also known as the *mast cell growth factor receptor* locus). This locus is associated with several different white patterns, including common white marks **classic roan**, **sabino**, and **white**. The *tobiano* allele is caused by an inversion of the genetic material about 70 kilobases downstream from the *KIT* locus, which means that the change is 70 000 DNA building blocks away from the gene itself. This change likely affects the function of the *KIT* locus, resulting in the white pattern. The consequences of this inversion are logical, because it is located close to the locus responsible for multiple types of white patterns. Homozygous **tobiano** horses do occur and are fully viable, in contrast to homozygotes of other patterns such as **frame** and some **dominant white** alleles.

Most homozygous **tobianos** can be distinguished from heterozygous **tobianos** by the presence of **ink spots**, **paw prints**, or **bear paws** (Figure 7.9). These roan or dark colored areas are typical of homozygous **tobianos** and are very rare in heterozygous horses. The amount of white in the overall pattern does not seem to be reliable in making the determination of homozygosity. Homozygotes as well as heterozygotes span the range from minimally white to maximally white.

Occasional horses with the *tobiano* allele are so dark as to not have white body patches. These minimally marked horses usually have white hooves and extensively white legs, but a minimally marked head. This is an unusual combination and is a subtle but important indication of the horse's true genetic makeup. The specific combination of extensive leg white and minimal head white is consistent with the action of the *tobiano* allele and is not consistent with the leg and face marks that are otherwise common in horses. The extent of the more common leg and face marks tends to vary in tandem, so that it is rare for a horse to have extensive marks on the legs and minimal marks on the head if these are caused by the genetic mechanism responsible for the common marks in horses. Although these minimally marked horses are genetically **tobiano**, they are usually missed as being such because they lack white patches on the body. These horses can produce **tobiano** offspring as reliably as any other, more obviously patterned, **tobiano**.

Although most minimal **tobiano** horses do give hints of their status, a few are so completely suppressed that no external observation could detect these. **Tobiano** horses without body patches have been called **crypto-tobiano** in the Huçul breed. While precise genetic mechanisms of the suppression are uncertain, the **crypto-tobiano** horses do tend to produce occasional **crypto-tobiano** foals along with the expected **tobiano** and nonpatterned foals. This suggests at least some dominant tendencies for the suppression. This has been proposed as a *Cp* locus (the "*Cp*" standing for "crypto") acting to cause the suppression. Aside from these rare minimally marked horses, it is very unusual for the *tobiano* allele to be present and to not betray its presence in the coat. **Tobiano** is completely suppressed very rarely, in contrast to the more frequent suppression of several other **paint** patterns.

The *tobiano* allele's location close to the *KIT* locus links it genetically to a few blood-typing protein loci (including the *Vitamin D binding protein* locus *Gc*, as well as *Esterase* and *Albumin*), and to the *Extension* locus (at which *chestnut* resides). Its closeness to *KIT* also links it to *Roan*, and this explains unusual ratios of foal colors when breeders use horses that express both **tobiano** and **roan**.

Genetic testing is possible for *tobiano* so that breeders can be sure of its presence. They can also document horses as heterozygous or homozygous for the allele, which can help in the development of breeding strategies for the production of a high percentage of patterned foals.

7.2.2   Calico Tobiano

A very few **buckskin** and **palomino tobiano** horses have colored areas that consist of irregular patches of red or dark tan as well as the expected yellow of those colors (Figures 7.11, 7.12, and 7.13). The white pattern is the usual **tobiano** but the colored areas interact with it to give an appearance somewhat resembling a calico cat. These are called **buckskin calico tobiano** or **palomino calico tobiano** depending on which background color is present. The extent of the dark patches is variable, and on minimally affected horses could be easily overlooked. The horses with more pronounced expression are very distinctive and unusual.

Calico tobiano horses are very rare, and occur occasionally in the American Paint Horse and Tennessee Walking Horse, as well as in some families of Choctaw Horse. The segregation data in these families indicate that this pattern is due to a dominant modifier,

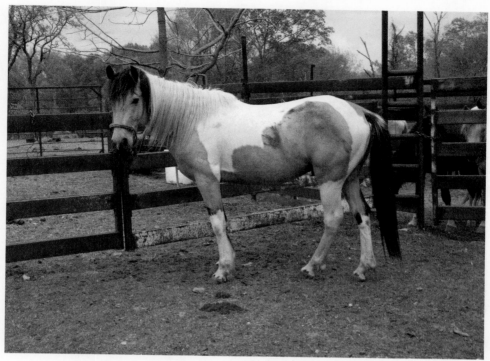

Figure 7.11 This **buckskin calico tobiano** shows the typical interplay of dark and light colored areas. In addition, he has the unmarked head consistent with the **tobiano** pattern. *Source:* courtesy of Jeannette Beranger.

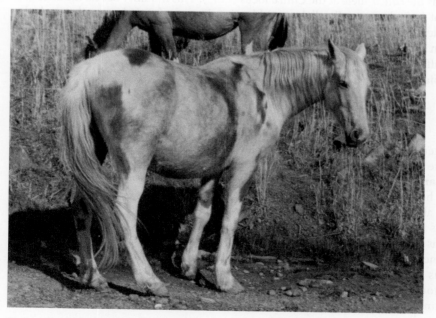

Figure 7.12 This **palomino calico tobiano** mare has a minimal **tobiano** pattern, but a pronounced expression of the **calico** interplay of pale and dark pigmented areas.

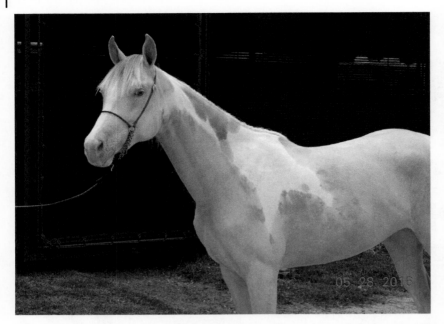

Figure 7.13 This horse is a combination of **tobiano, calico, cream,** and **champagne** (all on a **bay** background) leading to an unusual final appearance, but one that expresses each of these components. The **calico** interplay of dark and light areas is most evident close to the white patches from the **tobiano** pattern on this horse. *Source:* courtesy of Sarah Murray.

proposed as the *calico* allele at the *Calico* locus (*Cal^C*). This modifier has no influence on horses that lack the *cremello* allele, and likewise does not affect horses that lack the *tobiano* allele. It is therefore difficult to manipulate in breeding programs because the production of **calico** foals depends on the specific combination of three dominant alleles at three different loci. The sex of the foal seems to have no effect on the expression of **calico tobiano**, in contrast to the situation with calico cats.

7.2.3 Overo

Paint patterns other than **tobiano** are usually lumped together as **overo** (oh VAIR oh). **Overo**, like **tobiano**, has a Spanish derivation. In North America it has come to mean "non-**tobiano**," whereas in South America it is used in a loose sense to mean any patterned horse. In South America, **tobiano** as well as **leopard complex** patterns were originally all considered subtypes of **overo** in addition to those patterns that North Americans currently refer to as **overo**. In South America the patterns historically grouped as **overo** long ago included **tobiano, sabino** (one specific subtype of what North Americans call **overo**), or one of the **leopard complex** colors (which South Americans also call **overo**, although specifically *overo pintado*). Within this complicated history and confusing usage, horse fanciers somehow need to fit at least four non-**tobiano paint** patterns that are distinct from one another both phenotypically and genetically.

The genetic differences between most of the various distinct **overo** patterns have only recently been investigated, although the **frame** pattern was the first of any colors or patterns to be documented by DNA analysis. Part of the confusion over these patterns results from the fact that all of the more common three (**frame**, **sabino**, and **splashed white**) are frequently lumped together, when, in fact, each is distinct. The most prudent course is to rely on the specific name for each pattern, relying on **overo** only to mean "non-**tobiano**," which is what the term has come to mean in North America.

7.2.3.1 Frame

7.2.3.1.1 Definition and Classification

The **frame** pattern is one of the patterns usually called **overo** in North America. The usual progression of the **frame** pattern is illustrated in Figure 7.14. **Frame** horses generally have dark hooves and legs (or markings no more than expected of solid-colored horses). The heads are usually extensively marked with white. White patches usually occur on the middle of the sides of the body and neck and only rarely cross the topline. The patches tend to have clean edges, but are sometimes more ragged than **tobiano** patches. The patches also have a horizontal arrangement rather than the more vertical tendencies of **tobiano** patches. The name "**frame**" for this pattern comes from the distinctive horizontal arrangement of the white patches, leading to the appearance of a pigmented frame around central white in the intermediate range of expression of the pattern (Figure 7.15). Many **frame** horses have a pigmented upper lip on an otherwise very white head, and this is sometimes called a moustache. Blue eyes are very common on **frame** horses, even when a colored patch rather than a white patch surrounds the eye.

Minimally marked **frame** horses can fail to get white body patches (Figure 7.16). Such horses usually have **bald faces**, but dark legs and no body patches. This is somewhat the reverse of minimally patterned **tobiano** horses with white legs and unmarked heads. The combination of extensive white on the head and solid-colored legs is unusual, because usually face and leg white vary in tandem so that extensively marked heads occur along with extensively marked legs. The **frame** pattern contrasts with this trend and allows for the **bald face** along with solid-colored legs. Maximally marked **frame** horses tend to have nearly white heads, pigmented lower legs and feet, and extensively white sides (Figure 7.17). The white on the sides in these maximally marked horses can extend over the topline of the horse (generally somewhere in the mane), but still retains its horizontal character. Maximally marked **frame** horses are never entirely **white**.

The **frame** pattern has a fairly limited geographic distribution. It is most common in North America or in horses of North American ancestry. It also occurs in South America

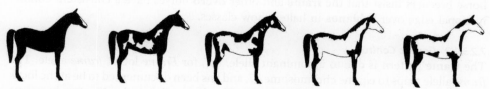

Figure 7.14 The **frame** pattern has a very regular progression from minimal to maximal that helps to distinguish it from other patterns. **Frame**, if no other white pattern is involved, is distinguished by dark legs, facial white, and white patches that are horizontal on the body and neck.

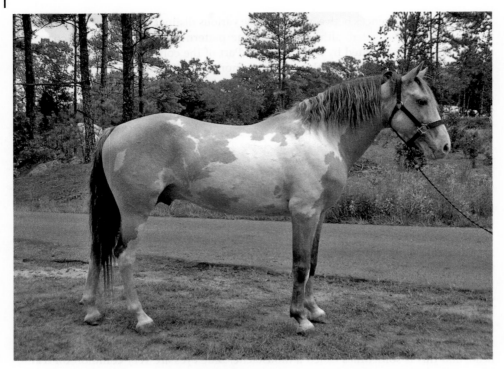

Figure 7.15 The middle range of expression of **frame** usually has facial white, and white patches on the center of the body or neck. The coat color of this horse is **amber champagne**. The pigmented areas "frame" the white patches on the horse, and these can be of any base color or diluted color. *Source:* courtesy of Gretchen Patterson.

as a rare variant. In both continents it seems to have originated in Spanish horses, and it is now nearly restricted to these Spanish breeds or to their derivatives such as the Paint and Pinto. A few recent occurrences of the **frame** pattern in the Thoroughbred breed indicate that the allele is present, if rare, in a number of breeds. The occurrence in the Thoroughbred may indicate that it can lurk for generations under the cloak of suppression. **Frame** also occurs in Miniature Horses and in feral horses in Ethiopia. It is ironic that the **frame** pattern is one of the patterns usually associated with the general name **overo** in North America, because it clearly is not what is usually called **overo** in South America, where the name originated.

Frame horses have few specific traits attributed to them by horse owners. Some Paint horse breeders insist that the **frame** and other **overo** horses have a consistent conformational edge over **tobianos** in halter show classes.

7.2.3.1.2 *Genetic Control*
The **frame** pattern is due to a dominant allele, Fr^F, for *Frame* locus, *frame* allele. The *frame* allele maps to equine chromosome 17, and has been documented to be at the locus that controls *endothelin receptor B* (*EDNRB*). The *frame* allele is due to a two base-pair change in this gene that results in a change in the protein sequence, and thereby a change in the protein's function.

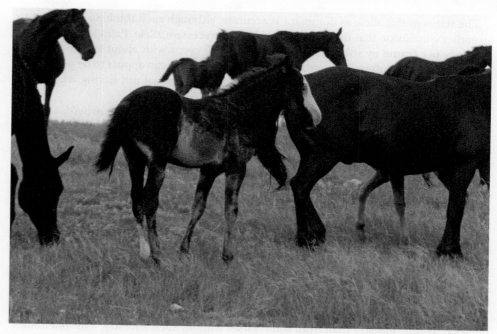

Figure 7.16 The minimal expression of **frame** lacks patches of white on the body, but the combination of extensive facial white and dark feet is a good indicator of the allele's presence. This foal is **black**, but has the typical ashy-grey foal coat so common with that color.

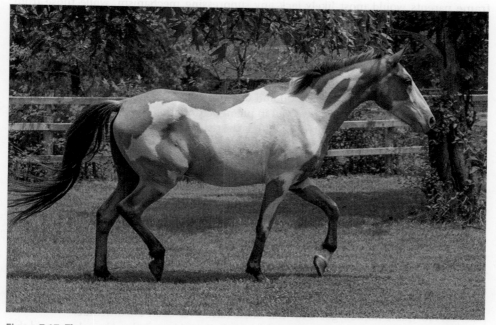

Figure 7.17 The most extensive expression of the **frame** pattern has white patches that can involve the topline of the horse, but it is still common for feet to be dark. *Source:* courtesy of Neil Chapman.

The status of this allele as dominant is accurate, although such thinking is counter to an earlier conclusion that this pattern was due to a recessive allele. Paint horse breeders routinely use **frame** by solid matings to achieve foal crops with about half of the foals having the **frame** pattern. In some instances the *frame* allele can appear to be passed as a recessive, but usually this is due to a minimally marked animal not having white body patches and thereby being misclassified as a nonpatterned horse.

Occasionally, the *frame* allele does indeed seem to pop up out of nowhere, as it did recently in the Thoroughbred and seems to do occasionally in other breeds, such as the American Quarter Horse. This implies that the simplistic interpretation of **frame** as a single dominant allele might not tell the whole story. Such "crop-out" horses do go on to reproduce the **frame** pattern as a dominant allele, and the **frame** pattern is very certainly due to a dominant allele. This allele is the same in all **frame** horses, and crop-out horses test positive for this usual *frame* allele. This fact makes *de novo* mutation in crop-out horses an unsatisfactory explanation because an identical mutation that recurs repeatedly is essentially impossible. The presence of the allele has been documented in some unpatterned horses, and this is good evidence for a mechanism that can suppress expression of the allele. Some of these suppressed horses give no hint of the presence of the allele. Others have the unusual combination of a **bald face** and unmarked legs, which should alert observers to their true status as **frame** horses.

Some breeders insist that they have more success in getting patterned foals from solid horses of **frame** ancestry than from solid horses without such ancestry. This phenomenon can also be explained by a genetic mechanism for masking of the pattern in some horses. Such a mechanism would not be present in patterned horses, but could be lurking undetected in solid-colored horses. The result is that solid-colored horses with **frame** parents would most likely lack any suppressing mechanism, while those from non-**frame** breeding would essentially be untested for this mechanism, and might well have it. The mechanism would only betray itself by suppressing **frame** expression following introduction of this allele by appropriate matings.

While exceptions do occur frequently enough to require attention, it is still true that the dominant allele hypothesis does the best job of explaining the transmission of the **frame** pattern from generation to generation and does this for all but very rare exceptions.

In addition to *EDNRB* being involved in pigmentation, this gene has other important functions in the developing embryo, and this is the reason that homozygosity for the *frame* allele is lethal. The *frame* allele, when homozygous, is responsible for the production of **lethal white** foals. These foals are entirely or largely white and die within a few days of birth because innervation of portions of the intestinal tract is faulty and food cannot be passed through the lower digestive tract. In early embryos this gene controls an increase in numbers of both melanocytes and nerve cells. Both of these come from the embryonic neural crest. In homozygous embryos the multiplication of these cells is incomplete, leaving the foal with no melanocytes (and therefore **white**) and also with no nerve cells in the large intestine, which impedes gut mobility. The situation with **lethal whites** is complicated, though, because some foals produced by mating **frame** horses to nonpatterned mates are in fact **lethal white**. In these cases the nonpatterned parent was probably either minimally patterned or one in which the expression of the Fr^F allele was masked. No viable homozygotes for this allele have ever been documented.

Direct DNA tests are available for the *frame* allele and have helped breeders avoid the mating of two carriers. These tests have also detected a few solid (with no white pattern) horses that have the *frame* allele, documenting that it is indeed possible for horses to have the allele but not the white patches associated with it. Whatever mechanism causes this suppression of white on horses with the *frame* allele contributes to the confusing exceptions to the generally dominant transmission of this pattern.

7.2.3.2 Sabino and White

7.2.3.2.1 Definition and Classification
Another of the **overo** patterns, called **sabino** (sah BEE no) in this guide, has a hopelessly confusing terminology. This pattern is what is usually intended when South Americans use the catchall term **overo**, and it is one of the three patterns commonly called **overo** in North America. In northern Europe this pattern is called **sabino**. Unfortunately, by a strict definition, **sabino** is Spanish for "pale red" or sometimes "roan." **Sabino** in some parts of South America specifically means **fleabitten grey**, especially **greys** on which flecks are red and not black. **Sabino** has a connotation in Spanish for pale colors and specifically for a pale red or pink color. The result of history and usage of **sabino** and **overo** is that the terminology surrounding the distinct patterns in the **overo** group is confused and at this point is a bit hopeless.

The specific pattern referred to as **sabino** in this guide is variously called **sabino**, **calico**, **speckled**, **flecked**, or **particolored** (in the Arabian breed this last term is favored). In a few cases the more highly flecked and roan manifestations of this pattern are called **buttermilk roan** or **Spanish roan**. Flecked and roaned **sabino** Welsh Ponies with minimal pattern on the body are called "**with roaning**," as in "**bay with roaning**." Welsh Ponies with the **sabino** pattern have also been called **blagdon**, after a stallion that sported this pattern. Not all horses of this pattern are speckled or flecked, but because the term **sabino** is already well accepted in North America for identifying this pattern it should continue to be used despite the shortcomings of its strictest Spanish definition.

The **sabino** pattern usually involves extensive leg white and facial white (Figures 7.18, 7.19, 7.20, 7.21, 7.22, 7.23, 7.24, and 7.25). Areas of white are usually on the belly and can either occur as roan areas, speckled areas, or, rarely, as white patches with clean, crisp edges. Most **sabinos** are flecked or roaned, and this is especially true in horses with extensive patterns. On extremely white **sabinos**, color remains as roan or speckled areas on the ears, tail base, flanks, and chest. Some **sabinos** are solid white, although most have at least some color on the ears. A few **sabino** horses have wholly or partially blue eyes, though most have brown eyes. Blue eyes are especially common on horses with unpigmented skin and white hair around the eyes. Partially blue eyes are most common when the border between unpigmented and colored areas runs through the eye.

The minimal **sabino** pattern is simply extensive white marks, and this is easily missed as being a **paint** pattern. These white marks differ from usual white markings in that they tend to have narrow extensions up a leg or down the throat. Some people call these extensions "**lightning strikes**." On the front legs, these extensions are usually on the rear aspect of the leg, while on the rear legs the extensions tend to go up the front aspect (Figure 7.19). In addition, many minimally marked **sabinos** are very lightly **roaned**, and while this characteristic can help identify some minimally marked **sabinos**, it is equally true that not all lightly **roaned** horses are indeed **sabino**. Many minimally marked **sabino** horses have **roaned** flanks, and can be easily confused with horses that have **ticking**.

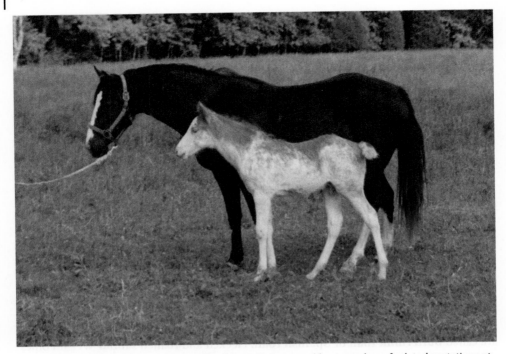

Figure 7.18 **Sabino** patterns vary considerably, and are caused by a number of related mutations at the *KIT* locus. The minimal pattern is generally white marks easily confused with the usual markings on horses, but the more extensively marked horses are easily identified. **Sabino** does interact with base color, so **black** horses are likely to be less extensively marked than are **chestnut** horses, as clearly evidenced by this mare (**black sabino**) and foal (**chestnut sabino**).

The maximal **sabino** pattern is variable. Some **sabinos** have small flecks of color scattered over the coat, some are entirely white with colored ears, and occasional horses are entirely **white** (Figure 7.25). Another relatively common maximal pattern is white with colored ears, chest, tail base, and along the back (Figures 7.23 and 7.24). The colored areas in these manifestations are generally, but not always, roan or speckled.

The **sabino** pattern is widespread in nearly all types of horses, although it is frequently overlooked when minimally expressed. **Sabinos** with very crisp, clean white patches can be easily confused with **frame** horses, although generally the white leg marks help to accurately classify such individuals because those are lacking on most **frame** horses. A few crisply marked **sabinos** can be confused with **tobianos** because the patches can extend vertically. Such horses are rare, and fortunately most of them usually have at least some flecking at the edges of white patches. The flecking or roan aspect of the patches helps distinguish these horses from **tobianos**. Extensive facial white on these horses also helps make that distinction, because **tobiano** by itself does not yield white marks on the face.

Extremely roan **sabinos** can be confused with **classic roan** horses, but white on the legs and faces, as well as roan areas on the head will give these away as **sabinos** and not **classic roans** (Figure 7.21). Roan areas on **sabinos** are also less even and uniform than

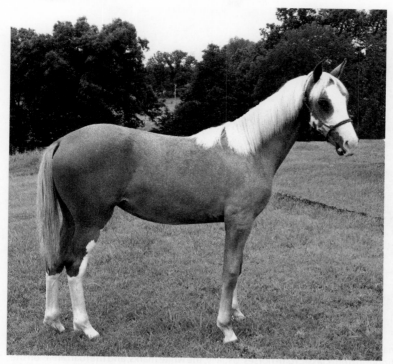

Figure 7.19 Lower grades of **sabino** pattern can usually be detected by the tendency for the white leg marks to extend upward on the front aspect of the hind legs, as well as the rear aspect of the forelegs. Facial white also tends to be more extensive than usual white marks. *Source:* courtesy of Dyan Westvang.

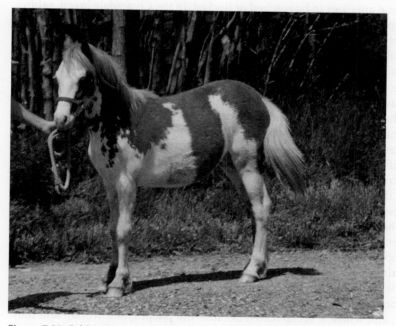

Figure 7.20 **Sabino** horses with very crisp borders to the white patches are unusual and can make it difficult to accurately identify all horses with this pattern.

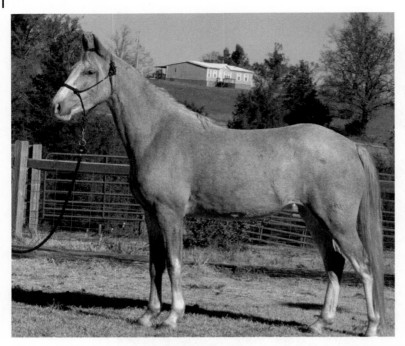

Figure 7.21 While many **sabino** horses have roan or speckled areas, the very most **roan** examples can be difficult to distinguish from **classic roan** horses. Usually, the white marks, and the roan areas on the head, can help to accurately identify these. *Source:* courtesy of Dyan Westvang.

are **classic roans** and are likely to be patched or flecked. In the Clydesdale breed, **sabino** is a very common pattern and frequently is very roan or flecked (Figure 7.22). Clydesdale breeders mistakenly refer to the pattern as **roan**, although it is a **sabino** pattern and not **classic roan**. While both **sabino** and **classic roan** patterns occur in the Tennessee Walking Horse, most horses registered as **roan** in this breed are indeed **sabino** and not **classic roan**. The popular foundation sire, "Roan Allen," is an example of a **sabino** registered as a **classic roan**.

The extent of the white patterns on **sabinos** of various background colors somewhat parallels that of white face and leg marks: most extensive on **sorrels**, less so on **chestnuts**, less still on **bays**, and usually minimal on **blacks**.

Accurate identification of minimally marked **sabino** individuals can be difficult and has contributed to confusion about the pattern. Minimally marked individuals lack white patches on the body and have only white **socks** and abundant facial white. Such animals are almost never classified as **sabino**, but are capable of producing **sabino** offspring. This phenomenon is fairly common in American Quarter Horses, Welsh Ponies, and Warmbloods. More extensive levels of white with this pattern are fairly obvious and are not easily misidentified. The higher levels of expression of this pattern overlap with **dominant white**, in which case horses are mostly **white**. Some few horses are indeed solid **white** with pink skin and dark eyes. The hair coat is entirely white except for occasional small dark spots in skin or hair. The relationship between **sabino**, **dominant white**, and **white** is complicated because the phenotypes overlap and they

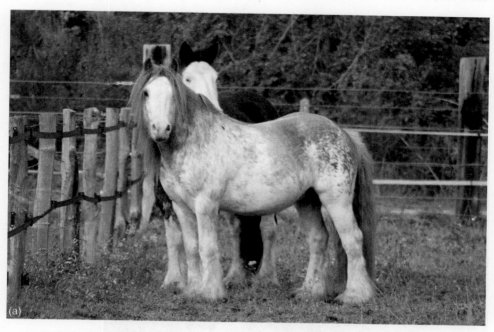

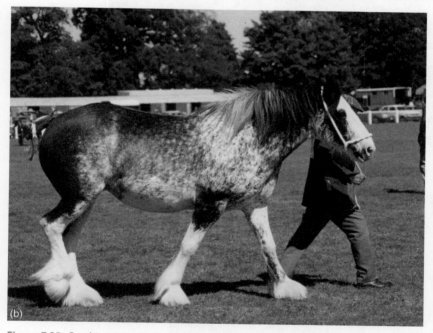

Figure 7.22 Combinations of white patches and speckled roan areas are typical of **sabino** Clydesdale horses, and the pattern is usually called **roan** in that breed. This Gypsy Cob has a pattern similar to the one common in Clydesdales. *Source:* (a) courtesy of Laurence Viala.

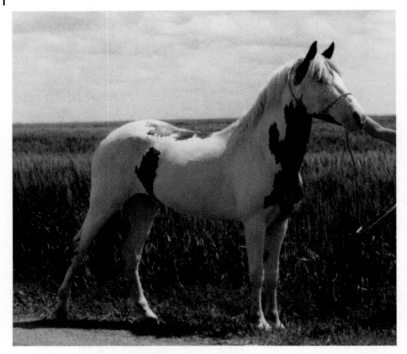

Figure 7.23 Extensively marked **sabino** horses are often the **medicine hat** pattern with colored ears, chest, and flanks. *Source:* courtesy of Marye Ann Thompson.

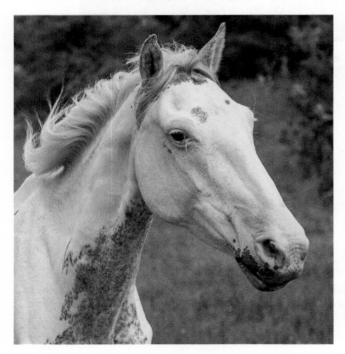

Figure 7.24 Many "nearly white" **sabino** horses retain speckles of color over the ears, lower neck, and chest. *Source:* courtesy of Neil Chapman.

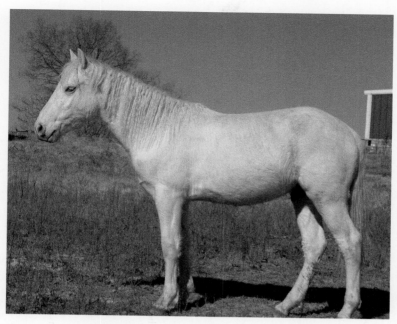

Figure 7.25 The most extreme expression of many of the alleles at the *KIT* locus is a fully **white** horse. *Source:* courtesy of Dyan Westvang.

are also genetically related. They are somewhat easier to understand when discussed as a single group.

White horses used to be favored by some European royal families for use as flashy coach horses, but this use is no longer routine because they show dirt so well. Other than the preference (or avoidance) of the pattern itself, **sabino** carries no other implications in folk wisdom concerning horses.

7.2.3.2.2 Genetic Control

Genetic studies into the control of the **sabino** pattern have revealed a complicated and fascinating situation. Multiple distinct alleles cause the patterns that are grouped together as **sabino** or (**dominant**) **white**. These all occur at the *KIT* locus, which is involved in several white patterns, including **tobiano**, white markings, and **classic roan** (Table 7.1). The variability of color distribution in maximally patterned horses has long suggested that multiple patterns existed, and the genetic findings have now confirmed this. **Sabino** and **white** are therefore most accurately seen as a group of patterns rather than a single one, but the separate types have overlapping phenotypes that defeat any attempt to neatly separate them out from one another. **Sabino** and **white** overlap and are genetically related, so any discussion of them goes best when they are considered together.

One mutation leading to **sabino** horses is called *sabino-1* (*Sb1^{sb1}*). This was the first of the **sabino** patterns to have its genetic cause documented, which accounts for it being number one. The *sabino-1* allele is due to a single base-pair change in intron 16 of the *KIT* locus on equine chromosome 3. The change in the locus by the *sabino-1* mutation makes exon 17 functionally absent from the protein coded by the locus.

Table 7.1 Mutations at or near the *KIT* locus.

Mutation compared with reference genome	Position	Allele	Heterozygous phenotype	Homozygous phenotype	Breeds
Inversion in chromosome		*ToT*	**Tobiano**	**Tobiano with ink spots**	Widespread
Undocumented		*RnRn*	**Classic roan**	**Classic roan**	Widespread
A>T	Intron 16	*Sb1sb1*	Minimal to extensive **sabino**	Extensive **sabino** to **white**	American Paint Quarter Horse Missouri Fox Trotter Shetland Pony Spanish Mustang
G>C	Exon 15	*W1*	**White**	None detected	Franches-Montagnes
C>T	Exon 13	*W2*	**White** (3 horses)	Unknown	Thoroughbred
T>A	Exon 4	*W3*	**White** (2 related horses)	Unknown	Arabian
G>A	Exon 12	*W4*	**White** (3 horses)	unknown	Camarillo White
Deletion of C	Exon 15	*W5*	**Sabino** to **white** especially when with *W20*	Thought to be lethal	Thoroughbred
C>T	Exon 5	*W6*	Flecked all over (1 horse)	Unknown	Thoroughbred
C>G	Intron 2	*W7*	Nearly **white** (1 horse)	Unknown	Thoroughbred
C>T	Intron 15	*W8*	Flecked all over (1 family)	Unknown	Icelandic
C>T	Exon 12	*W9*	**White** (1 family of horses)	Unknown	Holsteiner
Deletion of 4 bases	Exon 7	*W10*	**Sabino** to **white** especially in combination with *W20*	Thought to be lethal	Quarter Horse

Mutation	Location	Allele	Phenotype		Breed
C>T	Intron 19	W11	**White** (1 family)	Unknown	South German Draft
Deletion of 5 bases	Exon 3	W12	Extensive **sabino** (1 horse)	Unknown	Thoroughbred
C>G	Intron 17	W13	**White** (2 horses)	Unknown	Quarter Horse
Deletion of 54 bases	Exon 17	W14	**White** (1 horse)	Unknown	Thoroughbred
A>G	Exon 10	W15	**Sabino** (1 horse)	Unknown	Arabian
T>A	Exon 18	W16	Nearly **white** (1 family)	Unknown	Oldenburger
T>A and A>G	Exon 14	W17	**White**, 1 dark and 1 blue eye (1 horse)	Unknown	Japanese Draft
C>T	Intron 8	W18	Extensively flecked **sabino** (1 horse)	Unknown	Swiss Warmblood
T>C	Exon 8	W19	Intermediate **sabino** (3 related horses)	Unknown	Arabian
C>T	Exon 14	W20	Minimal **sabino**	Minimal **sabino**	Widespread
Deletion of G	Exon 17	W21	Medium **sabino**, with mixed blue/brown eye color (1 horse)	Unknown	Icelandic
Unpublished*[a]		W22			
Unpublished[a]		W23			
Unpublished[a]		W24			

a) The specifics of these have not been published, but their identification was graciously provided by Dr Bianca Haase.

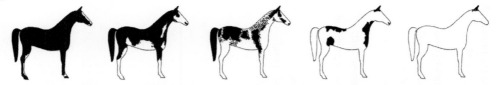

Figure 7.26 Progression of the **sabino-1** pattern. The *sabino-1* allele results in white on the face and legs, and also patches and roan areas on the body.

The progression of white patches caused by *sabino-1* is illustrated in Figure 7.26. The *sabino-1* allele is incompletely dominant and causes homozygotes to be nearly white, while heterozygotes usually have extensive white markings and most often have typical **sabino** body patches with speckling or roaning. This allele has been documented in Tennessee Walking Horses, American Miniature Horses, American Paint Horses, Aztecas, Missouri Fox Trotters, Shetland Ponies, Spanish Mustangs, and others. Notably, it is absent from Arabian and Clydesdale horses that are phenotypically **sabino**. This indicates that multiple genetic mechanisms can cause similar patterns. The absence of *sabino-1* has now been documented for a variety of breeds worldwide despite horses in these breeds having the typical **sabino** phenotype.

In Franches-Montagne horses a single base-pair nonsense mutation in exon 15 at the *KIT* locus causes a truncated protein that reduces the number of melanocytes and thereby produces the white pattern. This mutation has been called *dominant white-1*, or *W1* for short. The phenotype of horses with this allele is almost always entirely **white**, as illustrated in Figure 7.27. The extensively white horses retain pigment on the ears, and sometimes along the topline. This distribution of white and pigmented areas in the extensively white horses is an important common thread for several of these related patterns that are each caused by different mutations at the *KIT* locus. The breeding practices in the Franches-Montagne breed discourage the use of **white** stallions, and as a result all **white** and **sabino** horses so far documented in the breed are heterozygous. Consequently, while the likelihood of this mutation accounting for lethal **dominant white** is certainly present, the specific breeding tests to prove this have not been done.

Investigations into the occurrence of **white** or nearly **white** patterns in several breeds have documented 25 different mutations at the *KIT* locus (including *SB-1* and *W1*), and this number is certain to go up even more (Bianca Haase, personal communication). These additional alleles all cause different levels of **sabino** expression, but most of these result in completely **white** horses. The alleles have been given the *white* name, followed

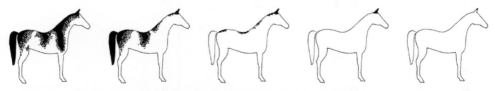

Figure 7.27 Progression of the **dominant white** pattern. The phenotype of horses with *dominant white* is nearly always **white**, with the more heavily pigmented end of the range only rarely seen. It is more extensively white than *sabino-1* horses. **Sabino** and **dominant white** can easily be confused phenotypically. In its strictest sense, *dominant white* is reserved for those *KIT* alleles thought to be lethal to homozygous embryos.

by the number indicating the sequence in which they were discovered. These mutations are all dominant, and each has a typical range of expression that covers a portion of the range of expression from extensive white marks up to an entirely **white** horse. These are a family of mutations all at a single locus, and they have overlapping phenotypes.

In general, each of these *white* mutations is limited to a specific breed, with the exception of *W20* (a single base-pair change in exon 14), which is widespread across many breeds. The *W20* allele is also unusual because the patterns related to it are much less extensive that those caused by the other alleles. The multiple alleles at *KIT* include several different genetic changes, outlined in Table 7.1. Most are single base-pair changes; a few are multiple base deletions. Each of these mutations either changes the amino acid sequence in the protein product or shortens the protein. For example, the allele in the Camarillo White breed (*W4*) is a single base-pair change in exon 12 that results in changing the amino acid sequence of the protein product. A four base-pair deletion in exon 7 is the basis of the *W10* allele in Quarter Horses and results in a protein product with a shortened amino acid chain. The multiple alleles have overlapping phenotypes, so that prediction of a specific allele causing a specific pattern is often impossible when based on physical appearance alone. Genetic testing is now available for some of the documented mutations.

While each of these mutations changes the resulting protein, some of them have more severe consequences. Several of the most extreme of these mutations appear to be lethal to homozygous embryos, and these are the ones that likely cause the heterozygous phenotypes toward the more extensively white end of the range. The homozygous embryos are lost early in gestation, in contrast to the **lethal white** foals caused by the *frame* allele that are born fully formed but die soon after birth. The homozygous *dominant white* embryos are lost so early that they are never noticed.

The most extreme alleles within this group, therefore, fit the definition of *dominant white*, with **white** heterozygotes and no homozygotes produced. The less extreme mutations, such as *sabino-1*, cause less extensive white regions in heterozygotes, while homozygotes are more extensively white and also are fully viable. Even though the actions of these *KIT* alleles vary greatly, they are all thought to reduce *KIT* signaling, which leads to a reduction in the number of melanocytes during development.

Relationships between the alleles can be complicated. The *W20* allele is found in multiple breeds, and by itself has a fairly minimal effect on the phenotype. It causes low levels of white markings easily confused with the common white marks in many breeds. This is true even when the allele is homozygous. When combined with other alleles at this locus, the horses are nearly completely **white**. This situation is called "compound heterozygous" due to the horse having two different mutated alleles. An example would be a *W20* allele on one chromosome 3 and a *W5* allele on the other. The *W20* allele can therefore be thought of as a modifier allele instead of a *dominant white* allele on its own merits.

Clydesdales, some Gypsy horses, some Arabians, and some American Paint Horses have a pattern of **sabino** inheritance that is more consistent with a polygenic mode than a single allele. The resulting patterns are easily confusable with **sabino** horses caused by *sabino-1* or *dominant white* alleles and are illustrated in Figure 7.28. In some families, horses produce obviously patterned **sabino** foals roughly in proportion to their own degree of whiteness. This is consistent with a polygenic mode of inheritance, and the lack of the *sabino-1* allele in these breeds points to a potentially independent genetic

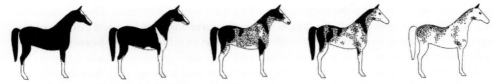

Figure 7.28 Progression of the polygenic **sabino** pattern. The phenotype of polygenic **sabino** is very similar to that caused by *sabino-1*.

mechanism leading to the **sabinos** in these breeds. In these breeds the interaction of extent of white on **sabino** horses with base color tends to follow the same trend as for **white marks: chestnut** horses are whitest, followed by **bay** horses, with **black** horses being least white.

Some few instances of **lethal white** foals have occurred from the mating of two **sabinos**, although in other instances **white** foals produced by such matings have been viable. The **lethal white** foals produced by **sabino** horses are most likely due to the **sabino** parents also having the **frame** pattern, but being classified as lacking it due to the compound pattern (**frame** plus **sabino**) more closely resembling **sabino** than **frame**. Genetic testing for the *frame* allele could quickly sort out the issue. Nomenclature gets to be a headache at this point, because **lethal white** is usually reserved for foals homozygous for the *frame* allele. Some *dominant white* homozygotes, likewise, are lethal, but in this case the loss is of early embryos, so these foals are never born to be noticed or counted.

Some very obviously and loudly marked **sabino** horses have very plainly marked parents. These obviously patterned horses then go on to reliably transmit the pattern and are something of an enigma because they can be accounted for neither by the polygenic hypothesis nor by the single dominant alleles. Some few of them have new mutations at *KIT*, but not all do. They occur frequently enough that it is likely that a specific mechanism is capable of masking the expression of **sabino** in some horses. This suppression is likely genetic, although the details are uncertain. A suggestion of simple single-gene suppression has been proposed, although the extensive data necessary to document such a mechanism have not been reported. Some such horses have minimally marked **black** or **bay** parents, while they themselves are more loudly marked **sorrel sabino**. In some of these cases the minimal marking of the **sabino** pattern on the **bay** or **black** parents has been missed, only to become more obvious on the **chestnut** or **sorrel** offspring. This is subtly different than true suppression of the pattern.

The extent of expression of the **sabino** pattern in some breeds seems to be under genetic control. This is most evident in breeds or families with the **sabino** that is polygenic in origin. Breeders trying to minimize white patches on the body while retaining flashy high white stockings and blazes can take advantage of the genetic control over the extent of the pattern. Breeds noted for this are the Clydesdale and Welsh Pony, but a similar tendency is present in at least portions of other breeds, such as the Arabian. In these breeds it is wise to mate horses with extensive white to those with at least one dark foot in an effort to control the amount of white on the legs and body. This strategy tends to produce horses with the desired white marks but without white body patches.

In contrast, if the goal is to produce white patterned foals (such as in the Paint breed), then using very extensively white **sabinos** mated to solid-colored horses will usually accomplish a high percentage of the desired obviously patterned foals. The few **sabino** horses that are entirely white, or nearly so, tend to transmit the pattern to their foals more reliably than do **sabino** horses that are more conservatively marked. Using **sabinos** with either *sabino-1* or the *dominant white* alleles can also be useful if white patches are the goal of the breeding program, although the *dominant white* alleles are likely to produce a large proportion of entirely **white** foals.

The documentation of multiple genetic controls for the **sabino** pattern points to the fact that the **sabino** classification does indeed include a handful of distinct patterns. In that sense, **sabino** is now serving as a catchall designation for distinct genetic mechanisms. The evidence for this is mostly genetic, but also has some subtle phenotypic aspects as well. The more extensively white horses within the **sabino** classification do not all converge on a single pattern, but instead vary from all **white** to patched, to flecked, speckled, or roan. Many are nearly **white** but retain pigmented ears, and occasionally spots along the topline. These differences in maximal patterns may well be related to different alleles causing each distinct manifestation.

The **paint** patterns other than sabino all exhibit the trend that the whitest individuals converge on a consistent array of colored patches that is reasonably repeatable for all horses with the same pattern. In many **sabino** horses the convergence is on the **medicine hat** pattern. In others, the horses are simply speckled all over. In yet others, areas of color remain dorsally, but the pigmented areas on chest and flank, typical of **medicine hat**, are missing. These visual characteristics have long suggested that the **sabino** classification included several different genetically distinct patterns. The DNA evidence is now supporting this hypothesis. The problem remains that in the middle portion of the range of expression the overlap of phenotypes is great, so that complete separation of the genetic mechanisms by phenotypic evaluation is likely to remain elusive.

White occurs as a distinct and separate pattern in several horse breeds, and most of these are related to the *KIT* mutations. Many of the other distinct white patterns can occasionally produce horses that are white enough to be confused with truly **white** horses, and these include **grey**, some **medicine hat** and **war bonnet paints**, sabinos, and **splashed whites**, as well as the **few-spot leopard complex** pattern (discussed in Chapter 8), as well as horses with combinations of these patterns. All of these **white** horses are exceptions to the rule that the base color is usually evident on all horses. For these horses it is only possible to note their whiteness.

White as a distinct pattern occurs in a few breeds, such as the Tennessee Walking Horse, American Albino (although **white** horses are not albinos because they have dark eyes instead of pink eyes), and also rarely in the Thoroughbred, Arabian, and many other breeds. Most of these are related to the *KIT* locus alleles discussed earlier, although a few families of **white** Thoroughbreds have proven negative for *KIT* locus mutations, so there may be other sites at which mutations code for completely white coats.

7.2.3.3   Splashed White

7.2.3.3.1 *Definition and Classification*
Another pattern usually lumped in with **overo** is called **splashed white** by Europeans. The progression of white areas on **splashed white** horses is illustrated in Figure 7.29. Horses with this pattern usually have white legs, and the body is white ventrally. The head is extensively, and most often completely, white. The edges between colored

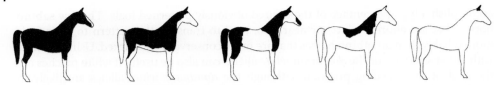

Figure 7.29 Progression of the **splashed white** pattern. **Splashed white** horses can be confused with the less roan variants of **sabino**, but also with **frame** horses when those have **white marks** on the legs. One useful key to distinguishing these is the tendency for **splashed white** horses to have belly white, as well as the more vertical arrangement and clean sharp edges to the white areas on **splashed white** horses.

and white areas are usually very crisp, similar to the edges of the **tobiano** pattern. Blue eyes are the rule and accompany moderate to extensive levels of expression of white areas. This pattern is much more rare in North America than the **frame** and **sabino** patterns.

The minimal **splashed white** pattern is a solid-colored horse with facial white markings that are distinctive both by shape and location. The muzzle usually has a teardrop shaped **snip**, while the **star** is above the level of the eyes and has a rounded upper edge, making it look like a hot-air balloon. Leg white may be minimal but is usually present and greater on the front legs than the hind legs. The eyes may be **blue** or partially blue with blue "chips" in the lower half of the iris.

At moderate levels of expression horses are obviously patterned, and usually have a **blaze** that is broader on the lower aspect than on the top aspect. The top of the **blaze** is usually high and round, often narrowing halfway down the face. Most of the legs have white markings, and eyes are usually **blue** or partially **blue** (Figures 7.30, 7.31, and 7.32).

At more extensive levels of expression, the head and legs are generally white, and white extends up the belly onto the body. The most usual pattern resembles an "inverted **tobiano**." It is common for **splashed white** horses to have a colored upper lip, much like the common moustache marking in **frame** horses. The maximal **splashed white** pattern is occasionally all **white**, but usually has residual dark areas on ears or topline.

Splashed white has a somewhat restricted range and occurs in only a few breeds, such as Welsh Pony, Finnish Draft Horse, Icelandic Horse, and Paint Horse. It can occur as a very rare surprise in a number of other, generally solid-colored breeds, including the Thoroughbred and Morgan. It also occurs in the Appaloosa as a heritage from the influence of a few founders of the breed that had this pattern. **Splashed white** can be confused easily with minimally roaned or minimally speckled **sabinos**. In North America most horses that appear to be **splashed white** are more likely to be cleanly marked **sabinos**, but lacking the roaning and speckling that usually accompanies common manifestations of **sabino**. Differences between **splashed white** and **sabino** horses can be subtle, and the result is that some horses are nearly impossible to identify accurately unless parents or progeny are inspected for additional evidence as to which pattern is present.

7.2.3.3.2 *Genetic Control*

Splashed white is historically rare, although it is experiencing an increasing incidence in the Paint breed in North America due to selection in favor of it. Early studies in some European populations, including the Welsh Pony and the Finnish Draft Horse, led to the

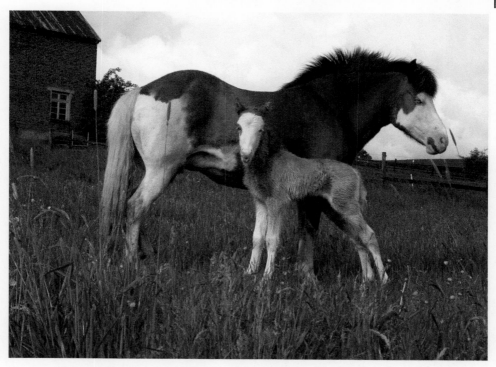

Figure 7.30 **Splashed white** horses generally have crisp white markings on the head, legs, and lower body. *Source:* courtesy of Henriette Smit-Ariens.

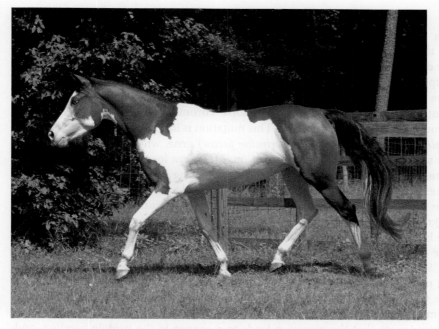

Figure 7.31 The middle range of **splashed white** expression usually leaves pigment on the dorsal portions of the body, neck, and the ears. *Source:* courtesy of Laura Hornick Behning.

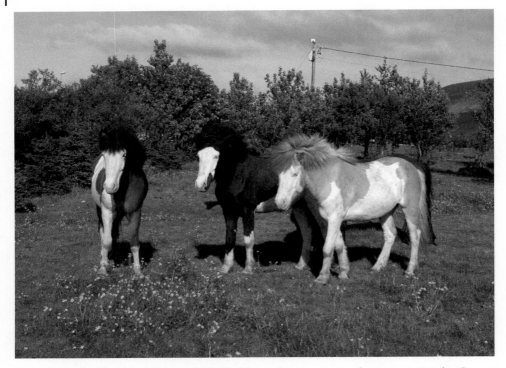

Figure 7.32 As with other patterns, **splashed white** can be superimposed over any coat color. *Source:* courtesy of Henriette Smit-Ariens.

hypothesis that it was a recessive pattern. Later investigations into **overo** patterns suggested that the **splashed white** pattern is actually due to a dominant allele (Spl^S). Molecular data have proven that the situation with **splashed white** is more complicated, with multiple mutations at different loci able to cause the phenotypes that are so similar as to all be classed together as **splashed white** (Table 7.2).

One mutation is $MITF^{prom1}$ located on horse chromosome 16. This allele occurs widely throughout several horse breeds. This mutation is in the promoter portion of the *MITF* (*melanogenesis associated transcription factor*) gene, which is the region in the DNA that signals for the gene to be turned on. *MITF* is a locus also implicated in the usual white marks of horses, and is involved in regulating the number and function of melanocytes. The mutation is an insertion of 11 nucleotides that replaces a single thymine in the normal genetic code. The presence of this mutation in many different breeds (Quarter Horse, Thoroughbred, American Paint Horse, Shetland Pony, and Miniature Horse) suggests that it is an old mutation. Horses homozygous for this allele have more extensive white than those heterozygous for the allele. This is designated "*SW1*" or "*Splashed White 1*." Many homozygotes for this allele have been documented, indicating no tendency for lethality.

In some Quarter Horse families the **splashed white** pattern is due to a single base missense mutation in *paired box 3* (*PAX3*) (*PAX3:c.209G>A*). This is symbolized as $PAX3^{C70Y}$ to denote that the mutation leads to a change in the protein product, and

Table 7.2 Mutations associated with **splashed white** and **macchiato** patterns.

Mutation	Position	Allele	Action	Breeds
Insertion of 11 bases	Promoter region	MITFprom1 (or *SW1*)	Heterozygotes darker than homozygotes	Quarter Horse Thoroughbred American Paint Shetland Pony Miniature Horse
Small deletion	Exon 5	MITF^{C280fs*20} (or *SW3*)	Likely lethal in homozygotes	Quarter Horse American Paint
A>G	Exon 6	MITF^{N31S}	Macchiato	Franches-Montagne (1 horse)
G>A	Exon 2	PAX3^{C70Y} (or *SW2*)	Likely lethal to homozygotes	Quarter Horse American Paint
C>G	Exon 2	PAX3:c.95C>G (or *SW4*)	Contributes to **leopard complex** expression	Appaloosa

that this change occurs specifically at the 70th amino acid in the chain. This mutation likely arose in a mare born in 1987, and its presence seems limited to Quarter Horses. This is a missense mutation that affects the amino acid sequence in the protein product. *PAX3* is involved in melanocyte proliferation early in embryonic development. Mutations in this gene are thought to alter protein function and to reduce the number of melanocytes, leading to white patches. In common use this is designated the "*splashed white 2*" or "*SW2*" allele. No homozygotes for this allele have been documented, and comparative mouse data suggest that homozygous embryos would not be viable but would be lost as embryos.

The phenotypes of these two alleles are similar, and horses that bear both mutations are generally more extensively white than those with only one or the other. Horses bearing a mutation at both genes appear to have additional consequences, and at least one horse homozygous for *MITF^prom1* and heterozygous for *PAX3l^{C70Y}* was deaf.

A third allele, "*splashed white 3*" or "*SW3*," is *MITF^{C280fs*20}*, which is due to a small deletion in exon 5 that causes the protein to be truncated early. This essentially inactivates the *MITF* protein product. This allele is likely lethal to homozygotes. One completely white horse was a compound heterozygote for *MITF^{C280fs*20}* and *MITF^prom1*.

A fourth allele has only been noted in the Appaloosa breed (*SW4*). This is a single base change in *PAX3* (name *PAX3:c.95C>G*) that alters the amino acid sequence in the protein. This mutation has been found in one family of horses with **leopard complex** patterns and is believed to contribute to the broad **blazes** observed in this family (see Chapter 8 for more details on this pattern).

Many **splashed white** horses are deaf. Also, many have normal hearing. Some breeders contend that the **splashed white** horses with white around the eyes are more likely to be deaf than those with color around the eyes. The details of the relationship of deafness to the **splashed white** pattern are not known with certainty, although breeders and owners should be aware of the potential for these horses to be deaf. Deaf horses can become useful and reliable mounts, but training and management procedures obviously must rely on something other than audible cues.

7.2.3.4 Manchado

A relatively rare and obscure pattern of white has appeared in Argentina in several breeds such as Arabian, Criollo, Thoroughbred, and Hackney Horse. These horses are remarkable for their similarity of pattern, and also for their rarity.

The rarity of **manchado** makes generalizations difficult, but the range of pattern that has been described is illustrated in Figure 7.33. Most **manchado** horses have large crisp white areas, but also have a host of smaller very round or smoothly contoured spots of pigment in the white areas. These are unlike any other pattern, although a casual glance could leave the observer convinced that these were **leopard complex** patterns. They are not, and the character of the pattern is very different from the patterns of the **leopard complex**, not least because it lacks the symmetry expected of those patterns.

Minimally patterned **manchado** horses tend to have white on the top of the neck, involving the mane (Figure 7.34). From there the white tends to encroach on the neck and body, usually leaving the head and legs colored. The pattern appears to progress from top to bottom, so that the bottom of the neck and the belly tend to be colored. The interplay of larger and smaller pigmented spots in the white areas makes this a very distinctive pattern (Figure 7.35).

The genetics of this pattern have not been investigated. It is unusual because it has appeared repeatedly in Argentina and does not appear to occur very often elsewhere. This, however, may be a consequence of a widespread Argentine fascination with horse color and its classification. In Argentina, any peculiar or new phenomenon of horse color tends to be noticed and discussed more widely than would similar occurrences in most other countries. The repeatability of the **manchado** pattern does suggest a genetic cause, though the range of breeds in which it occurs is awkward as they are not related nor are they commonly crossed one with the other to produce breeding stock (Thoroughbred, Criollo, Polo Pony, Arabian, Hackney). Paintings of Hackney horses from the 1800s suggest that the pattern has been around at least since then, if only rarely. The sporadic occurrence of **manchado** suggests that it might be due to a recessive mechanism, and, moreover, that the allele is rare.

7.2.3.5 Overo Crop-Out Horses

A major impediment that undermines the recognition that the **frame**, **sabino**, and **splashed white** patterns arise from dominant alleles (or a polygenic origin for some **sabinos**) is that these patterns frequently pop up in foals from parents that do not have

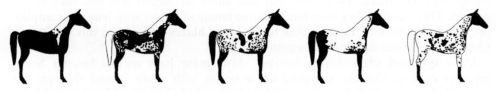

Figure 7.33 Progression of the **manchado** pattern. **Manchado** horses are very rare, and close inspection usually reveals their unique combination of dark legs and head, and body white that starts dorsally and contains small colored areas.

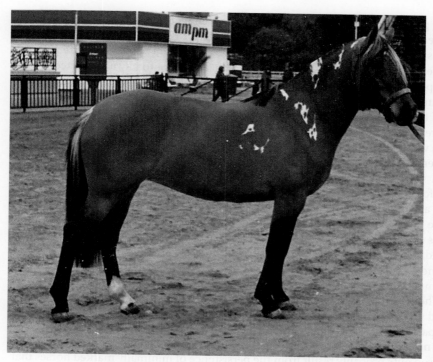

Figure 7.34 **Manchado** has the unusual characteristics of being clean and crisp, but with smaller pigmented spots inside white patches. *Source:* courtesy of Luis Flores.

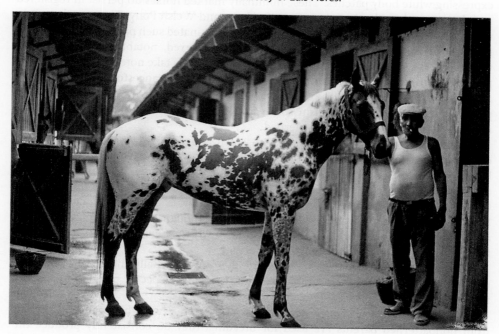

Figure 7.35 More extensively marked **manchado** horses are usually quite uniquely marked. *Source:* courtesy of Luis Flores.

white body patches. Patterned foals from nonpatterned matings are called "crop outs" by several breed associations, such as the American Quarter Horse and the American Paint Horse. This phenomenon occurs with the **frame**, **sabino**, and **splashed white** patterns frequently enough that such surprising patterned foals are not totally unexpected. While it does happen, it is much more rare for an unexpected **tobiano** foal to occur than it is for one with an **overo** pattern.

Some of these unexpected crop-out horses are possibly due to new mutations in the loci that are already documented. This is most likely for the notoriously numerous *KIT* mutations, which include both the **sabino** and **dominant white** patterns, but mutations in other genes have also been found. A few instances have been proven to be novel mutations. One example is *dominant white 12* (*W12*) (Table 7.1) in which a white patterned foal was produced from two minimally marked Thoroughbred parents. This horse had a novel mutation that was not detected in either parent, and the mutation likely arose during egg or sperm formation. Another example occurred in a Franches-Montagnes colt from two **bay** parents with no white pattern. The colt had white patches on the head, legs, and body. The pigmented areas were also diluted. The combination of dilution and white pattern led to the distinctive name **macchiato** for this color. The causative mutation is in *MITF* gene that also causes both *splashed white 1* and *splashed white 3*. The mutation in this case is missense mutation that leads to a change in the amino acid sequence in the protein, denoted as $MITF^{N31S}$. This change was not present in either parent. This colt was deaf, and it had low progressive sperm motility and, therefore, no fertility.

Other crop outs probably result from the persistence of minimally marked horses that have the genetic machinery for one of the white patterns, but are not themselves expressing white body patches. These minimally marked horses do persist in registered populations such as the American Quarter Horse and Welsh Pony. These are breeds in which white body patches would have historically eliminated such patterned horses from registration. Some of these rules have now been relaxed, notably in the American Quarter Horse. When white body patches appear, breeders take note, at which point the patterns seem to have come from nowhere. A closer look at ancestors, though, usually reveals an extensive leg or head mark that betrays the presence of one of these white pattern alleles. By this mechanism some crop outs are arising from parents that are misidentified as genetically nonpatterned.

An additional mechanism can arise in which some horses do indeed betray no evidence of a white pattern allele and yet can be proven to have such alleles either by progeny testing (for most patterns) or by direct DNA evidence (the **frame**, **sabino-1**, and **dominant white** patterns). This is a type of suppression that happens rarely with all the patterns, but occurs consistently enough that it is a verifiable phenomenon. Suppression is probably genetically conditioned, although the details of the genetic action are undocumented. Likewise, it is unknown whether such suppression is general for all patterns or specific for only one at a time.

Suppression of white patterns can result in some unusually marked horses (Figures 7.36 and 7.37), and these can be difficult to assign to specific patterns due to the masking of some of the areas expected to be white.

Regardless of the mechanism allowing for crop outs, when white patterned horses from nonpatterned parents are used for breeding, they do consistently produce the patterns in the same manner as would be expected from dominant alleles. Earlier work

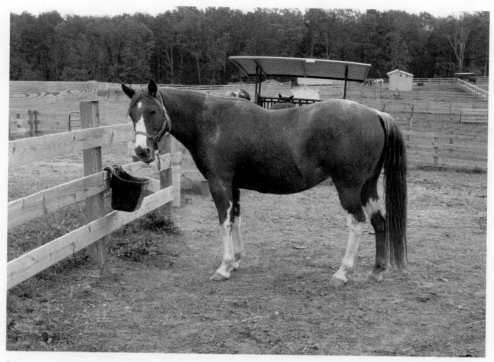

Figure 7.36 This **sabino** mare shows evidence of a mechanism to suppress **sabino** expression. She has pigmented areas superimposed over what should have been white on the face, as well as on the right rear leg.

noted their occurrence from nonpatterned parents and assumed that the patterns were recessive. However, if the crop-out patterned horses are used for breeding, they generally perform as though the patterns are indeed dominant.

7.2.4 Combination Paint Patterns

Some horses have patterns that result from various combinations of two or more of the **paint** patterns (Figures 7.38, 7.39, and 7.40). These horses further confuse the nomenclature issue because some of them are difficult to categorize. This is especially true when breeders mate the various types together to produce loudly patterned offspring. All combinations can exist, and it is not always possible to be certain which components are present on an extensively white horse. Combinations are additive, so that the white areas of each pattern are added together with the result that horses with multiple patterns generally have more extensive white than do horses with only a single pattern. The combination of **tobiano** with any of the **overo** patterns is usually called **tovero**, especially in the Paint horse breed.

A few combination paint patterns have a pronounced tendency to produce horses that are entirely white or nearly so. Some of these very white patterns have special names. One of these is the **medicine hat paint**, which is largely white but has pigmented areas

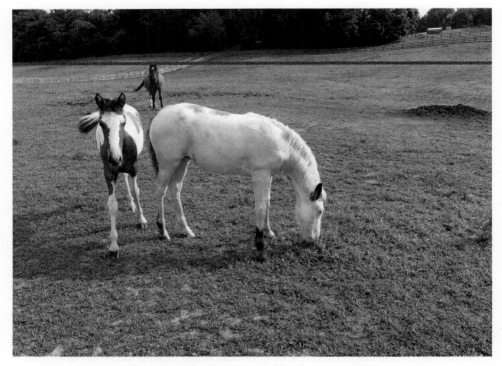

Figure 7.37 This **sabino medicine hat** foal has an unusual dark lower front leg, consistent with some process that can mask white pattern.

over the ears and perhaps eyes, chest, flank, and base of the tail. These horses were held to be magical or sacred by some Native American plains tribes. The Lakota and Comanche called these **brown-eared** horses (or **black-eared**, or **yellow-eared**, whichever was appropriate). **Medicine hat paints** can result from very white **sabinos**, **frame** and **tobiano** combinations, **sabino** and **frame** combinations, or **sabino/tobiano** combinations. Horses that exhibit even more white than **medicine hats** retain color only on the ears and have minor pigmented body spots. These are called **war bonnet paints** (or also **brown-eared** horses by the Lakota and Comanche) and are usually pale **sabinos** or combinations of the various patterns.

Combination **paints** are especially common in breeds such as the Paint, Pinto, and Gypsy breeds, where these patterns are avidly sought after. In any such breed or population many individual horses have two or three of these patterns. Such combination horses can be useful in a breeding program because they produce a preponderance of white patterned offspring, even following mating to solid-colored horses. The foals have white patches consistent with the various types of patterns present in the composite parents. In other breeds, such as the Spanish Mustang, where **paint** patterns occur in a minority of horses, such combinations are more rare. These patterns then tend to occur only as one pattern on a horse unless an individual breeder is selecting in favor of white patterns of various types.

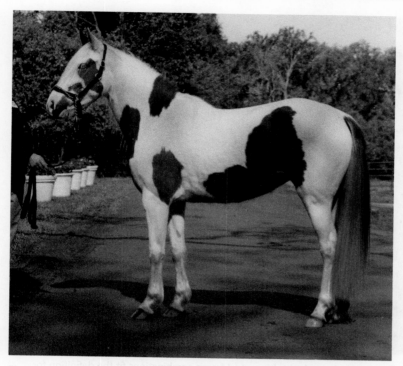

Figure 7.38 Combinations of **tobiano** with **frame** superimpose both white patterns so that the final pattern does not overlap with any single pattern but instead reflects the presence of both.

Homozygotes of the various alleles are especially useful if production of patterned foals is the goal. Homozygotes appear to be limited to the **tobiano, sabino-1, W20** and perhaps some of the **splashed white** patterns. Very white **sabinos** from the polygenic mechanism reproduce nearly as reliably as would a homozygous horse, although these still tend to produce the occasional unpatterned foal. The **frame** pattern cannot exist in the homozygous state, because such foals are **lethal white**. In addition, those alleles located at or near the *KIT* locus (*tobiano, roan, sabino-1,* and *dominant white*) can occur as composites of any two of these alleles, but due to linkage the production results will be nearly the same as for a homozygous horse because the alleles do not segregate independently.

Three of the **paint** patterns are due to dominant alleles (*tobiano, frame, splashed white*), a fourth (**sabino**) is variably dominant or polygenic, and the fifth (**manchado**) is rare and its mode of transmission is undocumented. Owing to the dominance of most of the patterns, a horse heterozygous for any one of the patterns would generally be expected to produce about 50% patterned offspring following mating to nonpatterned horses. A horse with two different pattern alleles at unlinked loci would produce about 75% offspring with white patches. If these loci were linked closely together, or if they were truly compound heterozygotes with two mutant alleles at the same locus, then breeding these individuals results in 100% foals with white patches. Compound heterozygote horses are very interesting and are useful in breeding programs focused

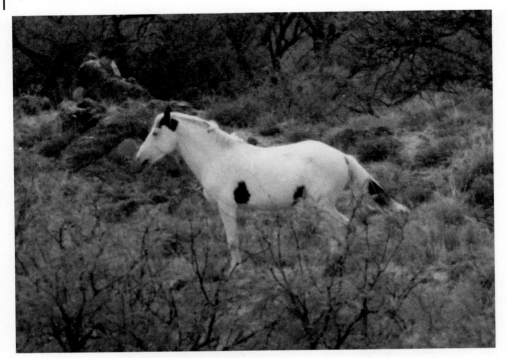

Figure 7.39 The more extensively marked **tobiano** and **frame** combinations fit the definition for **medicine hat** paints, but have clean and crisp markings in contrast to the usual speckled or roan areas of extensively marked **sabino** horses.

upon producing foals with white patches from nonpatterned mates. Most will be nearly white as the patterns are superimposed additively.

Many breeders who desire foals with **paint** patterns tend to favor outcrosses to nonpatterned horses; as a result, they mate patterned individuals to solid-colored horses. Many breeders tend to use solid-colored horses with extensive white marks in their breeding programs. The thinking behind this strategy is that horses with white marks are more likely to throw patterned offspring than are unmarked solid horses. This approach probably has some merit when considering **sabino** and **splashed white** patterns, because some horses express the alleles minimally as high white stockings and a lot of facial white. Using this same approach with **tobiano** or **frame** patterns probably is not warranted because these occur as single alleles independent of the polygenic white marks, and horses with these two alleles are less easily confused with horses having only white marks. In support of this strategy, though, is the diminished likelihood of an extensively marked horse having modifying alleles that might suppress white patterns.

Paint patterns are highly valued by owners of some breeds and by some entire cultures. Many Native American tribes (at least those in North America) selectively bred their horses for these patterns. This was related in some instances to religious belief, as exemplified by **medicine hat** and **war bonnet** color phases. Gypsies also have an affinity for patterned horses used to pull their wagons. The drum horses of some British

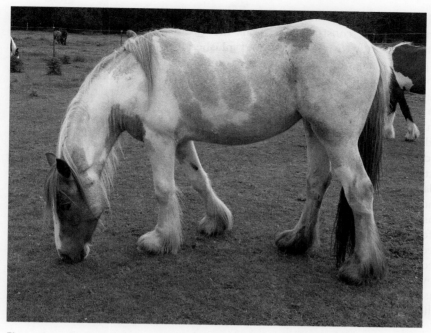

Figure 7.40 This horse has a combination of **tobiano**, **sabino**, and **classic roan**, leading to a final appearance that depends on all three patterns. *Source:* courtesy of Debbi Jenson.

regiments are **tobiano** horses. These are essentially **tobiano** Shire horses, the result of many generations of mating these **tobianos** back to registered Shire horses.

Frontier days' North American cultures that were based on Anglo-Saxon influences usually disparaged horses with **paint** patterns, perhaps because they were so characteristic of the herds belonging to Native Americans. These patterns are now becoming less controversial and even seem to be countenanced in some breeds in which they were disparaged in the past, such as the Arabian, Saddlebred, and Tennessee Walking Horse. While once very common in breeds of Iberian ancestry, they are now very rare in most of these, as well as in most of their descendants.

7.2.5 Paint Summary

The five paint patterns have a very confusing nomenclature, and include **tobiano**, **frame**, **sabino** (which itself includes **sabino-1**, **white**, **dominant white**, and polygenic **sabino**), **splashed white**, and **manchado**. An important detail is that these patterns are indeed genetically separate, and so they should each be recognized as distinct patterns. A good way to think of these is to remember that **tobianos** are dripped with white, **frame** horses have white sides, **sabinos** are flecked with white (one is tempted to say "splashed with white", but that only compounds the nomenclature problem), as if they trotted through a shallow pool of white paint, **splashed whites** are dipped in white as if lowered feet first into a vat of white paint, and **manchado** horses have dark feet, dorsal white, and small round spots in the white areas (and most people will never see one of these anyway!).

A very close examination of large numbers of "**overo**" horses reveals some families with patterns that have consistent variations that are distinct from the usual three patterns within the group (**frame**, **sabino**, and **splashed white**). This suggests that a few more such patterns may yet be undocumented and that probably these are genetically separate from the others. These would generally be lumped in the **sabino** classification because they are generally flecked and roaned. Most of these are flecked to some extent, but tend to lack the dark chest, ears, flank, and tail base patches that are retained by horses with extensive expressions of the **sabino** pattern.

Folk wisdom tends to hold fairly consistently that the various **paint** patterns interact somewhat differently with different background colors. It is generally believed that it is easier to attain obvious patterns on a **chestnut**-based background than it is on a **bay**-based or **black**-based background. This has been shown to be true with the usual **white marks** of horses and by inference might likewise be true of the specific **sabino** pattern that is caused by the multifactorial inheritance pattern. For the other patterns, no tendency for **chestnut**-based colors to be more obviously marked has ever been documented. An argument for a **chestnut**-based advantage (when white patches are the goal) could be made in some families for patterns in which linkage plays a role. However, even in those situations the linkage phase can be disrupted frequently enough that the passage of the patterns along with specific background colors might be true of some families, while in other families the opposite color relationships would hold true.

8

Patterns with Symmetric White Patches: The Leopard Complex

Rebecca Bellone, Sheila Archer, and D. Phillip Sponenberg

8.1 Leopard Complex

8.1.1 Definition and Classification

The **leopard complex** of white patterns on horses tends to be remarkably symmetric. These patterns are breed characteristics for two specific breeds in North America: Appaloosa and Pony of the Americas. In addition, the patterns regularly occur in a wide number of international breeds, including Noriker, Tannu Tuva Pony, and Spanish Mustang. In most of those breeds the patterns occur alongside nonpatterned horses, although at least one, the Knabstrupper, has a strong preference for them. In several other breeds the patterns occur only rarely, and in many breeds they are completely absent. While rare in most breeds, these patterns and their genetic control are a very powerful example of the intricacies of the biology of color and pattern production, and offer many lessons in the basic biology of color in horses.

These patterns are called a "complex" because they are all genetically related, despite the fact that the phenotypes of some of the extreme expressions of the patterns would be difficult to relate to one another by visual inspection alone. This phenomenon makes these patterns distinct from the other patterns of white in horses, and can easily lead to confusion in classifying them together as members of a single group of patterns. The **leopard complex** includes several different basic patterns, but they all share a single genetic basis.

The complex was specifically named after the **leopard** pattern (Figure 8.1), which is the most distinctive of all of the patterns of the complex and is best described as a horse with a white pattern over the entire body with superimposed round or oval pigmented spots. Other patterns of the complex can be very visually distinct from the fully expressed **leopard** pattern. Several of the distinct manifestations have separate names, and to add to the confusion they can each occur separately and can sometimes be seen in various combinations. The fine details are discussed and illustrated later, after a more general discussion of the components of the complex.

Identifying the whole range of the **leopard complex** of patterns is complicated, although the process becomes easier by realizing that all of the patterns involve varying degrees of expression of three main basic components. These three building blocks are all related to the *leopard complex* (Lp^{Lp}) allele: white pattern, Lp^{Lp}-caused roaning, and

Equine Color Genetics, Fourth Edition. D. Phillip Sponenberg and Rebecca Bellone.
© 2017 John Wiley & Sons, Inc. Published 2017 by John Wiley & Sons, Inc.

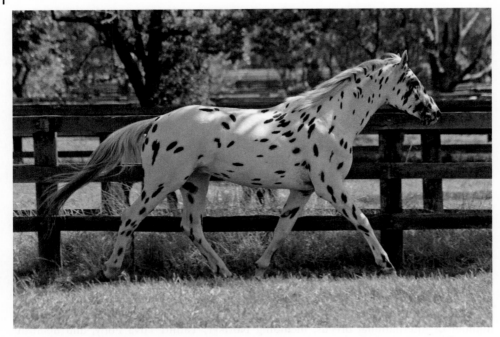

Figure 8.1 The **leopard** pattern, for which the entire group of patterns is named, is essentially a white horse with dark **leopard** spots. *Source:* courtesy of Petra Davidson.

round to oval pigmented spots (known as **leopard spots**). These three components tend to be distinct and reasonably consistent, although the degree of expression of each is highly variable. It is the variation in the expression of these three components that leads to the different extremes of **leopard complex** patterns.

One of the most easily identifiable components of the complex is the obvious distinct white pattern, which is present at birth. In the most minimally marked horses this may well be absent. The least extensive white pattern is symmetric white over the hips, and is usually present at birth. As the level of white increases, the white area expands to cover the body from the rear forward. In the most extensively white patterns a nearly white horse results, usually with residual color in flanks and throatlatch. The usual range of white patterns and **leopard spots** is illustrated in Figure 8.2.

The second component is known as Lp^{Lp}-caused **roaning** or **varnish roaning**. In some cases it is referred to as **snowflake** or **frost**, depending on the final visual aspect of the pattern. Unlike the white pattern component, the **roan** component is not present at birth and develops with age. This aspect is called **varnish roan** to distinguish it from **classic roan** described in Chapter 6. This type of **roaning** affects areas that are pigmented at birth rather than those that are white, and usually does not affect the pigmented **leopard spots** within the white pattern areas. As the degree of **varnish roan** increases over time, it can appear as though the white patterned areas are increasing in size. The extent of the white hairs added by **varnish roan** is variable, so that some horses have minimal roaning while on others this aspect of the pattern is dramatic and obvious. Both the extent and the rate of roaning in the patterns are highly variable. On some

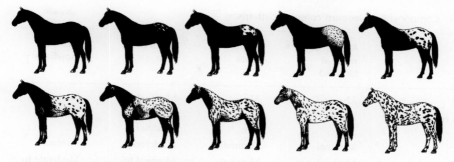

Figure 8.2 The **leopard complex** white pattern continuum showing some of the variability that can occur in horses with the pattern. The minimal pattern involves only the hip region, and then expands to cover nearly the entire horse.

horses the white increases as small patches rather than individual hairs. These are called **snowflakes**, but are part of the same process that increases **roaning** (or white hairs) in these patterns.

The third main component to the patterns is pigmented **leopard spots**, which are derived from the base coat color. The **leopard spots** are usually a single color for each spot, which depends on the base color of the horse. However, many horses with dark base colors show increasing variation in spot color over time. On **sooty** base colors these tend to segregate out into distinct black spots along with tan, red, or yellow spots. The uniformity of color within each individual spot suggests that each one comes from a single melanoblast (melanocyte precursor cell) early in embryonic life. These pigmented spots are superimposed over the white patterned areas. They can also extend into adjacent colored areas, in which case they appear as somewhat hyperpigmented dark spots against a somewhat lighter background color. The number of **leopard spots** that appear on an animal depends on how many copies of the Lp^{Lp} allele the horse inherits. The details are described more fully in Section 8.2.

Each of the three aspects of the **leopard complex** is variable and ranges from minimal to extensive. Table 8.1 outlines the interactions of these three components to produce the array of patterns in the complex that have distinct names. The variations are described in greater detail in the following.

The **leopard complex** has historically been explained as several distinct and independent patterns, and some horses do indeed exhibit only one of these patterns in isolation from the others (see Table 8.1). The patterns, going somewhat from minimal to maximal expression, include **mottled, frost, snowflake, varnish roan, speckled, blanket, snow cap blanket, near leopard, leopard**, and **few spot leopard**. While each of these variants does occur in isolation, it is also common for horses to exhibit combinations of two or more of the basic patterns within the complex. The individual patterns are all part of this complex of patterns and are all related to the same gene, even though some are remarkably distinct from one another visually. For example, the appearance of a horse with the **snowflake** pattern (Figure 8.3) is so different from that of a **leopard** horse (Figure 8.1) that it is difficult to imagine these as springing from the same basic mechanism.

Table 8.1 Components of **leopard complex** patterns.

Pattern	Amount of **white** at birth (%)	**Leopard spots**	Extent of **roan**	Extent of **snowflake**
Mottled	Absent	Absent	Minimal	Minimal
Varnish roan	Absent	Absent or rare	Moderate to maximal	Minimal
Frost	Minimal	Minimal	Moderate	Minimal
Snowflake	Minimal	Minimal	Minimal to moderate	Moderate to maximal
Speckled	Minimal	Minimal	Maximal	Moderate to maximal
White spots over hips	≤10	Present or absent	Moderate	Minimal
Lace blanket	10–20	Present or absent	Moderate	Minimal
Spotted blanket	20–40	Present	Moderate	Variable
White blanket	20–40	Absent	Moderate	Variable
Large spotted blanket	40–60	Present	Moderate	Variable
Large snowcap blanket	40–60	Absent	Moderate	Variable
Near leopard	60–80	Present	Variable	Variable
Near few spot leopard	60–80	Absent	Variable	Variable
Leopard	90–100	Present	Variable	Variable
Few spot leopard	90–100	Absent	Variable	Variable

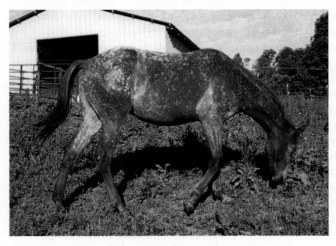

Figure 8.3 The **snowflake** pattern has distinct speckles that appear as small round patches of white on the coat. *Source:* courtesy of Sherry Bryd.

Part of the confusion of the past understanding of the **leopard complex** patterns is the presence of so many different manifestations within a group related by a single genetic cause. Each of the very distinct manifestations within the complex progresses from a minimal to a maximal expression that is reasonably consistent for each individual manifestation, especially when these occur in isolation. This orderly progression of visually distinct manifestations has made it easy to misinterpret this single highly variable complex of patterns as several distinctly different patterns. The actual situation of nested variability within a single group of patterns with a single genetic cause is quite different from the situation with the **paint** patterns, where the extremes of each distinct **paint** pattern tend to converge on a single narrow range of expression that is unique and distinct from the other **paint** patterns as a sort of visual clue to the underlying distinct genetic causing each pattern (Chapter 7, Figure 7.3).

One of the more common expressions of the **leopard complex** is the **blanket** pattern in which white areas occur over the croup and hips of the horse (Figures 8.4, 8.5, and 8.6). These white **blankets** can have crisp clean edges, flecked edges, or roan edges. The crisp solid-colored areas of most horses with **blanket** patterns become **roan** with age, although on some horses this aspect is minimal. Some horses with **blankets** have pigmented **leopard spots** in them (Figure 8.4); others lack these pigmented spots (Figure 8.5). A clean white blanket with few or no spots is called a **snow cap blanket** (Figures 8.5 and 8.6).

When **blankets** are extensive they continue into the **near leopard** and **leopard** patterns (Figures 8.1 and 8.7). Horses with the highest level of white pattern are nearly completely white, and have pigmented **leopard spots** superimposed. These are the "nose

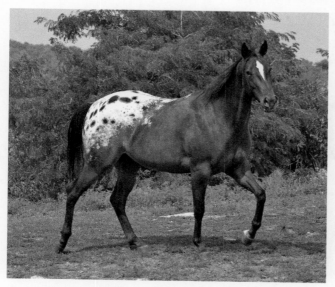

Figure 8.4 This **brown** horse has a **blanket** with **leopard spots**. As is common in horses with the **sooty** overlay, the **leopard spots** are darker than most of the body color. This pattern was present at birth, and no **varnish roan** aspect is yet present, but could develop with increasing age. This **spotted blanket** pattern derives its name from the symmetric character of the white pattern that looks like a white blanket draped over the horse. "**Spotted**" is added to indicate the presence of the dark **leopard spots**. *Source:* courtesy of Elizabeth Estridge.

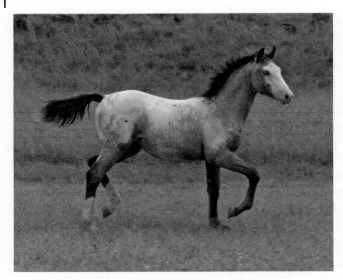

Figure 8.5 As some **blanket** horses develop **varnish roan** the resulting pattern can extend as vertical stripes over the barrel. This is most common in extensive **snow cap blankets** that lack **leopard spots**. The white mark on the face of this horse is unrelated to its **leopard complex** pattern. *Source:* courtesy of Petra Davidson.

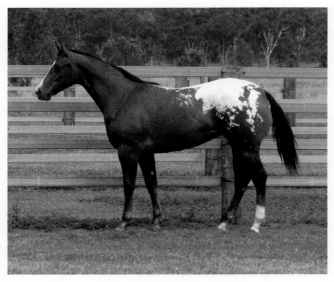

Figure 8.6 **Snow cap blanket** patterns lack the **leopard spots** of **spotted blankets**. While a few small **leopard spots** may be present, the white is generally clean and clear. This horse also has several small **pepper spots** at the edges of the **blanket**, and these should not be confused with **leopard spots**. *Source:* courtesy of Petra Davidson.

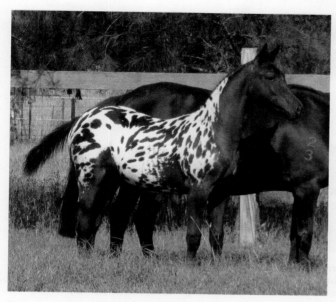

Figure 8.7 The **near leopard** pattern has white over most of the body but retains pigmented areas, usually on the front end as well as the legs and flanks. This pattern has **leopard spots**. Leopard spots on many horses have a distinct pattern in which they appear to flow out of the flank and then over the barrel as well as over the rear. *Source:* courtesy of Petra Davidson.

to toes" **leopards**. At birth, the **leopard spots** are usually the background color of the horse and can be any basic horse color. Most **leopard** horses retain the base coat color on the flanks, behind the elbow, and on some areas of the neck and head. On most horses these areas become roaned as the horse matures. The roaning process generally does not affect the **leopard** spots themselves, but only the residual pigmented areas remaining on the coat. **Leopard spots** on most horses have a distinct orientation that makes them appear to flow out from the flank and then over the rest of the body (Figure 8.7). Horses that are extensively patterned but not nose to toes are classified as **near leopards**. No distinct boundary exists between the different levels of white pattern that have distinct names, so that small **blankets, blankets,** large **blankets, near leopards,** and **leopards** all form a continuum rather than discrete groups cleanly separated from one another. Horses that are greater than 80% white at birth are usually called **leopards**, while those in the range 60–80% are called **near leopards**. Some of these horses have patterns with roan edges, which feather out into the solid-colored areas as a series of vertical roan stripes. This is especially true over the ribcage area.

    Few spot leopards are largely white, but can retain the areas of residual color on flank, neck, and head that often become roan with age (Figure 8.8). **Few spot leopards** are essentially **leopards** without pigmented spots. A few **leopard spots** may occur on these horses, and these are usually located very low on the body or somewhat peripherally on the horse, either on the head or a leg joint. They are very rare over the rump or back.

    On the other end of the spectrum a fairly minimal expression of the **leopard complex** is the **mottled** pattern (Figure 8.9). Horses with this pattern are often referred to as having "characteristics only," because they are born with no coat pattern but have other

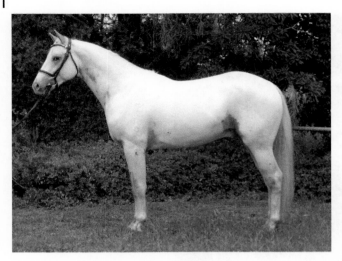

Figure 8.8 Most **few spot leopard** horses do have color remaining around the edges of the horse (legs, throat, head). These areas become roan with age. When the horse is a lighter color, such as **palomino**, these residual dark areas are subtle and can be easily missed. *Source:* courtesy of Petra Davidson.

minimal expressions that involve skin, hooves, and eyes. **Mottling** occurs as small dots on the skin of the anus, genitalia, mouth, and eyelids. On pink skin the dots are pigmented, and on pigmented skin the dots are pink or white. In addition, the sclera of the eye is frequently white as well (Figure 8.9). Striped hooves result from vertical bands of pigment on otherwise unpigmented hooves, and are common on all horses with **leopard complex** patterns (Figure 8.10). The trio of characteristics including mottled

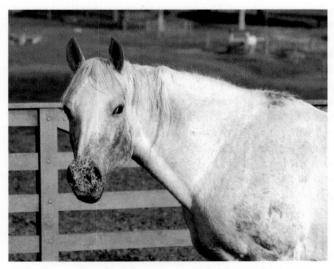

Figure 8.9 The **mottled** pattern is one of the least evident patterns within the **leopard complex**, and horses with minimal expression could be misidentified as lacking the pattern. This horse also has the white sclera around the eye that is typical of **leopard complex** horses. *Source:* courtesy of Petra Davidson.

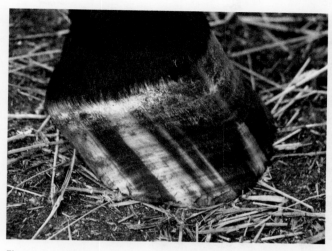

Figure 8.10 Striped hooves are another common characteristic of horses with **leopard complex** patterns. Striped hooves, **mottled** skin, and a white sclera of the eye are the trio of characteristics shared by most horses with the **leopard complex**, even those with minimal expression. *Source: courtesy of Petra Davidson.*

skin, white sclera, and striped hooves occurs on most horses with the **leopard complex**. Some horses within the complex lack one or more of them at birth. Over time they will gradually appear on nearly every horse within this complex of related patterns. This trio of characteristics can also occur on some horses lacking the **leopard complex**, so while they can be useful general indicators of the presence of the **leopard complex**, they should be used cautiously because they can be misleading in some cases as an absolute indicator for the presence of the gene responsible for the **leopard complex**.

The **leopard complex roan** pattern (also called **varnish roaning** as described earlier) is progressive from birth to maturity, and varies considerably in its extent as well as its development with age. It stabilizes at some point, so that most horses remain **varnish roan** and only rarely become completely **white**. The roaning occurs in two basic forms: **frost** and **snowflake**. **Frost** describes roaning that consists of single white hairs scattered over the coat (Figure 8.11). At moderate levels of expression, **frost** horses have roaning over the croup and hips and are not to be confused with the **frosty roan** pattern, which is not related to the **leopard complex**. In contrast, **snowflake** roaning occurs as rounded white patches that most often are between 1 and 3 inches (2–7 cm) in diameter (Figure 8.3). These are scattered fairly randomly over the body, but tend to be more profuse over the foreparts of the horse. They commonly vary in location and size from year to year. **Frosty roan** and **snowflake** horses are occasionally called **buttermilk roans**, which can be confusing because this term is also used for some **sabino** horses.

Frost and **snowflake** roaning often occur together. They may progressively affect so much of the horse that most of the body eventually becomes white or nearly so. When this occurs, unique dark areas called **varnish marks** remain. This pattern is also called **marble** due to its similarity to the pattern on some types of marble stone. **Varnish roan** is best described as a mixture of white and colored hairs, with the areas over bony prominences remaining darker than the rest of the coat (Figure 8.12). These areas

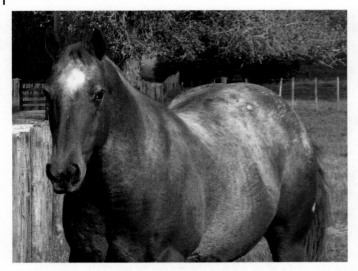

Figure 8.11 The **frost** pattern is a fairly even mixture of white hairs into the base coat color. It is concentrated over the back and hips. *Source:* courtesy of Petra Davidson.

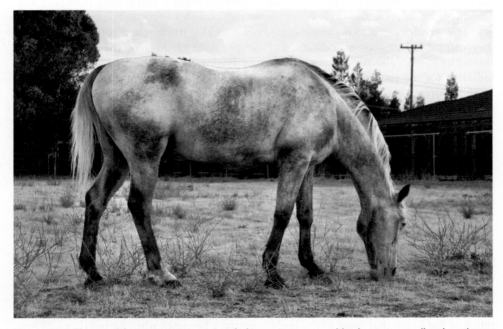

Figure 8.12 The **varnish roan** pattern retains dark areas over several body areas, usually where bone is close to skin on the head, hips, and lower legs, but also usually over the jaw, neck, and upper legs. *Source:* courtesy of Rebecca Bellone.

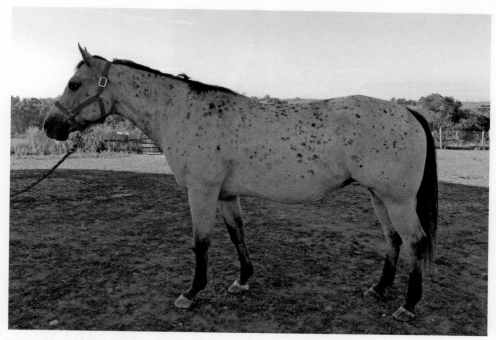

Figure 8.13 **Speckled** horses retain pigment on an otherwise **varnish roan** background. *Source:* courtesy of Elizabeth Estridge.

typically include the facial bones, shoulders, withers, hips, and stifles. These varnish marks in combination with the roaned head help to differentiate this pattern from the **classic roan** pattern that lacks these characteristics. In addition, **varnish roan** horses have the mottled skin and white sclera that are so common among horses with the **leopard complex** of patterns. The dark areas over bony prominences also differentiate **varnish roans** (a **leopard complex** pattern) from **frosty roan** horses (which are not a part of the **leopard complex**), on which the opposite holds true. The dark areas (**varnish marks**) can be seen in combination with many of the other manifestations of the **leopard complex** of patterns.

Horses that develop extensive roan patterns may show numerous small dark splotches on a white field. This pattern is called **speckled** (Figure 8.13). **Speckled** horses could be confused with **fleabitten greys**, except that the colored specks are larger and **speckled** horses also tend to have skin, sclera, and hoof characteristics of the **leopard complex** group. The **speckled** appearance can also develop on areas that were white patterned at birth. This process of repigmentation within white patterned areas can cause a horse that was born with a typical **leopard** pattern to end up resembling a horse born with a **spotted blanket** but that became heavily roaned with age (Figure 8.14).

The **leopard complex** of patterns often varies over the course of an individual horse's life, especially as the **roan** aspect increases with age. Some **leopard complex** horses are born with one of the patterns and then remain relatively unchanged for their lifetime, with the exception of some minimal roaning. Others are born nonpatterned, or with one of the minimal patterns, and then progressively acquire different component patterns of

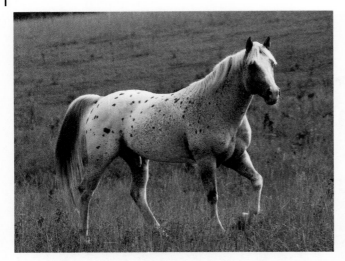

Figure 8.14 This **leopard** horse has a strong expression of repigmentation **specks**, which has changed the overall appearance from the original **leopard** to one much more like a **blanket**. *Source: courtesy of Elizabeth Estridge.*

the complex. This usually occurs with the **snowflake** and **varnish roan** patterns, but occasionally other patterns develop in the same progressive manner. Many horses combine various components of the **leopard complex** for a distinctive individual appearance (Figures 8.15 and 8.16).

Leopard spots can vary in their overall character, as can the white pattern and the type and extent of roaning. **Leopard spots** typically consist of hairs with concentrated pigment, so they tend to appear darker than areas of base coat color that are unassociated

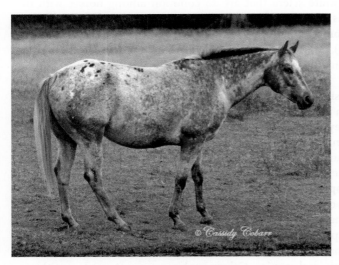

Figure 8.15 Many horses have a combination of components, such as this horse with **frost**, **snowflake**, **varnish roan**, and a small **spotted blanket**. *Source: courtesy of Cassidy Cobarr.*

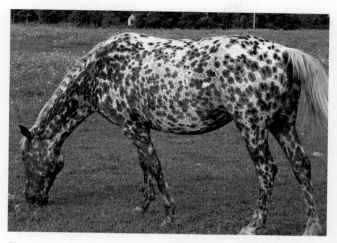

Figure 8.16 The combination of effects on some horses is striking. This **chestnut leopard** mare has numerous repigmentation **specks** in what were originally white areas, and then also distinct **roan** halos around the **leopard spots**. While now only subtle, the **leopard spots** also vary in color. *Source: courtesy of Sheila Kaminski.*

with the white pattern. On a few horses, the **leopard spots** are a different texture than the surrounding coat and can be felt in addition to being seen, especially when the horse is in winter coat (Figure 8.17).

On a few horses the exact location of the **leopard spots** changes somewhat with age, so that they move around and change position on the horse. This occurs only rarely. **Leopard spots** can also change over time in their intensity of color, usually becoming noticeably darker than the base coat color as the horse matures. For example, some of the **leopard spots** on a genotypically **bay** horse may become black (Figure 8.18).

On a few horses the **leopard spots** instead become lighter over a number of years. Spots that gradually become whiter are called **moldy spots** (Figure 8.19).

Leopard spots can be multiple colors on some horses. This is especially dramatic on **sooty** base colors, where combinations of colors are common. On **sooty** base colors, such as **liver chestnut** or **brown**, the black and red components tend to separate out and

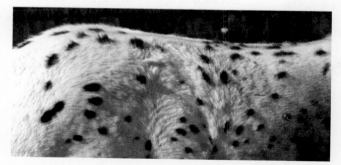

Figure 8.17 **Leopard spots** on some horses have a different texture than the rest of the hair coat. This is most noticeable in winter coat.

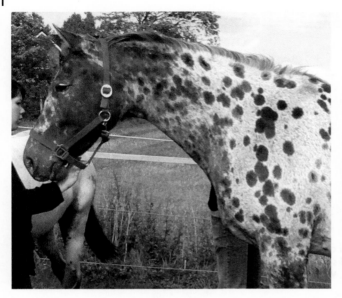

Figure 8.18 Some **leopard spots** on **bay** horses can become black over time.

occur as discrete spots of the different colors (Figure 8.20). A second mechanism leading to multiple colors of **leopard spots** is varying degrees of progressive dilution over time. On **black** horses this can result in a few spots becoming a dilute black or olive color (Figure 8.21). On **chestnut** horses, a few gold spots may appear.

    Leopard spots sometimes appear to be randomly distributed, but more commonly occur in an arrangement of elongated spots that seems to originate in the flank and then flow up and out over the front and rear of the body of the horse (Figures 8.5 and 8.6). On all **leopard complex** patterns it is fairly common for the dark pigmented spots to be rimmed by bands in which the skin is dark and the hair is white. The result is a **halo, ghost**, or **shadow** around the dark areas (Figure 8.22). **Halo spots** tend to develop over time, so that dark spots that originally had crisp edges develop a roan perimeter as the

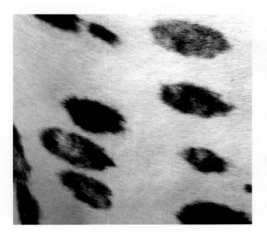

Figure 8.19 Some horses have **leopard spots** that become lighter with age, either becoming more **roan** or just a lighter color through dilution. Those that gradually lighten are called **moldy spots**.

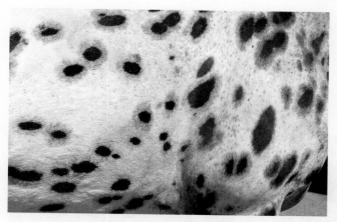

Figure 8.20 It is common for **leopard spots** on horses with a **sooty** color to separate out into distinctly different colors related to either the base coat or the blacker **sooty** characteristic. This horse likely has a **brown** base coat, and the **sooty** black areas as well as the more red **bay** base coat have separated into distinct **leopard spots** of these two colors. *Source:* courtesy of Rebecca Bellone.

horse matures. Some **halo** areas are truly roan rather than white hair over dark skin, but the effect is similar when viewed from a distance. Some people refer to these as **varnish marks**, although they are different in character and appearance from the dark areas over bony prominences of **varnish roans**, which are also called **varnish marks**. Another common name for **leopard spots** with a **halo** is **peacock spots**. On some horses the **halo** begins a short distance away from the edge of the **leopard spots** so that the dark **leopard spot** has a narrow rim of white and then a broader outer rim that is roan.

In addition to **leopard spots**, many horses with blankets also have several small spots where the white pattern meets the background color of the horse. These are called

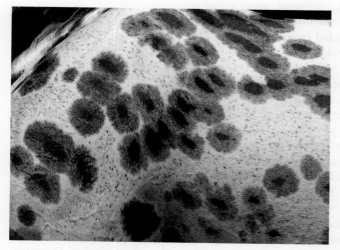

Figure 8.21 This **black leopard** horse has a gold spot, **halo spots**, and **repigmentation spots**. *Source:* courtesy of Petra Davidson.

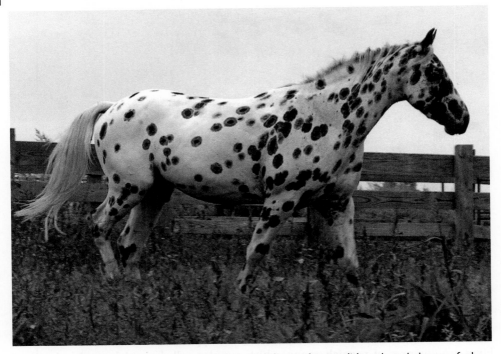

Figure 8.22 **Halo spots** develop with age. This horse's **leopard spots** did not have halos as a foal, but as he matured each spot developed a **roan** rim. The spots also began to vary in color, with some spots more brown and some more black. This is despite the horse's **black** background color. *Source: courtesy of Cheryl Wood.*

pepper spots, and are usually small spots that are dark or roan near the boundary of the white pattern area, and extend into the adjacent colored region as small round white patches. Most **pepper spots** are round; some are oval.

Other unique physical characteristics that occur on some horses can also help to identify horses with the **leopard complex**. The legs of **leopard complex** horses can be marked with the common white markings of all horses. However, when the **leopard complex** patterns occur on horses lacking these marks, the lower legs may be dark or, alternatively, they may display a dramatic interplay of white and pigmented regions. These white splashes are most strongly expressed on the inner and outer regions of the cannons, and are called **lightning strikes** or **lightning marks** by some people because they are often distinctly ragged and conspicuous. The coronary band associated with **lightning marks** is dark, unless normal white leg markings are also present. Anterior extensions of the dark into the white are common on **lightning marks** (Figure 8.23). Very extensive **lighting marks** wrap entirely around the cannon, but the coronet area remains pigmented with a distinctive upward pointing triangular shape on the front surface. On some horses common white leg markings combine with **lighting marks** to yield markings that have features of both. It is common for a horse with extensive **lighting marks** to have white-tipped ears. This is especially true when horses have a relatively extensive amount of white pattern, which is also the situation in which **lightning marks** tend to be maximally expressed.

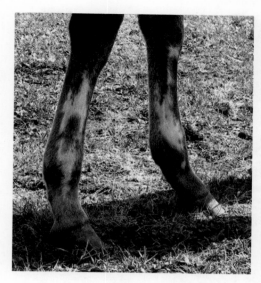

Figure 8.23 Some **leopard complex** patterned horses have **lightning marks** on the lower legs. These distinctive white areas are not the same as the usual **white marks** of horses, which can be noted by the presence of the pigmented regions just above the hooves.

Some horses with **leopard complex** patterns have round white patches in otherwise colored areas. These are called **snowball spots** and are unrelated to paint or other white markings. They occur on only a few horses, and are a rare manifestation of the complex.

A very few horses with **leopard complex** patterns have large, irregular patches of the base color that boldly overlie regions that are otherwise expected to be white. These patches are similar to patches on patterns of other species that are reversions away from the pattern and back to the original base color. These are called **mismarks** or revertant patches and are very rare in the **leopard complex** of patterns, but do occur on some horses (Figure 8.24).

The **leopard complex** patterns are also associated with sparse mane and tail growth on many horses. These are often referred to as "**rat tailed**" (Figure 8.25). As with other characteristics within this group, some horses are more strongly affected than others. Horses with black points and **leopard complex** patterns tend to have brittle mane and tail hair, so that these colors will tend to have **rat tails** more than will **chestnut**-based colors that lack black manes and tails. The key here is the color of the hair; black hairs appear to be more brittle than red hairs when Lp^{Lp} is present (detailed in Section 8.2). In horses with extensive amounts of white (either the white associated with **blankets** or **leopards**, or roaned) the tail and mane can be largely white, which is generally less brittle, and therefore more full. The effect of age on the **rat tails** is largely due to sexual maturity, at which point the pigmented hairs become more brittle and the mane and tail are more likely to be thin and sparse.

The **leopard complex** of patterns occurs in several breeds worldwide. In most breeds, the patterns occur in only a small number of individual horses and not as a breed characteristic throughout the entire breed. In these breeds the expression of the **leopard complex** patterns is variable, but usually when any of the patterns occur in a breed they all can be found. The minimal patterns, such as **frost** or **mottled**, are easy to overlook as **leopard complex** pattern. Minimal expression allows these patterns to persist in several breeds, if only at a low frequency. This occurs in breeds such as the Connemara Pony and

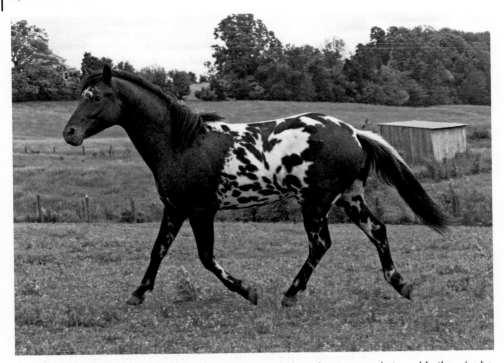

Figure 8.24 **Mismarks** are uncommon irregular pigmented patches in areas that would otherwise be white on **leopard complex** horses. This horse is basically a **leopard**, but the extensive **mismarks** have covered up most of the white on the rear quarter as well as the neck and forequarter. The residual **leopard** pattern can be seen on the head and lower legs. The **mismarks** have become roan, allowing the non-roan **leopard spots** to be seen. *Source:* courtesy of Elizabeth Estridge.

Welsh Pony, where the breed registry does not tolerate the more extreme expressions (such as **blanket** or **leopard**). Historically, this was also true of the American Quarter Horse, although recent rule changes now allow these patterns in that breed.

A few breeds highlight these patterns as a breed characteristic; for example Appaloosa, Pony of the Americas, British Spotted Pony, and Knabstrupper. In other breeds these patterns occur with full recognition by the breed registry, but only as one of several allowable colors or patterns within the breed. Such breeds include the Spanish Mustang, Noriker, South German Coldblood, Gypsy horses and a host of Asian breeds such as the Karabair and the ponies from Tannu Tuva and Mongolia. A few breeds that once had the patterns have now lost them, such as the Gotland Pony. It is a tantalizing fact that these patterns are generally rare in most populations, but also have a wide geographic distribution.

Leopard complex patterns were very popular in the European Renaissance period of history and generally had an origin in Spanish horses that were widely used throughout European horse breeding during that era. They were also popular among Native American tribes, especially the Nez Percé but also other mainly northern tribes. The patterns retain popularity with many breeders today, but usually in their association with specific breeds based around these patterns.

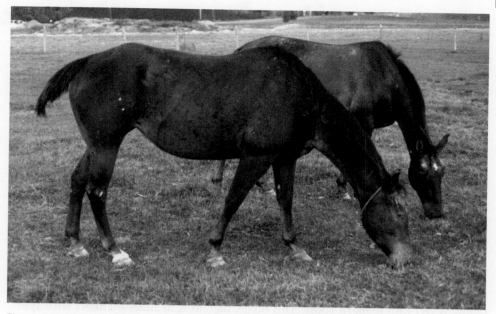

Figure 8.25 The **rat tail** of many horses with the **leopard complex** occurs over age and affects black pigmented hairs more than white ones. The tail hairs are brittle and tend to break. Although this horse has a minimal expression of the pattern, it does have a typical **rat tail**.

8.1.2 Genetic Control

The details of genetic control of the **leopard complex** are complicated. All three components of the **leopard complex** vary greatly from horse to horse (white pattern, **leopard** spots, and **varnish roaning**), making identification challenging in some instances. The main core of the control of these patterns is a two-locus system that accounts for a great deal of the variation in the amount of white pattern. Added to this are several other genetic interactions that all combine to give the final range of patterns from horses that are so minimally marked as to be missed as having a pattern, all the way to others that are nearly completely **white**. Although the system causing these patterns is complicated, it can be simplified by taking the components one at a time. The essential concept is that a single gene determines if a horse will express one of the patterns, and many other modifying genes then influence which specific pattern is likely to result.

8.1.2.1 The Leopard Complex Allele

The core cause of all of the **leopard complex** of patterns is a single allele (*leopard complex*, or Lp^{Lp}). Lp^{Lp} is the main genetic switch that determines if a horse will be patterned. Lp^{Lp} is inherited as an incompletely dominant trait, and homozygotes have a different phenotype than heterozygotes. Homozygotes of the *leopard complex* allele ($Lp^{Lp}Lp^{Lp}$) have few if any pigmented **leopard spots**, while heterozygotes usually have them. Both heterozygotes and homozygotes vary in the extent of white pattern, because the extent of white is under the control of other genetic information that is completely

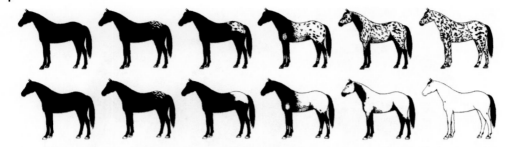

Figure 8.26 The Lp^{Lp} pattern continuum. The horses in the top row illustrate the range of pattern for horses that are heterozygous $Lp^{Lp}Lp^+$, while those on the bottom row illustrate horses homozygous $Lp^{Lp}Lp^{Lp}$. An important detail is that horses of either genotype can be born with characteristics only (mottled skin, striped hooves, and white sclera) and not show a white pattern at birth. Most of the minimally expressed horses will eventually show some roaning with age, in common with horses at higher levels of expression of the pattern.

independent of Lp^{Lp}. The pattern continuum for both heterozygotes and homozygotes is illustrated in Figure 8.26.

Heterozygotes typically vary from minimally white (on hips) to maximally white (entire body) with **leopard spots**. This range, therefore, includes **blankets with spots** and **leopard** horses. Homozygotes vary from minimally white to maximally white, but almost entirely lack **leopard spots**, so that the middle ranges of expression are **snow cap blankets** while the higher levels of expression are **few spot leopards**. Some horses with Lp^{Lp} have no white pattern at birth, and the only indication of the presence of the allele is other characteristics, such as mottled skin, striped hooves, and white sclera. Most of these horses with minimal expression at birth will eventually become **varnish roan** with age. The **roan** aspect of the patterns occurs on both homozygotes and heterozygotes, and is highly variable in either genotype. White-tipped ears occur in both heterozygotes and homozygotes, and as a result are not a reliable indicator of zygosity.

In addition to the obvious differences in the number of **leopard spots**, other phenotypic differences do distinguish homozygotes and heterozygotes. Homozygous horses have a condition known as congenital stationary night blindness and cannot see under low light conditions. This would rarely interfere with most modern uses of horses but should be noted if such animals are expected to negotiate unfamiliar territory in dark environments. For the safety of the animal, some owners choose to leave night-blind horses stalled at night with a light on, or in a pasture with other horses that can see in low light conditions.

Some homozygous horses also have somewhat smaller eyes than other horses. Their eyes occasionally show an upward tilt, causing them to appear to be looking upward. This trait is known as **sky eyes** and is most likely to occur in homozygotes, but has also been seen in occasional heterozygotes.

Hoof characteristics are different between homozygous Lp^{Lp} horses and heterozygotes. On legs with dark color on the coronary band (no **white marks**) the heterozygotes typically grow hoof wall that is generally pigmented but that has light vertical stripes. On some homozygotes this is somewhat reversed, so that the effect is a pale hoof with dark vertical stripes. However, many homozygotes have totally unpigmented hooves. The most accurate way to determine whether a horse is homozygous or heterozygous for Lp^{Lp} is by DNA testing rather than by relying on these variable external clues.

The specific locus involved in producing **leopard complex** patterns is the *Transient Receptor Potential Cation Channel, Subfamily M, Member 1 (TRPM1)* locus. This locus maps to horse chromosome 1. The specific character of the mutation at this locus that leads to the **leopard complex** patterns is a 1378 base-pair insertion into intron 1 of *TRPM1*. This insertion is thought to disrupt normal expression of this gene, causing both the white patterns (in both heterozygotes and homozygotes) and night blindness in those horses that are homozygous. Studying the genetics of this trait in horses has helped to unravel the essential role of *TRPM1* protein in night vision for horses, as well as in humans and mice. Humans with mutations in *TRPM1* are also night blind; however, they do not have any unusual pigmentation phenotype. Investigations are ongoing to determine how these extra bases of DNA in the equine *TRPM1* gene alter pigmentation in horses. This insertion originated from a retrovirus, and has been present in some horses since before their domestication. The mutation dates as far back as the Pleistocene era.

The *leopard* allele, Lp^{Lp}, allele is the single determining factor of whether or not a horse will have a **leopard complex** pattern. A horse must inherit this allele in order to display one of the **leopard complex** patterns and associated traits. Among patterned horses, each of the components of the patterns is subject to modification from outright suppression through minimal expression, and all the way to maximal expression. Many of the modifiers that account for these differences in expression are genetic and are therefore susceptible to selection by horse breeders (Figure 8.27).

8.1.2.2 Modifiers Affecting Extent of White Pattern at Birth

Loci known as modifier genes act to determine the extent of white pattern. Some of these add to the extent of the white, whereas others detract from it. The balance of these determines the final extent of white pattern at birth. Horses with Lp^{Lp} but lacking the positive modifiers that contribute to the presence of white pattern can easily be mistaken for truly nonpatterned horses that lack Lp^{Lp}. This is especially true of young horses with minimal expression of **varnish roaning, mottling, white sclera**, or striped hooves. Phenotypic research indicates that several modifiers work with Lp^{Lp} to yield the final pattern expressed at birth.

8.1.2.2.1 Pattern 1: A Major Modifier Locus

The modifier with the largest positive influence on the degree of pattern is *PATN1* (*first pattern modifier* or *Pattern-1*). Most of the molecular research to date has been on this one modifier. It is a dominant trait having a specific and necessary role in producing horses with greater than 60% white at birth, which includes both **leopard** and **near-leopard** patterns. Leopard and **near-leopard** horses are generally $Lp^{Lp}Lp^{+}$, $PATN1^{P}$—, while **few spot leopards** and **near few spot leopards** are $Lp^{Lp}Lp^{Lp}$, $PATN1^{P}$—. **Blanket** horses are similar with respect to the Lp locus, but usually lack $PATN1^{P}$, and if there are pigmented spots in the blanket they have the genotype $Lp^{Lp}Lp^{+},PATN1^{+}PATN1^{+}$,—.

Horses with $PATN1^{P}$ are usually between 60 and 100% white at birth, which includes larger **blankets** as well as **leopards** (Figure 8.28). Most are at least 80% white, although a few horses are exceptions to this rule and are **suppressed leopards** with decreased white pattern and other changes discussed in more detail later. $PATN1^{P}$ homozygous horses

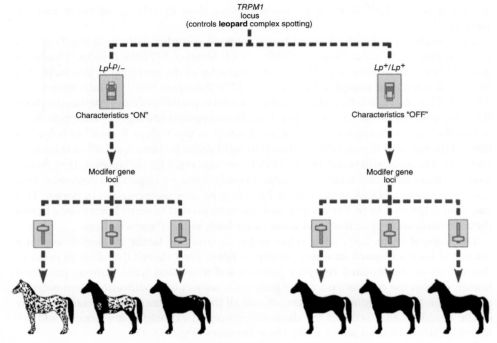

Figure 8.27 The control of the **leopard complex** of colors is related to the single major switch, Lp^{Lp}, which determines if the patterns are present or absent. Modifiers then act on those with the patterns to determine which specific pattern is expressed. Horses can carry the genetic alleles for modifiers, but without Lp^{Lp} no **leopard complex** pattern or characteristics are visible. *Source:* courtesy of Francesca Gianino.

are usually the "nose to toes" type of **leopard** pattern, while heterozygotes usually have slightly less white pattern.

Those horses with only $PATN1^+$ and without $PATN1^P$ are usually between 0% and up to 40% white (Figure 8.29). Horses with white pattern from 40 to 60% white at birth can be difficult to classify by phenotype alone because the degree of white on horses with $PATN1^+$ or $PATN1^P$ does overlap, especially in this middle range of **blanketed** horses. In a few rare cases horses have greater than 60% white pattern but do not have $PATN1^P$.

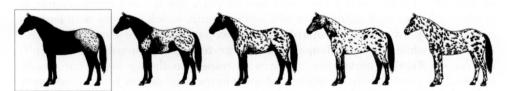

Figure 8.28 *PATN1* pattern continuum illustrating a **suppressed leopard** on the lowest end of the spectrum. All horses depicted in this figure are heterozygous $Lp^{Lp}Lp+$ but also have at least one copy of *PATN1*. The horse noted in the red box to the left is a **suppressed leopard**. The percentage of white is much lower than the usual 60%, but the area that is white has many more spots than the usual **spotted blanket** pattern.

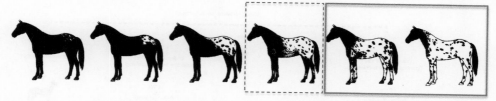

Figure 8.29 This is the continuum of patterns of $Lp^{Lp}Lp+$ horses that lack $PATN1^P$. Most horses with this genotype have patterns that are 40% white or less at birth. Horses in the middle range (40–60%) can be difficult to distinguish form horses with $PATN1^P$ (denoted by dashed box). Horses without $PATN1^P$ are only rarely above 60% white patterned at birth (boxed horses), and this genotype usually has fewer leopard spots in the same size white patterned areas than do $PATN1$ horses.

This is likely due to modifier loci that are yet uncharacterized. Despite these few exceptions, most horses can be fairly accurately identified as to which one of the $PATN1$ alleles is present.

Horses that have inherited $PATN1^P$ but do not inherit Lp^{Lp} (Lp^+Lp^+) do not show any white pattern, as they do not have the form of Lp that is required for **leopard complex** patterns (Figure 8.27). This detail can be confusing, because completely unpatterned horses can indeed have the $PATN1^P$ allele, unexpressed due to the lack of Lp^{Lp}. This is one reason for some breeders interested in the **leopard** pattern to use noncharacteristic breeding stock that comes from **leopard** background, because these horses are likely to provide $PATN1^P$ to their foals, and this can be paired with Lp^{Lp} by the breeder to result in the desired **leopard** foals.

$PATN1$ has been mapped to horse chromosome 3. A single nucleotide polymorphism (T > G) in the gene *Ring finger and WD repeat domain 3* (*RFWD3*) is associated with $PATN1$. This mutation is most likely regulatory, controlling how much of the gene product is produced. Its role in pigmentation is not yet known. This single nucleotide polymorphism is currently offered as a genetic test for $PATN1$ by several laboratories.

The basic phenomenon of these patterns being due to a single major switch (Lp^{Lp}) with a single major modifier ($PATN1^P$) can lead to some interesting results. Several years ago a "nose to toes" **leopard** appeared in the Connemara breed, which is noted for not having white patterns of any sort. The appearance of surprising **leopards** also happens occasionally in the Welsh Pony, although historic photographs do illustrate **leopards** in that breed. In these, and other, breeds it is likely that Lp^{Lp} passes along through many generations of horses that lack the modifiers that would allow it to be easily detected. This is especially likely with minimal expression of the patterns in **grey** animals (which are common in these two pony breeds) because the greying process would quickly mask any minimal expression of Lp^{Lp}. However, once matched up with $PATN1^P$ the result becomes very obvious, and very surprising to the breeders. The accuracy of the parentage of these cases can now be confirmed by DNA testing.

8.1.2.2.2 *Other Modifying Influences on White Pattern*

Aside from $PATN1$, other genes are speculated to have a role in modifying the extent of the white areas on **leopard complex** horses. These interact in complicated ways to produce the final pattern. It is likely that some modifiers enhance while others reduce the

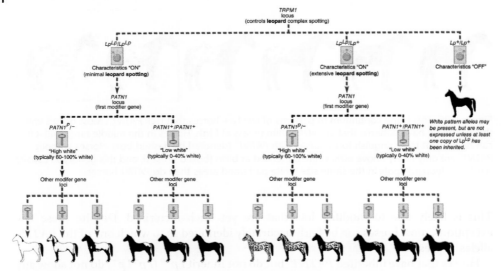

Figure 8.30 The variability in coat pattern of the **leopard complex** results from the interactions of several genes. *Lp* is the main switch that controls if a horse will have a pattern. The other switches determine the amount of white pattern and the extent to roaning. *Source:* courtesy of Francesca Gianino.

size of the white pattern, as exemplified by the range of patterns in those horses with and without $PATN1^P$ (Figure 8.30). For example, additional modifiers are thought to explain why some horses with Lp^{Lp} and $PATN1^P$ are only 60% white while others are 90–100% white. These additional modifiers also likely explain why horses in the range of 40–60% pattern level include some with and some without $PATN1^P$. Investigating these modifying genes, other than $PATN1^P$, has proven to be complicated.

Careful scrutiny of photographic records has helped to unravel some of the modifying interactions. Base coat color is one factor that helps to determine the extent of white on **leopard complex** patterns. **Chestnut** horses on average display a greater extent of white pattern, and **black** minimizes the extent. **Bay** is intermediate between these two. The general order of extent of white pattern, from least to most, is $A^aA^aE^+E^+$ (**black**, does not carry **chestnut**), $A^aA^aE^+E^e$ (**black**, carries **chestnut**), $A^AA^aE^+E^+$ (**bay**, carries **black** but not **chestnut**), $A^AA^aE^+E^+$ (**bay**, does not carry **black** or **chestnut**), $A^AA^aE^+E^e$ (**bay**, carries both **black** and **chestnut**), $A^AA^AE^+E^e$ (**bay** carries **chestnut** but not **black**), $— —E^eE^e$ (any **chestnut**). Dilutions of these colors do not seem to add any other influence to the underlying effect of these interactions.

Sex has also been shown to have an effect on the level of white pattern. Males are about 10–15% more extensively white than are females. This varies across different populations of horses, with some at the upper end of the range and others at the lower end of the range.

Horses with a **leopard complex** pattern that also have one of the **sabino** patterns tend to have larger areas of white pattern by about 10%. This may be evidence of a biochemical relationship of the genes involved, contributing to an additive effect.

A few families of **leopard complex** horses that lack **sabino** as well as $PATN1^P$ do have horses with obvious and large **blankets**, ranging up to 70% white pattern. This is a **near leopard** appearance, which is unusual for $PATN1^+$ horses (Figure 8.29). This suggests that other modifiers with lower gene frequencies than that of $PATN1^P$ can also play a major role in white pattern levels. These other modifiers have not yet been investigated, so the details of their occurrence are as yet unknown. They might be found in all breeds with Lp^{Lp}, might be breed specific to a few breeds, or might be limited to a few families. It is also uncertain if this level of modification is related to a single genetic locus.

One of the alleles ($SW4$) leading to **splashed white** ($PAX3{:}c.95C > G$) has so far only been detected in Appaloosa horses, and only in one family within that breed. In that family it accounts for white **blaze** markings on the head, and also likely contributes to somewhat enhanced levels of white pattern at birth.

The **lightning marks** that occur on the lower legs of some horses are usually an indication of modifiers that increase the amount of white. Horses with these marks usually have relatively high expression of white pattern on the body. The threshold for this effect appears to be 50%. Horses without $PATN1^P$ that exhibit large blankets often have extensive **lightning marks**, while horses that do have $PATN1^P$ but that show lower than average levels of expression tend not to have **lightning marks**. This suggests that some modifier other than $PATN1^P$ is causing both the **lightning marks** and the relatively high level of white pattern.

It is a general trend that Miniature Horses with **leopard complex** patterns express them to a reduced degree when compared with other breeds. This is likely due to a breed-wide suppression of expression of the patterns. This is genetically conditioned. As a result, horses in this breed that are expected by their genotype to be "nose to toes" **leopards** may only show an extensive **blanket**. Why this is the case in this breed is not known.

8.1.2.3 Modifiers Affecting Leopard Spots

The size and number of **leopard spots** depends on various factors. Base color, white face and leg markings, and sex each have an influence, as does the genotype associated with Lp^{Lp}.

Horses with a **black** background color tend to have the largest and most numerous **leopard spots**. In contrast, **chestnut** horses have the smallest and fewest spots. Those with **bay** or **seal brown** base color are intermediate between these two extremes.

The presence of white marks on the face and legs also reduces both the size and number of **leopard spots** (Figure 8.31). Similarly, **sabino** interacts with **leopard spots**, tending to reduce both the size and the number of the spots that are present in the white areas. This can result in some overlap of phenotype in heterozygous $Lp^{Lp}Lp^+$ horses that are also **sabino**, and true homozygous $Lp^{Lp}Lp^{Lp}$ snow cap horses. **Classic roan** can nearly completely remove **leopard spots** from some horses.

Males tend to have larger spots than females, while the females have smaller but more numerous spots. The reasons for these differences between the sexes are not yet known.

One strong influence on size and number of **leopard** spots is the Lp^{Lp} allele itself. Horses that are homozygous $Lp^{Lp}Lp^{Lp}$ have few to no spots of pigment in their white patterned area. Such homozygotes are classified as **few spot leopards** when they also have $PATN1^P$, and as **snow cap blankets** when that allele is not present. The final phenotype does vary with influences caused by base coat color. **Black**-based **few spot leopards** (homozygotes, $Lp^{Lp}Lp^{Lp},PATN1^P{-}$) tend to have relatively more **leopard spots** (still few) than do the **chestnut**-based colors, which usually have none. Those homozygotes with a **bay** base coat tend to have an intermediate number. The spots that

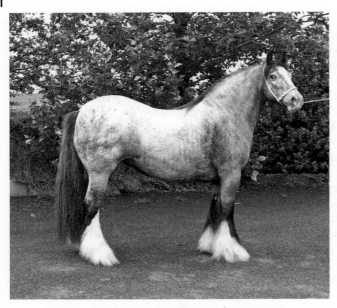

Figure 8.31 This Gypsy Cob mare has *PATN1^P*, and this along with her background color **black** should result in more obvious **leopard spots** than she has. The interaction with **sabino** (as evidenced by the white markings on feet and head) has reduced both the size and number of the **leopard spots**. An additional detail, unrelated to this interaction, is the subtle vertical striping on the barrel that is seen on many extensively patterned horses. *Source:* courtesy of Diane Butterfield.

do occur on these homozygotes are usually at the edge of a white patterned area near the stifle, throat latch, or elbow, and are rarely or never toward the center of the white patterned areas. The dilutions of base coat colors do not seem to have any effect on the size or number of **leopard spots**.

A few horses have an abundance of small **leopard spots** and have color rather than white on the head, parts of the barrel, and the legs. These horses occur in predominantly **leopard** families, indicating that they have *PATN1^P*, but they are expressing less extensive white than is expected of horses with that gene. This indicates that, in addition to the genes that increase the extent of white, other modifiers can actively decrease the extent of white. These horses have smaller white areas than expected of **leopard** horses, but they retain the same number of **leopard spots**. This pattern has been called **suppressed leopard** (Figures 8.28 and 8.32). The appearance suggests that the pigmented spots are crowded into the smaller white areas, almost like shrinking the entire **leopard** pattern into a smaller area of the horse. Most horses with this **suppressed leopard** pattern are white over the hips, back, and down the shoulders, leaving the head, neck, and barrel solid colored or roan. The details of the genetics of this suppression modifier are undocumented. The suppression does occur in foals of parents that lack the suppression, which may be an indication of some recessive tendencies.

8.1.2.4 Modifiers Affecting Varnish Roaning

The **roan** aspect of **leopard complex** patterns varies from **varnish roan** to **frost** to **snowflake**. These differences are generally due to differences in the extent and

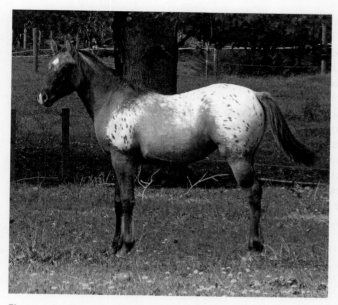

Figure 8.32 This is a **suppressed leopard**, illustrating the aspect of "shrinking" the entire pattern onto smaller portions of the horse's body. *Source:* courtesy of Petra Davidson.

organization of the white hairs that grow into the coat as the horse matures. Some horses with a **leopard complex** pattern develop minimal **varnish roaning**, and others become so extensively **varnish roan** as to be nearly **white**.

As with dark spotting, photographic record investigation supports the idea that the base color of the horse, the presence or absence of white face and leg markings, and the sex of the animal may all contribute to the final appearance. **Black**-based female horses that have no face or leg markings are the least affected by **varnish roaning** or **snowflake roaning**. In addition, horses that are homozygous $Lp^{Lp}Lp^{Lp}$ appear to **roan** more extensively than do those that are heterozygous. These differences result in dramatically different final appearances, but their control has not yet been investigated at the molecular level.

8.1.2.5 General Observations on Leopard Complex Pattern Expression

The few horses with revertant patches make it tempting to suggest that the *leopard* allele is genetically unstable with frequent back mutations to the *wild-type* (unpatterned) allele. This is certainly the case with somewhat similar patterns in other species (merle in dogs, as an example). However, no evidence for any instability of the *leopard* allele has been noted in any family of **leopard complex** horses, so the revertant spots likely have some explanation other than genetic instability of the allele. Melanocyte cultures established from a pigmented **leopard** spot showed the existence of the 1378 base pair Lp^{Lp} insertion, indicating that the pigmented spots are not caused by a loss of the genetic mutation in the cells that give rise to these spots. However, no pigment cells from revertant pigmented areas have been similarly studied.

A handful of breeds have Lp^{Lp} but are suspected to either completely or mostly lack $PATN1^P$ or any other major positive modifiers. The patterns in such breeds are either minimally expressed or unexpressed. This is because the extent of white pattern is limited by the absence of $PATN1^P$ or other positive modifiers. Some breeds, such as the Connemara, Welsh Pony, and American Quarter Horse, generally lack $PATN1^P$ or other modifiers. However, a tantalizing few boldly marked leopards do occasionally occur in these breeds. One explanation for this is the possibility that $PATN1^P$ (or other yet uncharacterized modifiers) on rare occasions matches up with Lp^{Lp} and can contribute to obvious levels of white pattern on such foals.

The presence of Lp^{Lp} allows for **leopard complex** white pattern, dark pigmented spots, and Lp^{Lp}-caused roaning. The action of $PATN1^P$ works to make the broad picture a multi-locus system. Lp^{Lp} works as a major determinant, with $PATN1^P$ and other yet undetermined modifiers (both increasing and suppressing) then determining the final pattern (Figure 8.30). The result is that horses with Lp^{Lp} but lacking modifiers can have little to no expression of the patterns. Similarly, horses with $PATN1^P$ but lacking Lp^{Lp} will have no pattern. Finally, those with both $PATN1^P$ and also Lp^{Lp} display an easily recognizable white pattern.

9

Overview of Patterns Adding White

In contrast to the complex interactions of color genes, alleles for white patches or white hairs all act independently of one another but in an additive fashion. They can occur on any base coat color, along with any dilute coat color. The white patterns can combine for some interesting effects, but in most cases the key components are still individually recognizable (Figure 9.1). The effects of the various alleles causing patterns of white are summarized in Table 13.4. An example summary for a **bay** base coat color is shown in Figure 9.2.

Patterns of white patches do tend to map to only a few loci, with some of the loci hosting multiple mutated alleles. The actual location of several of these mutants has important consequences for breeding programs in which the white markings are favored.

KIT has over 20 known mutants, most of which produce **sabino** or dominant **white** patterns. Close by this locus are the mutants for **tobiano** and **roan**. In addition, mutations involving *KIT* are thought to be an important contributing factor in the control of the usual **white marks** on the face and legs that are so common in many breeds. The presence of so much variation at or close to one locus means that these alleles will rarely or never recombine, and the alleles will segregate separately. So, for example, a **tobiano roan** horse is possible, but will produce 50% **tobiano** and 50% **roan** foals after mating to solid-colored mates. Passing along the parental combination, **tobiano roan**, would depend on crossover of very closely linked loci in order for the combination to appear in foals following mating to solid-colored horses. Such combination horses have not yet been described, and it is likely that they do not occur. If the crossover does occur, then those horses would produce 50% **tobiano roan** and 50% solid-colored foals following mating to solid-colored mates.

Other mutations are at other loci that are distant from *KIT* or are on other chromosomes. In this situation linkage is not an issue. These include *grey (STX17)*, *frame (EDNRB)*, *leopard complex (TRPM1)* and its modifier *pattern 1 (RFWD3)*, *splashed white 1* and *splashed white 3 (MITF)*, *splashed white 2* and *splashed white 4 (PAX3)*. Each of these could potentially combine with the different *KIT* alleles to provide for interesting and unusual final patterns.

Some of the mutations at a few loci (*KIT*, *EDNRB*, and *PAX3*) do have at least some deleterious effects in the embryo. This is logical when it is remembered that the white patterns tend to originate because of defects in the migration of the pigment cells from the neural crest. Not only is the migration aspect at risk, but so is the neural crest, and

Equine Color Genetics, Fourth Edition. D. Phillip Sponenberg and Rebecca Bellone.
© 2017 John Wiley & Sons, Inc. Published 2017 by John Wiley & Sons, Inc.

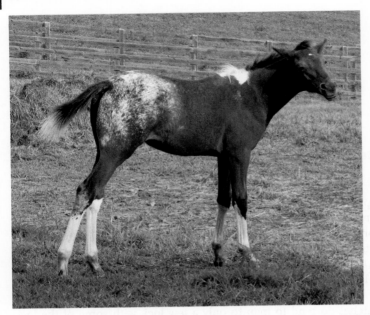

Figure 9.1 This foal has the combination of **tobiano** as well as a **small blanket**. Both of these independent patterns show very well in the combination on this foal, but on some combined patterns the overall whiteness precludes accurate designation of all the components that are present.

disrupting these too much can result in nonviable embryos or defective newborns. In some instances the addition of multiple subvital mutations at different loci can lead to some subvitality in the embryos bearing these combinations.

The interaction of the base coat color with these various patterns of white is also intricate. In some of these the base coat affects expression of the white pattern very little. In others, the base coat does matter. In general, for *leopard complex* and the various *sabino* mutations, **chestnut** is an easier target, and this results in phenotypes with greater amounts of white pattern than does **bay**, which is in turn more obviously patterned than **black**. This phenomenon is usually not all that important unless the goal is to minimize **white marks**, as is typical of several breeds. In those breeds it is easily possible for modestly marked **bay** and **black** parents to produce a **chestnut** foal that has extensive **white marks** that bar it from registration.

Each of the white patterns varies in extent, and in some families of horses this is consistent enough that it implies a genetic basis for the modification. In extreme cases the modification is sufficient to yield total or near-total suppression of the patterns, and this can upset expectations when white patterned foals occur from nonpatterned parents. While the details of the suppression of the white patterns are generally undocumented, suppression seems to occur more commonly in Miniature Horses than in other breeds. This suggests that suppression may be a general phenomenon affecting the expression of several patterns rather than a separate mechanism for each one.

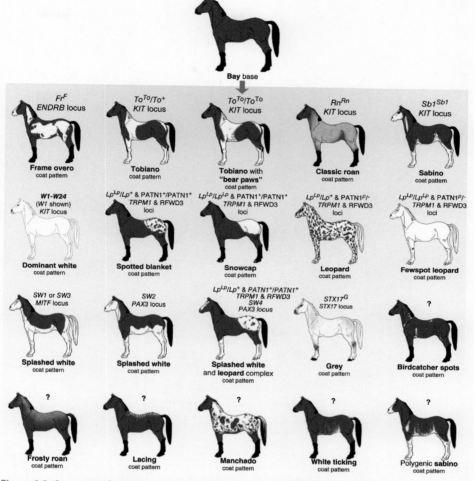

Figure 9.2 Summary of possible white patterns on a **bay** horse. White patterning can occur on any base color (and with any of the dilutions), but for simplicity this figure only illustrates each of the known white pattern mutations and some combinations on a **bay** horse. *Source:* courtesy of Francesca Gianino.

10

Horse Color and Horse Breeding

Horses occur in a wide variety of colors and patterns, and the relationship of color to horse breeding has several interesting details that relate to the complex interactions of horses, their breeding, and the culture surrounding their keeping and appreciation. It is noteworthy that many colors are limited to specific breeds or are otherwise rare. Some of the differences in distribution of horse colors among breeds are due to chance, some to historical events, while others are due to deliberate decisions taken by breeders now or in centuries past. Fashions in color can change over the years, such that colors can fall into or out of favor with horse breeders. The end result is that appreciation of color variation is inextricably woven into many horse breeding cultures.

Findings from fossil horse remains point to early variation in horse colors. **Bay** (most likely as its derivative **dun**) was present in the Siberian Pleistocene. Both **bay** and **black** were found in Iberia (likely modified to **dun** and **grullo**). The *leopard complex* allele was also found in horses before domestication, although the final pattern of these horses is undetermined and the multi-locus interaction behind those patterns is important in the final phenotype.

After domestication, Asian horse variation included **chestnut**, **bay**, **bay sabino**, and **black** by 1500 BC, then expanding to include **black silver**, **buckskin**, and **tobiano** by 300 BC. Eastern European sites include **bay**, **black**, **chestnut**, **sabino**, and **tobiano** by 1000 BC.

Throughout history horse breeders have practiced selection to influence the array of colors in their herds. Some color biases are positive and favor color variation. Others are negative and shun some colors as unacceptable or undesirable. Many of the biases concerning color have a somewhat regional basis. In modern Argentina a wide variety of colors are appreciated and cultivated; this was also the case in Spain 500 years ago, but is less true in Spain today.

In breeds of horses that are bred under the philosophy that "variety is the spice of life," it is possible to find nearly all colors and patterns of white known to occur on horses. In regions where color variation is valued, rare horse colors are favored due solely to their rarity. This assures that rare colors do not become extinct. The valuing of rarity for its own sake tends to keep some rare variants in breeds such as the Icelandic Horse, Miniature Horse, and also in many modern gaited breeds in the USA. Valuing rarity for its own sake is also occurring in the family of Gypsy breeds, so that novel combinations and colors are now appearing alongside the more traditional **black tobiano**.

Equine Color Genetics, Fourth Edition. D. Phillip Sponenberg and Rebecca Bellone.
© 2017 John Wiley & Sons, Inc. Published 2017 by John Wiley & Sons, Inc.

Historic practices in England and the USA favored somber-colored horses as saddle mounts, but odd or loudly marked horses for light harness work. This resulted in very different color arrays in these two classes of stock. In the 1918 Welsh Pony and Cob studbook very few photographs are included, and one of these is a **black leopard** cob stallion. While proudly advertised at that time, the color is now extinct in the breed due to later bias against white body patches on the ponies and cobs. It is easily possible that the *pattern 1* mutation still exists in the breed, and is just not evident due to the lack of the *leopard complex* allele.

Breeders in some regions, such as modern England and modern Spain, have attempted to standardize horse colors across several breeds in the region. They desire only a limited portion of the vast array that is possible. The result is that some colors become common and others become rare, and indeed can become extinct. In England the preferred colors for many horse breeds are generally **bay**, **chestnut**, **brown**, **black**, and **grey**. Ponies are allowed more variability, and the **linebacked dun** and **cream**-related colors are added to the mix, as is **roan**. White patches, such as in the **paint** and **leopard complex** patterns, are generally not favored, except in a very few English breeds. Those few are interesting from a breed perspective, because the patterns in them are ancient, local, and come from sources unrelated to the more modern breeds based on either **paint** or **leopard complex** patterns.

The philosophy that horses should all be some consistent and narrow range of colors results in a very narrow variability of horse color in many breeds. The Andalusian horse of Spain has nearly been standardized as a **grey** horse over the past century, although **bay** and **black** still occur. For at least a period in the recent past, whenever a color became rare in the Andalusian breed the registry would then bar registrations for that color. This had occurred with **chestnut**, though the current rules are more open to color variation than they once were. **Grey** in the Andalusian does hide considerable variability for color, and an occasional **linebacked dun**, **chestnut**, or **roan** foal is born in the breed, with **pearl** occurring rarely as well. These rare colors are currently more accepted than in the recent past. The modern Spanish attitude is interesting, because 500 years ago all colors and patterns occurred in Spanish horses, as they still do in the descendants of these horses in North and South America.

The Portuguese have taken a much more lenient approach to color, and consequently the Lusitano breed still has a considerable variability in color. This difference is interesting, because the Lusitano and Andalusian are such close cousins. Color is much less of a driving force in horse selection in Portugal. A detail of note is that some Portuguese stables that train high school dressage horses prefer **cream** and **ivory pearl** horses for this task, which puts some favorable selection pressure on these colors and the colors related to them.

Iceland has its own unique approach to color in the Icelandic Horse breed. The general tendency in Iceland is to ignore color altogether when selecting horses. Historically, the Icelanders have put no concerted effort into either increasing or decreasing specific colors. Colors that are unusual in most other regions of the world still persist in Iceland. This allows any breeder with a preference for specific colors the possibility of pulling horses of the desired color together from the general group for use in a breeding program. A slight preference among a minority of breeders does exist for rare colors, so no color or color allele is likely to drift to extinction. The color variability of Icelandic horses is especially noteworthy because Icelandic Horses have been isolated from all others for about 1000 years. The long isolation and old foundation of the Icelandic Horse provides a snapshot of the variation that once occurred in western European (Nordic and Celtic) horses a millennium ago. The wide color variation in Icelandic Horses indicates that great color variability has been typical of horses for a long, long time.

People who use and select horses sometimes change fashions both in types of horses and in horse colors, which can result in changes in color appreciation and designation. Many colors that are rare in any one region or time period simply have no distinctive name, while at the same time the more common colors have been meticulously named and split into various shades to facilitate the identification of horses as individuals.

Some horse colors are in or out of favor along breed lines. Some breed registries specifically disallow horses of some colors or patterns. Examples include various British pony breed registries that disallow white body patches on their registered horses. In the Connemara pony the slight preference shown for **grey** and **buckskin** (called **dun** in this breed) has resulted in the interesting detail that many of the **greys** have a **buckskin** base color. This can be forgotten as the horse matures to its final very white color, and the result is the production of **cream** foals from **grey** parents as generally unwelcome surprises.

Some registries, such as the Friesian, Haflinger, Suffolk, Cleveland Bay, Fjord, Buckskin, Exmoor Pony, and Palomino narrowly define the range of color allowed in the breed. In these breeds the whole concept of the breed also includes the color, an attitude that is common to other species of livestock but generally rare in horse breeding. The Appaloosa, Pinto, and Paint registries desire specific patterns in their horses, although they do accept (with restrictions) horses lacking the patterns. As a further complication in these breeds, the specific patterns wax and wane in popularity over time. In some cases this depends on which pattern is winning in the show ring.

The American Quarter Horse Registry has historically penalized white body patches in the breed, but has more recently enacted a rule change. Restrictions on the amount of white permissible in registered horses were eliminated, so that now registered Quarter Horses can sport white body patches. In the few years since this rule change it has been possible to find **frame**, **sabino**, **varnish roan** (a **leopard complex** pattern) and **splashed white** horses within the registered breed. It will be interesting to see if such patterns as **tobiano** have also been able to persist over the years. This is most likely through minimally marked horses, or those with complete suppression of patterns. For some patterns this persistence becomes unlikely for multiple generations, so that some patterns can indeed become lost forever in those breeds.

Other breeds encompass and encourage nearly the entire range of possible variants. Most notable of these are the Icelandic Horse, Spanish Mustang, the Gypsy breeds, and Miniature Horse. Some breed registries simply ignore the issue. The Thoroughbred is a good example of this, and while most Thoroughbreds exhibit common colors, some sport rare colors or white patterns, including **cream**-related colors, **sabino**, **roan**, **splashed white**, **frame**, and **white**. A fast Thoroughbred cannot be a bad color, and if a high-stakes winning Thoroughbred sporting an odd color comes along then that odd color is likely to increase in frequency as the winner produces foals.

A fairly recent phenomenon among many breeders and users of horses of several breeds in the USA is to favor unusual colors. This is a departure from the mainstream thinking of the past few centuries. This change in attitude will change the frequencies of colors in many breeds as well as across all horses as breeds fall into and out of favor. The favoritism shown the historically unusual colors, usually horses with white patches or with pale colors, has become more and more common among breeders of gaited horses. This trend can also be noticed among breeders and users of various Warmblood breeds. Acclaim for unusually colored individual Thoroughbred and Arabian horses is also more and more frequently encountered, and this is very much a departure from long-established tradition.

As the popularity of historically unusual colors progresses in some breeds, the frequency of those colors increases. As these increase it becomes more and more likely that individual horses will be produced that combine several of these previously rare colors. Some combinations become highly sought after, such as black and white **paints** of various patterns. This popularity changes gene frequency in some breeds, such as the Paint, in which other colors based on **black** also become more and more common. An example is **grullo** and white **paints**, which are now being produced more commonly than in the past.

Among the gaited breeds of the USA (Tennessee Walking Horse, American Saddle-bred, Rocky Mountain Horse, Mountain Pleasure Horse, Missouri Fox Trotter, and others) rare colors are highly desired, and the *silver dapple* allele has a reasonably high frequency. These breeds also have the *cremello*, *dun*, and *champagne* alleles. It can be nearly impossible to accurately determine which combinations of these alleles are present in some individual horses, which adds to the mystery of horse breeding as well as the surprises possible in foal crops. Breeders of these horses can become very anxious to know which specific combinations are present in young foals. Unfortunately, guessing the combinations of these alleles is difficult enough when observing adult horses and is nearly impossible when observing foals. Fortunately, the availability of genetic testing can reveal the component alleles before the horse matures.

The genetics of color and the power of selection for specific color variants are much better recognized now than in the past. This, along with increasingly numerous DNA tests, gives breeders powerful tools for manipulating the frequencies of colors within breeds. It must be remembered by all horse breeders that today's breeds all come to the present from a rich and intricate interaction of culture, genetics, use, and appreciation. In the quest for unusual colors it is important to remember that these generally occur in the context of a specific breed of horse with its own specific origin, providing both a genetic and a cultural resource. Guarding the genetic treasure of the breed is very important. The recent trend in horse breeding is to select horses to converge on only a very few common international types, while discarding several older, successful, and reasonably specialized types. It will be unfortunate if the quest for color contributes to the demise of these unique treasures, but will be a great boon for these breeds if the desire for the unusual equates into meaningful conservation, use, and appreciation of these important genetic resources.

11

Peculiarities of Hair Growth

In addition to the vast array of colors and patterns on horses, a few variations in hair type or hair growth also occur. On most horses the mane and tail are long and full, and the body hair is short and smooth. Some breeds, such as the Akhal Teke, have very fine hair that tends to lack the hollow core of the hair on most horses. This results in a metallic sheen to many colors in this breed. The genetic control of this peculiarity is unknown.

Among individual horses, as well as breeds, mane and tail length and abundance are variable. Some breeds tend to have sparse manes and tails, whereas others have full and abundant manes and tails. The sparse tails in the Appaloosa and other breeds with the **leopard** complex are related to that specific genetic mechanism, but in other breeds the sparse manes and tails have other causes.

In addition to the variation in the amount of hair, there is also variation in texture, and some horses have very wavy manes and tails. The diameter of the hair also varies, from coarse to fine. These differences loosely follow breed lines, so it is likely that they are under genetic control. Specific individual genes for these variations have not been documented.

Most horses have very clean lower legs, with short, smooth hair. This is the rule on most light horse breeds. Other breeds have longer hair on the fetlocks or pasterns, and this is referred to as **feathering, feather**, or **feathers** (Figure 11.1). **Feathering** can be either very fine or very coarse and also varies in extent from minimal to very highly developed. **Feathering** is a breed characteristic in Clydesdale, Shire, Friesian, Gypsy Cob, Gypsy Vanner, Mulassier, and some British pony breeds such as Fell Ponies and Dales Ponies. In some breeds (or populations) the amount of **feathering** is variable. An example is in Belgian horses. Those in Belgium are usually **feathered**; those in the American Belgian offshoot are usually clean-legged. Some groups, such as the Pryor Mountain Mustangs, have an interesting tendency for the horses in the feral, mountain groups to possess a small amount of feathering. When individual horses are moved into a domestic situation off the mountain they tend to lose **feathering** in the course of a few years. The genetics of **feathering** are unknown, but the differences among breeds in this trait do suggest some genetic control.

A rare variant in hair growth is the **curly** trait (Figures 11.2, 11.3, and 11.4). **Curly** horses have curled body and ear hair and also curly mane and tail hair. The winter coat of most **curly** horses is very, very curled. The summer coat is frequently only subtly curled, so horses could be misidentified as being noncurly. Another peculiarity of some **curly** horses is the shedding of the mane and tail along with the winter body coat

Equine Color Genetics, Fourth Edition. D. Phillip Sponenberg and Rebecca Bellone.
© 2017 John Wiley & Sons, Inc. Published 2017 by John Wiley & Sons, Inc.

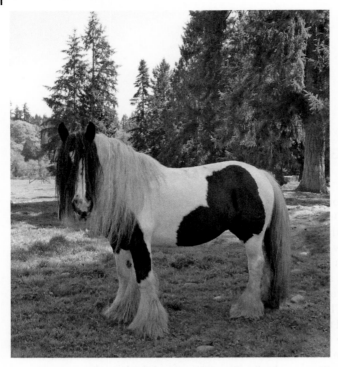

Figure 11.1 The Gypsy breeds tend to all have abundant manes, tails, and **feather** on the lower legs. In addition, most Gypsy horses have **paint** patterns, with **tobiano** the most common. **Black** is also a common coat color, so that **black tobianos** are especially common, but with the added feature of wide **blazes** from selection in favor of extensive white marks. *Source:* courtesy of Debbi Jenson.

each spring. The **curly** trait is the basis of a few registries, even though it occurs in several different breeds.

At least two independent genetic mechanisms can lead to **curly** horses. One of these is due to a recessive mutation and is symbolized CrR^c for *curly* at the *Curly Recessive* locus. This mechanism accounts for most curly horses that crop out of straight-haired breeds. This occurs in the Missouri Fox Trotter and the Percheron, among others. The other mechanism is dominant and is symbolized CrD^C for *curly* at the *Curly Dominant* locus. Horses homozygous for CrD^C are reputed to be more curled than heterozygous horses. This allele is likely responsible for most Asiatic **curly** horses (notably, the Lokai breed) and potentially the **curly** horses that occur in the Western Hemisphere, although genetic evidence is pointing to more than one dominant allele that causes **curly**.

Most **curly** horses in the Western Hemisphere descend from Spanish horses brought over during the conquest, and these occur in both North America and South America. Although the **curly** trait is dominant in these horses, it does have variable expression. Occasional horses with the CrD^C allele are minimally curly, do not shed the mane and tail, and could easily be missed as being **curly**. They are fully capable of passing the allele along to offspring, though, some of which will be fully **curly**. The two proposed genetic mechanisms (CrR^c and CrD^C) for curliness in horses appear to be totally unrelated, except that they cause a similar appearance.

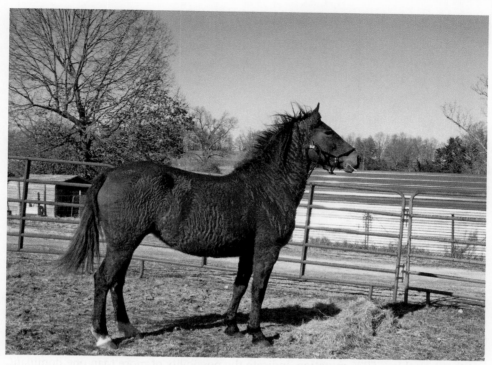

Figure 11.2 Curly horses have wavy body coats as well as wavy mane and tail hairs. These are most obvious in the winter. *Source:* courtesy of Dyan Westvang.

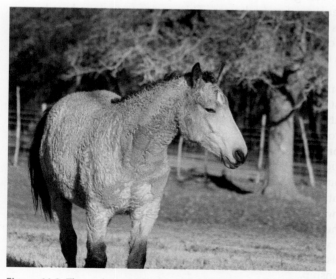

Figure 11.3 The curly coat is least obvious on the head, and most obvious on body and mane. The curliness is independent of body coat color. *Source:* courtesy of Barbara Carroll.

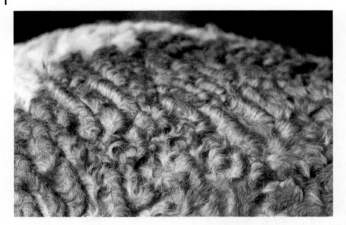

Figure 11.4 Some horse colors, such as this buckskin, have hairs with dark tips and light bases. This shows most dramatically when combined with a curly coat. *Source:* courtesy of Barbara Carroll.

A dominant allele has recently been investigated at the molecular level, and this may well represent what was initially proposed as CrD^C. A non-synonymous missense mutation in a keratin gene (*KRT25*) explains most, but not all, **curly** horses with a dominant mode of inheritance. Keratin genes are important components of hair and skin in all mammals. The few horses that were predicted to have inherited a dominant allele, but that lack this *KTR25* mutation, indicate the possibility of more than one dominant mechanism in horses. As of this writing, the recessive allele, CrR^c, has not been mapped or identified at the molecular level.

Another manner in which hair growth varies is in the persistence of a line of long, manelike hairs along the sternum of some horses. This occurs in various breeds as a subtle variation. Some horses have similar long hairs, even in the summer coat, along the underline of the head from chin to throatlatch. These are more common in breeds of draft horses but also occur in other breeds. A few horses have a "moustache" of long hairs on the upper lip. This is a rare variant that is found in some mustang populations descended from Spanish horses. It is unknown if this is due to a genetic mutation.

Most horses have at least some **whorls, rosettes,** or **cowlicks** where hair growth changes direction. These features are a permanent part of a horse's coat and are used in some regions as an adjunct to color in identifying horses. Most horses have a reasonably unique combination of **whorls**, which makes them a very useful and accurate characteristic for individual identification. The **whorls** have never been a main focus of horse identification in the USA, but in some regions of the world they are considered to be among the most reliable features to identify individual horses.

Folklore holds that the **cowlick** in the forehead can be a predictor of the character of a horse. Those horses with the **cowlick** between the eyes are reputed to be gentle and easier to handle than those with the **cowlick** in a lower position. It seems that many horses are exceptions to this rule, although research in cattle points to at least some credibility for such a relationship.

12

Donkey Color

Colors of donkeys are not as well characterized as the colors of horses. One reason for this is that interest in donkey breeding has generally lagged behind that generated by horse breeding throughout most regions of the world and throughout much of history. This difference in attention is probably related to the use of horses in building empires and the use of donkeys as subsistence animals. A few regions are notable exceptions to this rule. Despite being largely ignored by animal breeders, donkeys are very important worldwide, and include many interesting and useful breeds. Some of these breeds are used in their own right as riding or draft animals. Some breeds, such as the miniatures, serve as companion animals. Still others (usually the larger ones) are valued for their role in mule production. Saddle donkeys are also becoming more popular throughout many regions.

The general trend throughout all size classes of donkeys is increased demand and interest. Along with the demand has come an increased curiosity about the colors of donkeys and their genetic control. The American Donkey and Mule Society is spearheading important work into the description of donkey colors, and is also exploring the details of their genetic control. Additional support from the French National Donkey Institute and the Swiss National Science Foundation has aided in the discovery of the donkey coat color mutations that have now been documented. This guide largely follows the American Donkey and Mule Society nomenclature for donkey colors, although with a few departures from it.

12.1 Colors of Donkeys

Donkey color identification and genetics have several similarities to those of horses, but also several important distinctions. One important distinction is that the term "points" in donkeys refers to the usual light muzzle, eye rings, belly, and upper and inner aspects of legs of donkeys. These are similar to the same areas in horses described by **mealy** or **pangaré**, but in donkeys this aspect is called **light points** (Figure 12.1). In contrast, the term "trim" refers to mane, tail, and ear rims. Thus, donkey "trim" is somewhat analogous to horse "points" and has the same significance for color identification and biology. Various combinations of body color, trim color, and point color are summarized in Table 12.1 as they combine to give different color names.

Equine Color Genetics, Fourth Edition. D. Phillip Sponenberg and Rebecca Bellone.
© 2017 John Wiley & Sons, Inc. Published 2017 by John Wiley & Sons, Inc.

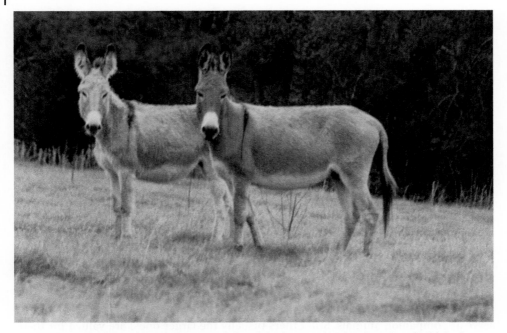

Figure 12.1 **Grey dun** is the most common color of donkeys, and is also the color of wild donkeys. Both of these donkeys have the usual **light points** (pale muzzle, eye rings, belly, and upper legs) typical of most donkeys. These donkeys also have the black trim that is usual on **grey dun**.

Table 12.1   Components and names for donkey colors.

Color name	Body color	Trim color	Points: light or dark
Grey dun	Ashy grey	Black or near black	Either
Charcoal	Dark grey	Black or near black	Either
Black	Black	Black (no contrast)	Either
Brown-black	Brownish black, or brown or tan areas on ears and face	Black or near black (some contrast)	Either
Smoky	Off-black over entire body	Black (some contrast)	Either
Brown	Brown	Brown	Either
Brown-grey dun	Ashy brown	Black	Either
Bay	Red	Black	Black legs
Russet	Red	Black	Light legs
Sorrel	Red	Flaxen, red, or brown	Either
Rose dun	Light red or light grey–red, some with pink skin	Flaxen, red, or brown	Either
Ivory	Off-white or pale beige	Cream	Either
Cameo (pale skin and eyes)	Pale	Pale	Either
No light points (NLP)	Any	Any	Dark

The basic color of wild donkeys is usually referred to as **grey dun** (Figure 12.1). **Dun** may be a better description, because **grey** has the connotation of progressive loss of pigment or whitening from its use in horses; however, **grey dun** has historical precedence for this donkey color and is the commonly accepted term. **Grey dun** donkeys are variably striped, with shoulder stripe, dorsal stripe, and leg stripes all being much more variable than are stripes on **dun** horses. While most **grey dun** donkeys have at least some of the stripes, some lack them altogether. The wild subspecies of donkey all have (or had, some are extinct) different striping patterns, and these are all evident in different combinations on their domesticated descendants.

The background color of **grey dun** donkeys varies from dark to light. The darkest ones are nearly black and are sometimes called **charcoal**. The middle range of color is most common, and is usually a flat bluish grey that is similar to **grullo** in horses. The lightest **grey duns** are a pale beige color. While most **grey dun** donkeys lack the reddish tones of **dun** horses, some in the middle range of shades do have a reddish or gold tinge. This is especially true on the face, and especially with heavy winter coats or foal coats. While the shades of color on **grey dun** donkeys vary from pale to nearly black, stripes are usually evident in all the various shades. **Grey dun** is the most common donkey color in most breeds and regions. This contrasts with the situation for nearly all other domesticated species in which the wild-type color is rare or nonexistent.

An important and obvious component of the wild-type color in donkeys is the pronounced pale points. This is similar to the **mealy** effect on horses (**pangaré**) but is much more distinct. The presence of pale points is very common on all donkey colors and is referred to as "**light points**" or "**white points**," although they are in fact a shade of cream and not truly white (Figure 12.1). The **light points** of donkeys usually have shorter and finer hair than that of the rest of the darker color body regions.

A few donkeys lack the **light points** that are so common among all sizes and types of donkeys. Sometimes only the muzzle is dark, while the belly and inner legs are pale. This is called a **black muzzle** or **dark muzzle**. When all points are dark the result is variably called **no light points**, **dark points**, or **black points**. These **dark-pointed** colors in mules were historically called **blue nosed** in some regions. The presence or absence of **light points** in donkeys does not change basic color names, the only difference being the notation of **dark points** (designated as "NLP" for "**no light points**") when they are present (Figure 12.2).

A common color of donkeys in several breeds is **black** (Figure 12.3). These do have the **light points** typical of most donkeys, but are still called **black**. However, it is also possible to have a black donkey with dark points (NLP), and these are also called **black**. On some **black** donkeys it is possible to see vestiges of the striping pattern, and some purists will not call these **black** but rather resort to **black with cross** or **smoky** for these "off-black" donkeys. **Black** is an especially common color in large, defined breeds of mule-breeding donkeys, such as the American Mammoth, Spanish Catalonian, Spanish Leonesa-Zamorano, and French Poitou. **Black** is indeed a breed requirement for several of them. The prevalence of black in these breeds traces back to a historical preference for dark mules, and a **black** jack is the best strategy for ensuring dark mules. **Black** donkeys can sometimes be difficult to assess by visual appearance because of the tendency for coarse, long winter hair to fade dramatically. This is especially the case in Poitou and Leonesa-Zamorano donkeys. Long hair is desired in

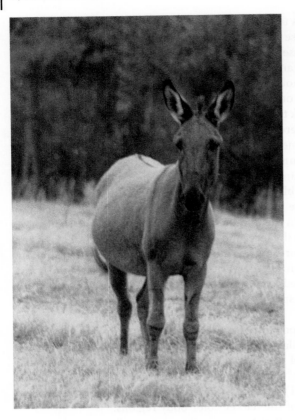

Figure 12.2 The absence of **light points** on donkeys is generally rare, and is noted as **"no light points"** on those that lack the usual light eye rings, muzzle, belly, and upper legs.

these breeds as a breed characteristic and is under genetic control as described in Section 12.5 (Figure 12.4).

Bay is occasionally encountered in donkeys. **Bay** differs from **black** by having reddish or brownish body color instead of the usual deep black body color of **black** donkeys. **Bay** is usually less red in donkeys than it is in horses and can be much closer to **black** than its counterpart in horses. **Bay** donkeys do have black or very dark trim. A few donkeys have a more red body color with black mane and tail (trim), but have light-colored legs. These donkeys are called **russet** if they lack white hairs in the body coat, or **bay roan** if they do have white hairs (Figure 12.5).

An annoying but common phenomenon of donkey colors is that donkeys with intermediate colors between two color classes are frequent (Figure 12.6). The colors of donkeys grade gradually from one to another, and while donkeys in the middle of the range are easy to identify, those at the intermediate edges are very difficult. Between **bay** and **black** are many donkeys that have black bodies, and tan or red on the head and ears and rarely over the back. These are variably called **black, brown-black,** or **dark brown**. These donkeys are lighter than **black**, but usually the lighter areas are regional so that the overall color approaches **black**. This color is common in breeds such as the Mammoth, in which selection has long favored **black** animals. A cross and back stripe are common, if subtle, on **brown-black** donkeys.

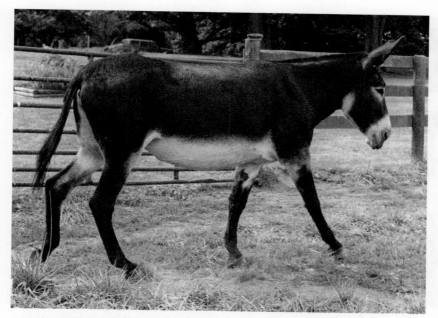

Figure 12.3 **Black** donkeys retain **light points**, but are still called **black**. This has long been a popular color for large mule-breeding donkeys like this American Mammoth. *Source:* courtesy of Mary Ellen Nicholas.

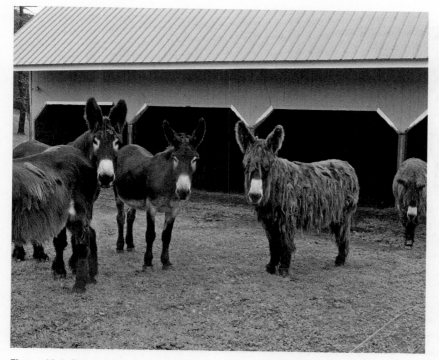

Figure 12.4 Despite their long hair, which tends to fade, Poitou donkeys are still **black. Black** is more easily seen in the younger animals of the group because they have shorter hair.

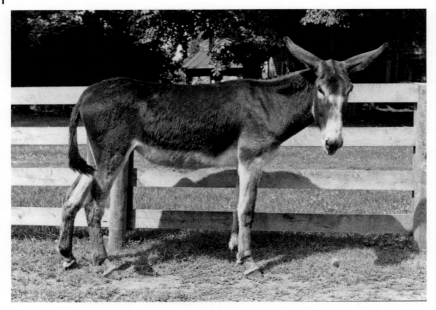

Figure 12.5 **Russet** and **bay** donkeys are closely related colors, but the **russet** (shown here) usually lacks the black legs that distinguish **bays**. *Source:* courtesy of Mary Ellen Nicholas.

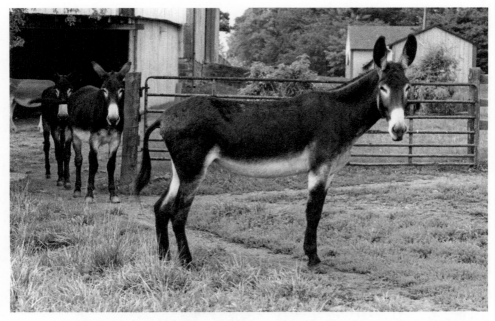

Figure 12.6 These three Mammoth jennies demonstrate the gradual progression of reddish tan areas that results in difficulty neatly separating out donkey color classifications. *Source:* courtesy of Mary Ellen Nicholas.

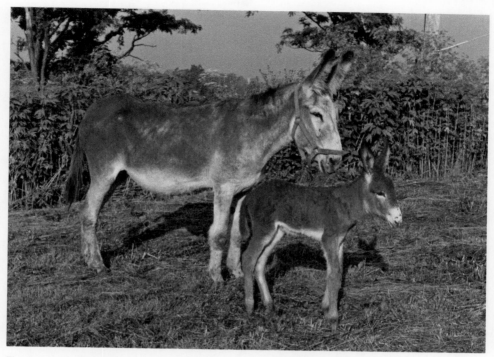

Figure 12.7 **Red**, or **sorrel**, donkeys usually do have **light points** and light or red trim. *Source:* courtesy of Mary Ellen Nicholas.

Donkeys with a red color are variably called **chestnut, sorrel,** or simply **red**. These are, logically, red instead of black and almost invariably retain pale points (Figure 12.7). The shade of red is variable. **Sorrel** tends to be used more widely than **chestnut** for these red shades of color, although people in different regions and different breeds associations vary on what to call this color. Trim on **sorrel** donkeys can be various shades of red or can be pale enough to be **flaxen**, and these are called **flaxen sorrels**. On some **sorrels** the mane and tail are very dark, nearly black, although the legs remain distinctly red or pale. In some instances it is difficult to clearly separate **russet** from these dark-maned **sorrels**. Most **sorrels** are striped like **duns**, and the stripes are usually red or brown and are darker than the body color (Figure 12.8). However, a few donkeys appear to be **red dun** instead of the more common **grey dun** with all the dun stripes (shoulder stripe, dorsal stripe, and leg stripes) on a pale red body color. A problem arises in naming this color, because nearly all reddish donkeys tend to have some striping, so the point at which to separate **sorrel** from **red dun** is arbitrary (Figures 12.8 and 12.9). A few breeders refer to the palest reds as **rose duns**, or occasionally as **pink** (Figure 12.9). These, as the names suggest, are pale reddish colors. Some of these animals have pink skin rather than black skin. This rare group of colors is very confusing due to the light skin color with the reddish base color.

A trend for the popularity of **sorrel** mules (especially in heavy draft mules) has made **sorrel** jacks increasingly popular, so that in the American Mammoth Jack breed this

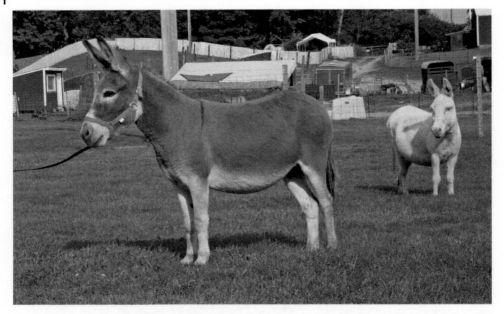

Figure 12.8 Many **sorrel** donkeys retain prominent striping, and are therefore difficult to distinguish from **rose** or **red dun**. *Source:* courtesy of Marlene Clark.

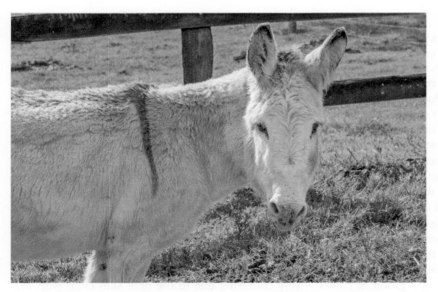

Figure 12.9 The lightest **red**-based colors are very pale, and likely a combination of **red** and **dun**, to produce **rose dun** or **pink**. *Source:* courtesy of BNA Photography.

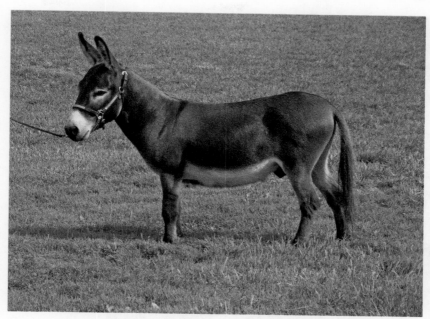

Figure 12.10 **Brown** and **chocolate** donkeys are dark, but distinctly brown rather than red or black. *Source:* courtesy of Deb Mix.

color has been displacing the previously popular **black** color. This is due to the reliability of producing **sorrel** mules from a **sorrel** jack and **sorrel** or **chestnut** mares.

Another relatively common color variant is **brown**, which is also called **chocolate** when it is very dark. In these donkeys the usual black body color is replaced by a brown color that can nearly be chocolate brown (Figure 12.10). This color is becoming more common due to selection favoring it in miniature donkeys. **Brown** donkeys usually have a foal coat that is red with a black mane, tail, and lower legs somewhat similar to adult **bay** horses. As adults they are nearly invariably a dark, uniform chocolate brown color with somewhat darker (and on some, black) manes, tails, lower legs, and striping. The red tones present on the foals nearly always vanish on the adults. The relationship between **brown** and **chocolate** is not obvious, and in practice these terms are used interchangeably for very similar colors.

Some donkeys are an intermediate color between **brown** and **grey dun**, having a brown tint to the **dun** color instead of the more usual bluish grey tint (Figure 12.11). These are called **brown-grey dun**.

Rarely are donkeys **ivory** colored, with pale color, pink skin, and blue eyes (Figures 12.12 and 12.13). This color occurs mostly in the Miniature donkeys, as well as in donkeys on Sardinia. **Ivory** has not been documented in the larger size classes. **Ivory** donkeys are commonly described as **white**, but do have faint striping. This is expected of a pale dilute color and not of **white**. Nearly all of these have blue eyes and pink skin, and appear to be very similar to **cream** horses. A few **ivory** donkeys also have white patches, and the subtle contrast between the cream color and the white patches is most noticeable in foals rather than adults. Some **ivory** donkeys are a darker color, as dark as a "coffee

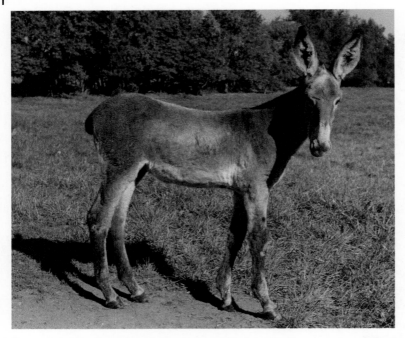

Figure 12.11 Occasional donkeys are very difficult to classify as to color, and **brown-grey dun** likely comes the closest to a good descriptive name. *Source:* courtesy of Mary Ellen Nicholas.

with cream" color, but these darker **ivory** animals still have the pink skin and blue eyes that characterize the more common pale shades of this group.

A very few donkeys are a **gold** color. **Gold** donkeys were once highly regarded on the island of Guernsey, where breeders also desired gold color in their cattle and goats. This strain unfortunately is now extinct, and exactly how gold they were is uncertain. A few donkeys are a somewhat **gold** color, and these might be close to what was on Guernsey (Figure 12.14). Another close approximation to this color might be darker **ivory** donkeys.

One family of donkeys in Australia has produced colors very similar to **champagne** or **pearl** horses (Figure 12.15). These donkeys have pale amber eyes, pale skin, and pale colors. Breeders are using **cameo** to describe these, in order to avoid confusion with the similar horse color. The **cameo** colors vary in much the same way as do **champagne** horses, and these differences are likely related to the different combinations of **cameo** with various background colors.

The interrelationships of donkey color are subtle and less distinctive than are those for horses. A few consistent phenomena do emerge, though, and these help to organize the colors into logical groups. The colors array themselves along a few axes of dark colors to light colors, with the intermediates blending into the extremes (Figure 12.16). One such axis is **black** to **charcoal** to **grey dun**. Another axis is **black** to **chocolate** to **brown** to **brown-grey dun** to **grey dun**. A third axis is **black** to **brown-black** to **bay** to **russet** to **sorrel** to **gold** to **rose dun**. The lightest colors (**ivory** and most **cameos**) tend to be more isolated on their own and are only rarely confused with other colors and do not blend into the other colors via intermediate shades.

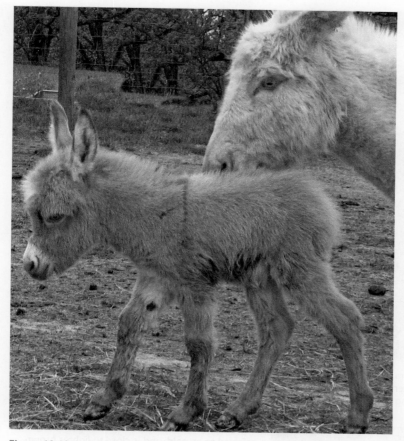

Figure 12.12 **Ivory**-colored donkeys vary from pale beige to nearly white. Most have striping, and all have pink skin and blue eyes. *Source:* courtesy of Connie Bonczek.

12.2 Patterns of White

Donkeys have fewer patterns of white than do horses, and while some are similar to horse patterns, most are very distinct from any horse pattern. Patterns of white on donkeys are summarized in Table 12.2.

Minor white marks are similar to the **star** marking of horses. In general, white marks are less common on donkeys than they are on horses. In most cases, any white markings on the legs, or extensive markings on the face, are caused by the same genetic mechanisms that lead to **spotted** donkeys, and usually affect the rest of the coat and not only the head.

The **roan** pattern in donkeys is commonly referred to by many observers as **grey** (Figure 12.17). This pattern is unlike either **roan** or **grey** in horses. The **roan** of donkeys is only moderately progressive, so that most **roan** donkeys are only slightly darker when young than they are when older. **Roan** donkeys usually rapidly stabilize at a lighter (but not white) **roan** at a few years of age. **Roan** usually affects the head, so that the dark

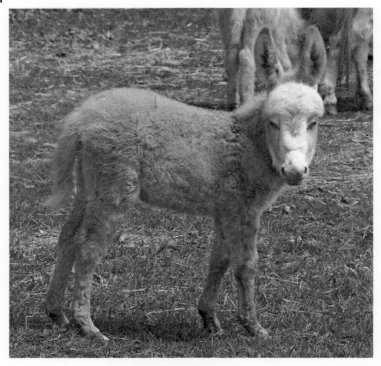

Figure 12.13 The range of shades of **ivory** is most likely related to the original base color that was subsequently lightened. This dark **ivory** foal is toward the darker end of the range of shades, and her white facial marking contrasts with the pale color. *Source:* courtesy of Lori Wargo.

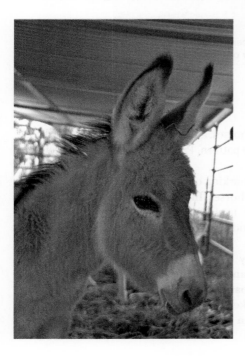

Figure 12.14 This may be the color previously referred to as **gold**, and is close to lighter **brown dun**. *Source:* courtesy of Bianca Haase.

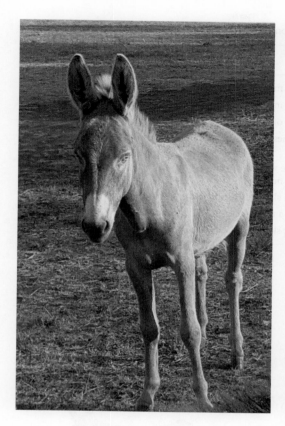

Figure 12.15 **Cameo** donkeys are very rare, and resemble **champagne** or **pearl** horses. *Source:* courtesy of Lyn Micallef.

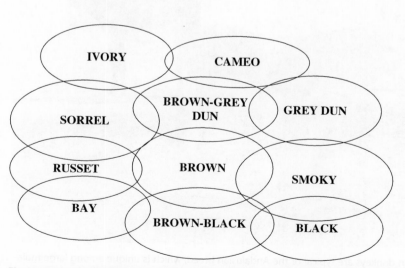

Figure 12.16 Relationships of donkey colors with regions of overlap. Donkey colors tend to overlap more profoundly than horse colors, making the border regions between color groups larger and potentially more confusing.

Table 12.2 Patterns of white occurring on donkeys.

Name	Description
Roan	White hairs mixed in with colored hairs on face and on body
Frosted	White hairs increasing with age
Frosty	White hairs on face and legs only
Spotted	White patches on body, minimum pattern is blaze on face or white on legs
Tyger	Nearly white with small round spots of pigment and usually pigment on neck
Dominant white	White, pink skin, with dark eyes
Fully frosted spotted white	White with a few small residual dark or roan spots, dark eyes
Albino white	White, pink skin, pale lashes, blue eyes

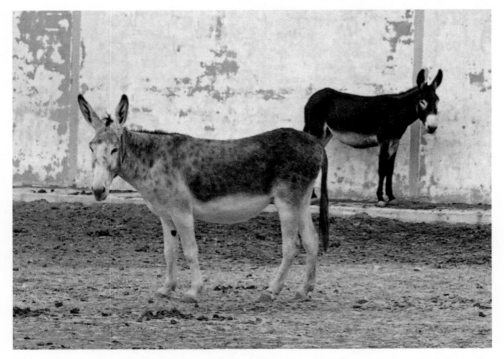

Figure 12.17 **Roan** donkeys are typical of the Andalusian breed, which is unique among large mule-breeding donkeys for not being **black**. The **black** jenny in the background is a Catalonian jenny, a breed that is consistently **black**.

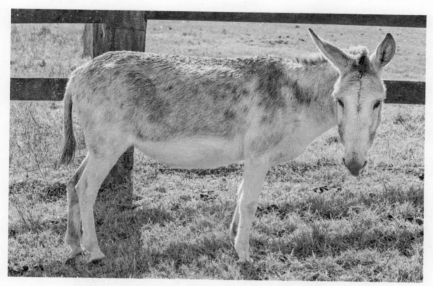

Figure 12.18 The interaction of **roan** with the base color can make some colors difficult to assess, especially if the final color is pale. *Source:* courtesy of BNA Photography.

areas that are characteristic of horses are lacking. **Roan** donkeys are commonly **dappled**, and these dapples are usually reversed, having dark centers and pale peripheries. **Roan** can be superimposed on any background color. **Roan** can act to make the legs pale and can therefore make color determination difficult when combined with certain background colors (such as **bay**) (Figure 12.18). **Roan** on a black background results in **blue roan**, which is the preferred color of the large Spanish Andalusian Donkey breed. **Roan** on a **bay** or **russet** background color is called **red roan** (Figure 12.19). On a **sorrel** background the result is **red roan** or **strawberry roan**. The result on **grey dun** is usually **grey roan**, and the interplay of white hairs in **grey dun** is frequently subtle and can easily be overlooked.

Subtypes of **roan** include **frosted** or **dappled**, in which the animals do become progressively whiter with age. Some of these animals end up **white** with dark skin, much as do **grey** horses. **Frosty roan**, in contrast, refers to animals on which the white hairs are limited to the head and legs only and spare the body (Figure 12.20). The exact interrelationships and boundaries between **roan, frosty roan**, and **frosted** are difficult to appreciate because many intermediate steps occur between these three different extremes.

Donkeys that have white patches are usually simply called **spotted** rather than having specific subtypes with different names, as is the case in horses. Most **spotted** donkeys have patterns consistent with a single basic design that varies in extent of white, even though a few donkeys sport somewhat distinct patterns that might lead to the conclusion that more than one pattern is possible. **Spotted** donkeys occur in a large number of breeds, and a registry specifically for **spotted** donkeys of any size does exist in the USA.

The most usual pattern of white patches on donkeys has characteristics distinct from any pattern in horses, and is illustrated in Figure 12.21. The white usually progresses

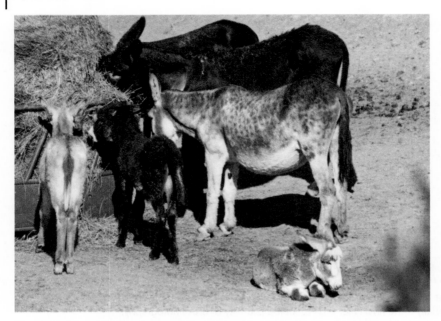

Figure 12.19 The shade of **roan** on donkeys varies with background color. The donkey in the middle has a **bay** or **russet** background color as betrayed by the black tail switch. The result is a **red roan**.

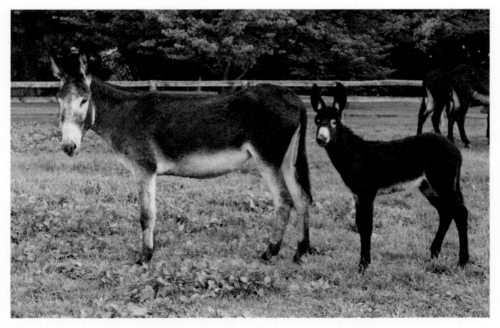

Figure 12.20 This jenny is a **frosty roan** donkey, with roaning limited to the head and legs. *Source:* courtesy of Mary Ellen Nicholas.

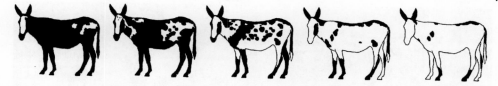

Figure 12.21 Progression of white, from least to greatest, on donkeys with the **spotted** pattern.

from the face and hind portion of the barrel. It is usually horizontal in character and also frequently crosses the topline. Most **spotted** donkeys have colored lower legs and feet. Many **spotted** donkeys have extensive white areas on the head, but do retain colored patches around the eyes and ears. Many also have isolated nearly round colored spots of pigment in the extensive white areas. On some donkeys these isolated colored spots are quite large and obvious; on others they are smaller. Small round ones that occur in white areas, like **blazes**, are sometimes called **medallion spots**.

Minimally **spotted** donkeys usually have a star or a blaze on the face (Figure 12.22). These facial marks often have a point that drops toward the nose. A small, round **star** is usually not associated with the **spotted** patterns, and these, while rare in donkeys, do occur in lines that never produce **spotted** foals. White patches on the body of **spotted** donkeys usually first appear in the hip area, as well as on the neck and face (Figures 12.23 and 12.24). Donkeys with intermediate levels of the pattern are usually very distinctively marked in a pattern different from any of the horse patterns (Figure 12.25). The most extensively white **spotted** donkeys usually retain color on the ears, back (other than top

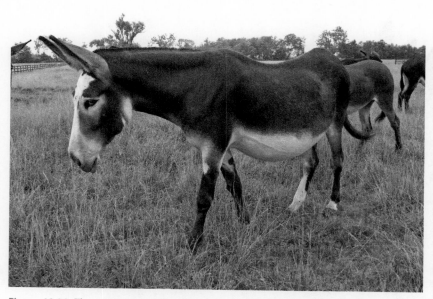

Figure 12.22 The minimal extent of **spotted** on donkeys is facial and leg white. *Source:* courtesy of Jeannette Beranger.

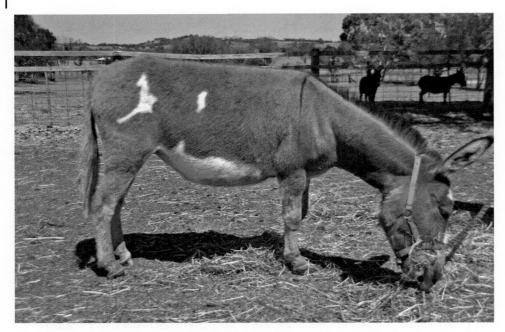

Figure 12.23 As the extent of **spotted** progresses, the white usually involves the rear portion of the body. *Source:* courtesy of Bianca Haase.

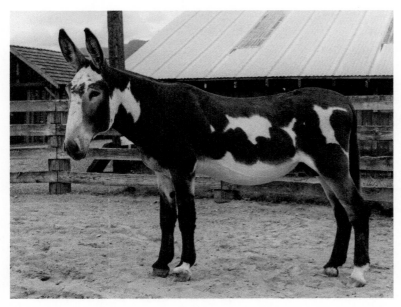

Figure 12.24 The middle extent of the range of **spotted** patterns has obvious white on the body, head, and neck, and often on the lower legs. *Source:* courtesy of Mary Ellen Nicholas.

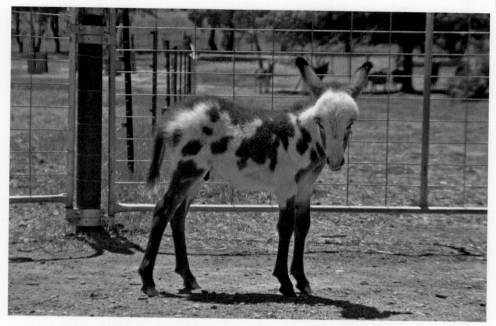

Figure 12.25 Many **spotted** donkeys have distinctively round colored areas within their white areas. The color tends to persist along the backline in most **spotted** donkeys. *Source:* courtesy of Bianca Haase.

of neck, which is white) and some on the tail. Generally the withers remain colored (Figure 12.26). Even the most extensively white **spotted** donkeys tend to have colored ears and eye patches (Figure 12.27).

Variants on the main pattern of white patches are rare. One of these is called **tyger**, which is illustrated in Figures 12.28 and 12.29. These donkeys are almost always predominantly white, with residual colored areas that are usually smaller and more round than in the usual **spotted** pattern. The spots on **tyger** donkeys also tend to have halos around them where pigmented skin or roan areas make them intermediate between the colored spot and the white background. Many **tyger** spotted donkeys have more color on the neck, and especially the top of the neck, than do **spotted** donkeys.

A few **spotted** donkeys have white lower legs and feet. This is an unusual finding in any donkeys, and so is noteworthy as a peculiar detail. These donkeys usually have extensive facial white as well.

Rarely are donkeys solid **white**, and recently the phenotype has been termed **dominant white** to reflect the similarity in genetics of this phenotype to dominant white in horses. Such animals are revered as good saddle mounts in some Middle Eastern countries. These have white hair, pink skin, and dark eyes. The name **white** is frequently but incorrectly applied to **ivory** animals as well as truly **white** animals. Both types exist in donkeys, and it is important to separate the two classes because they are genetically distinct from one another.

Some donkeys are born **spotted** with only a few pale-colored areas, and then usually these areas rapidly progress to nearly **white**. These animals are called **fully frosted**

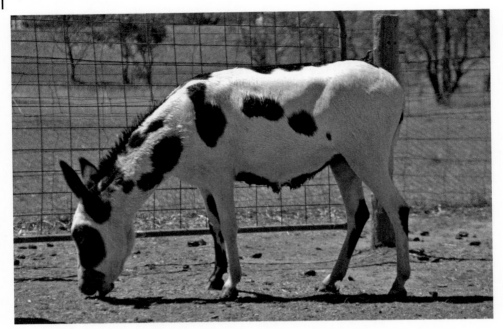

Figure 12.26 As the extent of white progresses, the characteristic roundness of the spots remains evident. *Source:* courtesy of Bianca Haase.

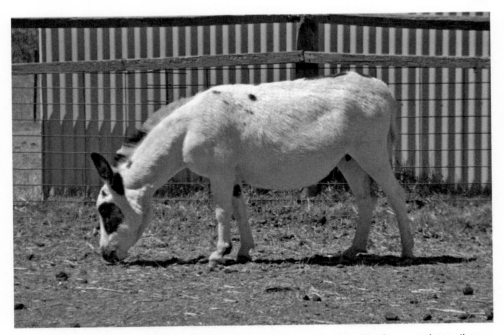

Figure 12.27 Extensively white **spotted** donkeys usually have enough colored areas to be easily recognized as **spotted**. *Source:* courtesy of Bianca Haase.

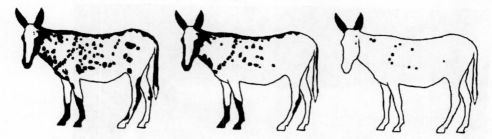

Figure 12.28 Progression of white, from moderate, to greatest, on donkeys with the **tyger** subtype of the **spotted** pattern.

spotted white because they combine characteristics of **spotted** donkeys and **frosted** donkeys. These can be easily confused with **white** donkeys if they are seen only at maturity.

Another type of all-white donkey occurs in a feral population on the Italian island of Asinara, northwest of Sardinia (Figure 12.30). These donkeys are completely **white**, lacking pigment in their skin, hair, and eyelashes. In contrast to **dominant white** donkeys, the eyes on these are light blue. These albino donkeys have low visual acuity, and are sensitive to sunlight.

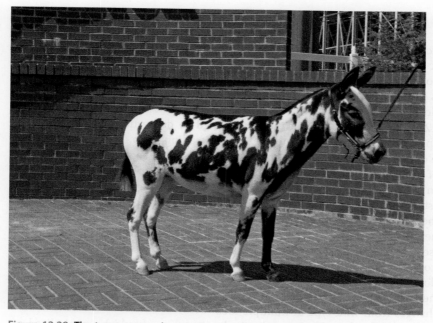

Figure 12.29 The **tyger** pattern has small spots of color within white areas. *Source:* courtesy of L. J. and Deb Mix.

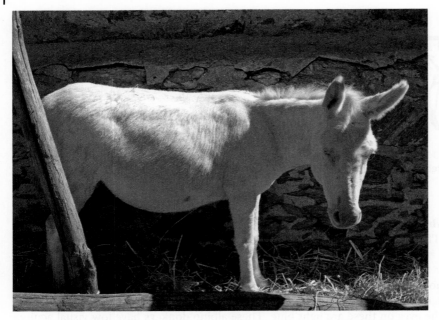

Figure 12.30 A white coat, pink skin, and pale blue eyes characterize **albino** donkeys. *Source:* courtesy of Valerio Joe Utzeri.

12.3   Genetics of Donkey Color and Patterns

The genetic transmission of donkey colors has not been extensively studied; however, five genetic mutations that help to explain donkey color variation have been identified. Evidence collected by the American Donkey and Mule Society indicates that the overall situation is generally analogous to that of horses. The genes proposed (and known) for donkey color are outlined in Table 12.3, and the interactions of these are summarized in Table 12.4. More studies of wild donkeys mated to domestic ones would clarify relationships between some colors and the loci controlling them. With the expanding knowledge of the genetics of horse coat color, comparison of genes identified in horse with that of donkey will likely unravel additional mutations contributing to donkey color variation in the near future.

The most common color in most populations of domesticated donkeys is **grey dun**, which is the wild-type color of donkeys. This is an interesting exception to nearly all other domesticated animals, where the wild-type color is very rare. **Grey dun** is very common, so it also happens that most deviations from **grey dun** are due to single-gene changes from the wild type. This phenomenon makes understanding the basics of donkey color somewhat easier than that of horses, but does little to document or explain some of the interesting colors that could result by assembling, all on a single animal, multiple changes from wild-type at multiple loci.

As is the case in horses, the **dun** color is dominant, so should be symbolized as *Dun* (Dn^+) at the *Dun* locus unless further research contradicts this proposal. *Dun* changes any dark color to a lighter color and maintains the distinctive and variable

Table 12.3 Proposed loci and alleles affecting donkey color. DNA mutations that have been identified are also noted.

Locus	Allele	Symbol	Action	Comment	Mutations identified
Agouti	bay	A^A	Dominant	Causes reddish body with black trim	
	brown black	A^b	Intermediate	Causes tan regions on head and ears	
	wild type	A^+	Recessive	Causes black with light points	
Ivory	wild type	I^+	Dominant	Full color expression	
	ivory	I^i	Recessive	Dilute with cream color, darker trim, blue eyes	
Cameo	cameo	Cam^C	Dominant	Dilute with pale skin, pale eyes	
	wild type	Cam^+	Recessive	Allows dark colors	
Dun	wild type	Dn^+	Dominant	Causes light body color, retains dark trim	
	nondun	Dn^{nd}	Recessive	Allows dark colors	
Extension	wild type	E^+	Dominant	Allows black in coat	
	chestnut	Ee	Recessive	Red throughout coat	c.629T>C in MC1R
Agouti	wild type	A^+	Dominant	Light points	
	no light points	A^{nlp}	Recessive	Dark points	c.349T>C in ASIP
Spotted ass	spotted	KIT^A	Dominant	Causes spotting, likely lethal to homozygotes	c.1978+2T>A in KIT
Dominant white	White	KIT^{Y221S}	Dominant	White coat, pink skin and dark eye	c.662A>C in KIT
	wild type	KIT^+	Recessive	Pigmented coat and skin	
Albino white	wild type	TYR^+	Dominant	Pigmented coat, skin, and dark eyes	
	albino	TYR^{H202D}	Recessive	White coat, blue eyes, white lashes	c.604C>G in TYR

striping patterns on donkeys. The effect of *Dun* on a black background is to give the familiar **grey dun** color of donkeys. Most donkeys are either **grey dun** or **black**. Despite being common, the mutation responsible for the dun phenotype in donkeys has not been identified.

Donkeys have an allele homologous to *chestnut* in horses at the *Extension* locus; and like in horses, the allele in donkeys is recessive. This eliminates black in the coat, similar to the action of the *chestnut* allele in horses. The mutation has recently been identified to be a single base change in the *MC1R* gene and is noted as c.629T>C. This change in the DNA is predicted to alter the function of the protein. If two copies of this allele are present (and therefore no functional protein is produced) this results in **red**, or **sorrel**, animals, usually with light points.

Table 12.4 Theoretical relationships of various donkey colors, showing the component effects present or absent in various colors.

Color	E^+	E^e	Dn^+	Dn^{nd}	A^a	A^+	A^A	C^d
Grey dun	+		+			+		
Black	+	−		+		+		
Sorrel	−	+	− or +?	+		−	−	
Rose dun	−	+	+			−	−	
Dun, dark points	+		+		+	+		
Black, dark points	+	−		+	+	+		
Sorrel, dark points	−	+	−	+	+	−	−	
Red dun, dark points	−	+	+		+	−	−	
Bay	+	−		+			+	
Ivory								++

The combination of *dun* and *chestnut* is undocumented, but is probably very close to **sorrel** in most animals. In the Mammoth breed *dun* is rare, and most animals are either **black** or **sorrel** because segregation at *Extension* is responsible for most color variation in that breed. In Miniature Donkeys the usual color is **grey dun**, and **sorrel** segregates from it as the expected recessive. These Miniature **sorrels** vary from dark to light, and most, if not all, of them have the Dn^+ allele as well. Their final color is frequently close to that of the Mammoth sorrels, nearly all of which lack Dn^+. This indicates that the combination of *Dun* and *chestnut* is not always a distinctively lighter color than *nondun* and *chestnut*. As a result of this, the few obviously **rose dun** or **pink** donkeys are unexplained, although these might well be combinations of Dn^+ and E^e, but probably have additional genetic information to yield the final light color.

Donkeys that are intermediate between **grey dun** and **black**, **black** and **sorrel**, and **grey dun** and **sorrel** are relatively common. These tend to be sought after in the Miniature Donkey breed. These colors are difficult to accurately identify, so genetic mechanisms for their production have not been documented. **Black with cross** and **brown** appear nearly **black** in most cases, and genetic distinctions between these and **grey dun** or **black** have been difficult to document. The mating together of these colors (like to like) tends to produce mostly the same color as the parents, but with enough variation in the other directions (both lighter and darker) that no repeatable dominance relationships emerge.

Bay donkeys are so distinctive that it is tempting to suggest that these are at the *Agouti* locus similar to analogous alleles in horses. However, unlike horses, a mutation responsible for the difference between bay and black donkeys has not been reported. **Russets** are sometimes difficult to cleanly separate from either **bay** or **sorrel**. In at least one case the mating of **sorrel** to **russet** has produced a **black**, which indicates that the control of these two colors is different and probably resides at two separate loci. In contrast to this, some **russet** animals in the Mammoth breed reproduce as if they were **sorrel** genetically. Additionally, **russet** occurs relatively frequently in Miniature Donkeys when **sorrels** are mated to either **blacks** or **grey duns**, indicating a potential relationship to a *chestnut*-based mechanism for this color. It may well be that some **russets** are essentially **sorrels** with very dark trim, while others are **bay** with lighter legs, either through extensive **light points** or from being **frosty** or **roan**. The phenotypic distinctions between the two types appear to be subtle, and these distinctions usually miss detection by most observers.

Detailed studies of **brown** and **brown-black** have not been documented. In at least a few families of Mammoth Jacks the **brown-black** color is passed consistently to offspring from **brown-black** parents, suggesting that this might be a dominant allele. If so, it is likely at the *Agouti* locus and intermediate between *wild type* and *bay*. The **brown-black** animals of this breed are distinctive and stand out from the more usual **black** Mammoths.

Ivory behaves differently than **cream** in horses. Homozygous donkeys are **ivory** with blue eyes. However, the expected yellow color of heterozygotes is not evident on donkeys as it is in **palomino** and **buckskin** horses. This absence of yellow donkeys could possibly be due to the rarity of **sorrel** and **bay** and the inability of the genetic mechanism of **ivory**, in a heterozygous state, to act on colors based on **black** (such as **black** and **grey dun**), which are so common among donkeys.

Most **ivory** donkeys occur in the Miniature breed as a single recessive deviation from **grey dun**, so the appropriate and elusive combinations to determine heterozygous effect on red-based colors may simply not have arisen. Alternatively, **ivory** may be due to a true recessive and therefore be unlike the *cremello* allele in horses. The distinct allele name *ivory* is appropriate, because DNA tests on **ivory** donkeys have demonstrated that these lack the same mutation as *cremello* in horses. The **ivory** color on a **black** background has been documented in Miniature Donkeys and is a much darker tan color than the usual off-white that is characteristic of the combination of **ivory** with **grey dun**. It is possible that *ivory* is analogous to *pearl* in horses.

The **dark points** (also called **no light points** or **NLP** for short) condition is recessive to the more usual light points. This variant occurs in Miniature Donkeys, feral burros, and very rarely in Mammoth Jackstock as well as Normand Donkeys. **Dark points** usually occur on a **grey dun** or a **black** body color, although they can occur on any color. The lack of **dark points** appears to be homologous to the case in horses. Recent molecular work identified a single nucleotide polymorphism at the *Agouti* locus (c.349 T>C) that explained **NLP** in Normand and miniature donkeys. Phenotyping studies have shown that the *nlp* allele varies in its penetrance, with some donkeys having only a dark nose and still retaining some pallor in the legs. Thus, the extent of the **light points** is variable in donkeys and is probably controlled by multiple genes (polygenic) so that some donkeys have minor **light points** while the **light points** on others are very extensive. The "no light points" characteristic has never been noted on a **red** or **sorrel** background, which is consistent with the *Agouti* mutation identified.

Cameo is a rare color in donkeys that has not been directly investigated, but it does occur in directly succeeding generations. This implies that it is due to a dominant gene, which may make it analogous to **champagne** in horses. The two jacks known to have the **cameo** dilution have both produced dilute and nondilute foals when mated to unrelated jennets, which also indicates that a dominant gene is likely involved.

The mating of **spotted** donkeys results in foal production consistent with **spotting** being due to a single dominant allele (KIT^A for *spotted* at the *KIT* locus). The production of **spotted** foals from **spotted** to **spotted** matings is about two **spotted** foals to one **nonspotted** foal, which indicates loss of homozygous embryos similar to the situation with the *dominant white* allele of horses. In no cases have **spotted** donkeys been documented as being homozygous, so it is a reasonable conclusion that all **spotted** donkeys are heterozygous and that homozygotes never survive the embryonic period. A mutation in the *KIT* gene (the same gene responsible for many white patch patterns in horses) has been identified in **spotted** donkeys and termed c.1978+2T>A (KIT^A allele). The four spotted donkeys in the study were all heterozygous for this mutation while all of the solid donkeys were homozygous for the *wild-type* allele (KIT^T allele). These data are consistent with embryonic lethality for the homozygous condition (KIT^A/KIT^A), and investigating additional donkey breeds will help to determine if all spotted donkeys are caused by the same mutation.

The extent of **spotting** varies from minimal to maximal. Minimally **spotted** animals consistently have at least a blaze on the face. These animals reproduce as if they were **spotted** even though they lack white body patches. Donkeys with only a **star**, in contrast, do not have the *spotted* allele and fail to reproduce the **spotted** pattern. It appears that all **spotted** donkeys have this single major gene, though it is likely that future investigations will provide evidence for major modifiers that produce the **tyger** and white-legged variants.

One possible additional and distinct white pattern occurs in a few families, most often in Miniature Donkeys. These tend to have a large forehead **star**, and sometimes a **snip**. A few of these also have white **socks**.

The **roan** pattern is genetically confusing. When **blue roans** are crossed, the result is usually **blue roan** or occasionally **black**. **Black** to **black** matings do not produce **blue roan** foals. These results indicate that **roan** is most likely dominant. Strangely, though, **strawberry roans** are produced from non**roan sorrel** parents, indicating a recessive tendency for **roan** on *chestnut*-based colors. This is a confusing result and is consistent enough that it cannot be attributed to misidentification of the animals. It might be that the dominance relationship is reversed depending on the remaining color genotype, or it might be that multiple types of roaning occur in donkeys. A third explanation is that low grades of expression of **roan** are more easily overlooked on red than on black backgrounds. No reports investigating the roan phenotype at the molecular level have been reported.

Donkeys that are genetically both **roan** and **spotted** are generally **white** or nearly so. They may be born with some residual small spots of color, but these quickly fade to white. These animals are called **fully frosted spotted white** and can produce **roan**, **spotted**, **fully frosted spotted white**, and solid-colored foals when mated to solid-colored mates.

White-born donkeys (all white coat, pink skin, and dark eyes) are rare. The mode of inheritance has not been investigated by family studies. In conjunction with studying the molecular genetics of the white **spotted** phenotype, a mutation explaining this rare phenotype has been discovered in the *KIT* gene (c.662A>C). In this study, one donkey with this phenotype was heterozygous for this mutation. The mutation is in the same gene as that in horses, and the white phenotype is similar to that of **dominant white** in horses, so this **white** phenotype in donkeys has been designated **dominant white**. It will be interesting to see if other **dominant white** donkeys also carry this same missense mutation, or if the molecular control is more variable, as is the situation in horses with **white** phenotypes.

Albino white has been investigated in a feral donkey population with this phenotype on Asinara Island. Because of the resemblance to albinism in other species, specifically oculocutaneous albinism type 1 in humans, the gene *tyrosinase* (*TYR*), was investigated. A single change in the DNA at this locus (c.604C>G) results in a change in the protein that is believed to disrupt its function. The 82 albino donkeys all tested homozygous for this mutation, while the grey donkeys in this study from the same population where either homozygous *wild type* or heterozygous. This indicates that the **albino white** phenotype has a recessive mode of inheritance. Determining the origin of this mutation and how it has been maintained in a feral population despite the adverse effects associated remains to be investigated.

12.4 Summary of Donkey Color and Patterns

Color attributes of donkeys have generally played less of a role in selection than has color in horses. In regions where donkeys are used as essential partners in a subsistence setting, the luxury of selecting for color has simply not been possible. In other regions, where donkey breeding has not been tied to subsistence, some selection for color has been undertaken. Colors in donkeys can be subtle, and the overlap between neighboring color designations can be confusing.

Color has been highly selected in some of the large, mule-breeding donkeys from the Mediterranean region. These tend to have fairly consistent color, such as **black with light points** in the Poitou, Leonesa-Zamorano, and Catalonian, and **blue roan** (along with other **roans**) in the Andalusian. The American Mammoth Jack, with roots in these and other large European breeds, was selected for years to be **black with light points**, but also include **brown-black** as an acceptable variant. This color bias came from the desire of mule buyers to have dark-colored mules, which could be produced consistently from **black** jacks mated to mares of nearly any color.

More recently, the market for mules has changed, and buyers of large draft mules prefer **sorrel** mules. As a consequence, selection in the American Mammoth has now switched from **black with light points** to **flaxen sorrel**, because **sorrel** jacks routinely produce **sorrel** mules from **blond sorrel** mares that are so common in the American Belgian breed. Many breeders note that **sorrel** jacks tend to be larger and more heavily boned than are **black** jacks, even within the same family. This could be a pleiotropic effect of the allele causing the **sorrel** color.

Coupled with this change in the draft mule market has been a resurgence of interest in saddle mules as well as saddle donkeys. For buyers of saddle mules and donkeys no specific single color is preferred, but rather any unusual colors are avidly sought. This has relaxed restrictions for color in the jacks producing these mules as well as in jacks used for producing donkeys. The jacks serving this purpose are usually American Mammoth Jacks or Large Standard Jacks. In the past, **roan**, **grey dun**, **spotted**, and **white** jacks were severely penalized, but some mule breeders now avidly seek them.

Most of the white patterns (in horses or donkeys) are passed to mule offspring as expected by their inheritance in either species. That is, most are dominant. **Tobiano** is an interesting exception, in that **tobiano** mules usually do not have body patches, but rather have only four white legs as if they only minimally expressed the **tobiano** pattern. Moderate **sabino** patterns are another exception, so that mules from mares with moderate to extensive face, leg, and belly white rarely express as much white as their dams. Usually, these foals have a star as a maximal marking and have no leg white. **White mules do occur**, but the exact genetic makeup of these is uncertain as to the alleles they have inherited from either the jack sire or the mare dam.

In Miniature Donkeys the recent trend has been for buyers to prefer rare and unusual colors. This has greatly increased variability of color in this size class of donkeys. In the past, most Miniature Donkeys were **grey dun**. Recent selection has favored **sorrel**, **spotted**, **ivory**, **white**, and **brown**. **Black with dark points** has also increased in popularity because an entirely black donkey is unusual. Most of the variations in color of Miniature Donkeys arise from changes from wild type at only a single locus at a time. As a result, most of these colors segregate from **grey dun** parents. As the less common colors are increasingly produced and mated among themselves (as opposed to back to **grey dun**), they will produce new combinations of mutant alleles simultaneously at several loci. This is similar to the situation in Miniature Horses, and the result is the wide array of colors in that breed. These new combinations will continue to shed light on the intricacies of genetic control of donkey color.

12.5 Hair Growth in Donkeys

Donkeys vary in the amount and texture of their hair. In general, donkeys have much less mane and tail hair than do horses. Mane hairs are coarser in donkeys than in horses, and tend to be upright on most donkeys. The body coat of donkeys is quite variable and ranges from very short and slick in breeds such as the American Mammoth, to very long and corded in the Poitou. It is generally true that the winter coat of donkeys is very shaggy. Many of these shed off slick in the summer. Some donkeys maintain a relatively fuzzy coat throughout the year with a longer summer coat than is typically seen, which can make subtle differences in color difficult to appreciate. In addition, some individuals display a long hair coat throughout the year without any change.

A study investigating long hair in Poitou donkeys determined a recessive mode of inheritance. The *fibroblast growth factor 5* gene (*FGF5*), a gene known to cause long-hair phenotype in other mammals, has two mutations associated with the long-hair phenotype in donkey: c.245G>A and c.433_434delAT. These alleles have been termed $FGF5^{l\text{-}donkey}$ and $FGF5^{l\text{-}poitou}$ respectively. Long-hair Poitou donkeys were either homozygous for the deletion mutation ($FGF5^{l\text{-}poitou}$) allele or were compound heterozygotes having one copy of each of the mutated alleles. It is possible that these mutations also explain long hair in other donkey breeds, because carriers for these mutations have been identified in the other short-haired breeds.

While most horses have at least one whorl in the flank region, whorls are rare in donkeys. Leg feathering is also rare in donkeys, even in those used for draft mule production. Mules produced from feathered horse breeds, such as Shire, Clydesdale, or Mulassier, usually have minimal feathering. Thus, while donkeys and horses have many similarities in phenotypes, there are differences that make studying both species interesting and important to unravel the molecular mechanisms of their beauty.

13

Summary Tables

Horse color names are summarized in Table 13.1. The names for main color category designations are usually used in a narrow sense for a specific color within the category, as well as for the category as a whole.

The main features of each pattern of white hairs are summarized in Table 13.2.

The results of genes affecting colors are listed in Table 13.3. The loci and the various alleles are outlined, with the mechanism of action if it is known. Alleles that are only proposals are indicated by question marks. *Wild-type* alleles are the original sequences for the locus, and are called "reference type" because the various mutated alleles are compared with this sequence.

The results of genes affecting patterns of white hairs are outlined in Table 13.4. The loci and the various alleles are outlined, with the mechanism of action if it is known. *Wild-type* alleles are the original sequences for the locus, and are called "reference type" because the various mutated alleles are compared with this sequence. For most loci the *wild type* has no DNA test, but for a handful a test is available.

Table 13.5 is a list of the usual genotypes of major colors. This table assumes accurate and reasonably detailed identification of horse colors, so that **brown** is separated out from **sooty bay**, **sorrel** from **mealy chestnut**, and **smoky** is never misidentified as **black**. In addition, **brown, seal brown,** and **brown-black** are assumed to be reliably identifiable, Table 13.5 includes only alleles at the *A, C, Ch, Dn, E, Mu, Pa,* and *Z* loci. Other effects (including shade, **sooty, mane color** on **chestnuts,** and **brindle**) are generally trivial or are so poorly understood genetically that they do not belong here. E^B is included as the cause of **sooty** colors with black points, even though this is unproven. **Dominant black** is assigned to E^D, though this is likewise unproven. Genotypes are presented as alleles that are usually present and responsible for the colors listed.

Alleles that are present in several breeds in the USA are listed in Table 13.6. Each breed has alleles that are usual for the breed and also has alleles that are somewhat unusual by virtue of being rare or having been the target of negative selection. This list is by no means complete and is meant only as a guide to the overall genetic machinery within the various breeds. Alleles coding for white patterns are only noted if present; the neutral allele (that for no pattern) is not listed because these occur in nearly all breeds. The *cremello, dun, champagne, mushroom, pearl,* and *silver dapple* alleles are likewise only noted if present, and their absence is not noted.

Table 13.7 includes the expected foal colors resulting from crossing various parental colors. Exact percentages for different colors always depend on the specific parental

Equine Color Genetics, Fourth Edition. D. Phillip Sponenberg and Rebecca Bellone.
© 2017 John Wiley & Sons, Inc. Published 2017 by John Wiley & Sons, Inc.

Table 13.1   Color names by major categories.

Color group	Color name	Body color	Point color	Comments
Bay	Bay	Red, tan, or brown	Black	
	Mahogany bay	Dark red brown	Black	
	Blood bay	Dark clear red	Black	
	Cherry bay	Bright red	Black	
	Red bay	Red	Black	
	Sandy bay	Tan red	Black	
	Gold bay	Gold red	Black	
	Honey bay	Light tan	Black	
	Mealy bay	Red with light flanks, muzzle	Black	
Black	Black	Black	Black	
	Raven black	Shiny black	Black	
	Jet black	Dark black	Black	Nonfading
	Summer black	Faded black	Black	Fading
	Smoky	Black or off-black	Black	Carries **palomino**
Brown	Brown	Sooty red or sooty tan	Black	
	Seal brown	Black, light flanks, muzzle	Black	
	Brown black	Uniform dark brown	Black	
	Light brown	Sooty tan–red	Black	
Buckskin	Buckskin	Yellow	Black	No stripes
	Sooty buckskin	Sooty yellow	Black	No stripes
	Golden buckskin	Gold yellow	Black	No stripes
	Silvery buckskin	Silver or white	Black	No stripes
Champagne	Champagne (classic)	Light pinkish brown, shiny	Brown	Pale skin, pale eyes
	Amber champagne	Yellow or beige, shiny	Brown	Pale skin, pale eyes
	Gold champagne	Gold yellow, shiny	Yellow or white	Pale skin, pale eyes
	Pale champagne	Pale beige, shiny	Light brown	Pale skin, pale eyes
	Ivory champagne	Nearly white, shiny	White	Pale skin, pale eyes
	White champagne	White, shiny	White	Pale skin, pale eyes
Chestnut	Chestnut	Red	Brown, red, or flaxen	
	Black chestnut	Nearly black	Usually dark	Fetlocks are red

Table 13.1 (*Continued*)

Color group	Color name	Body color	Point color	Comments
	Liver chestnut	Dark red	Brown, red, or flaxen	
	Red chestnut	Deep red	Brown, red, or flaxen	
	Golden chestnut	Gold red	Brown, red, or flaxen	
	Copper chestnut	Bright medium red	Brown, red or flaxen	
	Light chestnut	Light red	Brown, red, or flaxen	
	Yellow chestnut	Yellow red	Brown, red, or flaxen	
Cream	Cream	Pale	Pale	Blue eyes, pink skin
	Smoky cream	Dark cream	Light brown	Blue eyes, pink skin
	Perlino	Cream to off-white	Light brown	Blue eyes, pink skin
	Cremello	Cream to off-white	White	Blue eyes, pink skin
Dun	Dun	Light	Variable	Primitive marks
	Zebra dun	Tan	Black	Primitive marks
	Peanut butter dun	Rich medium tan	Black	Primitive marks
	Coyote dun	Sooty tan	Black	Primitive marks
	Golden dun	Clear gold	Black	Primitive marks
	Dusty dun	Flat beige	Black	Primitive marks
	Silvery dun	Very light tan	Black	Primitive marks
	Cream dun	Nearly white	Black	Primitive marks
Grullo	Grullo	Slate to beige, dark head	Black	Primitive marks
	Mouse dun	Slate beige, dark head	Black	Primitive marks
	Blue dun	Slate beige, dark head	Black	Primitive marks
	Lobo dun	Dark blue or sooty blue, dark head	Black	Primitive marks
	Slate grullo	Medium slate blue, dark head	Black	Primitive marks
	Olive dun	Tan beige, dark head	Black	Primitive marks
	Silvery grullo	Light slate blue, dark head	Black	Primitive marks

(*continued*)

Table 13.1   (*Continued*)

Color group	Color name	Body color	Point color	Comments
Mushroom	**Mushroom**	Flat uniform tan, dark to light	Light tan	Rarely dappled
Palomino	**Palomino**	Yellow	Pale	
	Golden palomino	Gold yellow	Usually white	
	Linebacked palomino	Gold yellow	Pale	Primitive marks
	Sooty palomino	Gold with sooty black overlay	Pale, or silver	
	Isabelo	Light beige or nearly white	White	
Pearl	**Pearl (classic)**	Pale pinkish brown	Medium brown	Pale skin, pale eyes
	Amber pearl	Light yellow or tan	Medium brown	Pale skin, pale eyes
	Gold pearl	Gold yellow	Light or cream	Pale skin, pale eyes
	Ivory pearl	Ivory or nearly white	Pale	Pale skin, pale eyes
Red dun	**Red dun**	Medium red	Usually darker red	Primitive marks
	Muddy dun	Medium flat red, brown head	Dark red or brown	Primitive marks
	Orange dun	Medium to light red	Medium to light red	Primitive marks
	Apricot dun	Light red, light shading	Medium to flaxen	Primitive marks
	Claybank dun	Light yellowish red	Variable	Primitive marks
Silver dapple	**Blue silver**	Bluish brown	Flaxen, mixed, or dark	
	Chocolate silver	Brown, often dappled	Flaxen, mixed, or dark	
	Black silver	Nearly black	Flaxen, mixed, or dark	
	Brown silver	Brown with red tone	Flaxen, mixed, or dark	
	Red silver	Red	Flaxen, mixed, or dark	
	Yellow silver	Yellow or gold	Flaxen, mixed, or dark	
	Pale silver	Light	Light	
Sorrel	**Sorrel**	Shaded red	Dark, red, silver, or flaxen	Light flanks, belly
	Blond sorrel	Yellow red	Flaxen	Light flanks, belly

Table 13.2 Patterns of white hairs.

Pattern	Subtype	Defining characteristics
Birdcatcher spots		Small random white spots over body
Frame		Dark feet, white on head, body spots horizontal
Frosty roan	**Squaw mane**	Individual white hairs in mane
	Squaw tail	Individual white hairs in tail
Grey		Progressive whitening with age. Specific variations are as follows
	Porcelain grey	Nearly white over dark skin
	Dappled grey	Dapples with light centers, darker peripheries
	Fleabitten grey	Retains small flecks of color which can increase with age
	Rose grey	Grey on a reddish base coat
	Iron grey	Nondappled medium grey
	Bloodmarked grey	Red areas grow in and enlarge with age
Leopard complex		Symmetrical white patterns typically centered over the rump, along with white sclera and striped hooves. Specific variations are as follows
	Mottled	Small flecks of white/pink on skin, some in haircoat
	Snowflake	Small irregular white spots scattered over coat
	Speckled	Small irregular colored areas remaining in largely roan or white coat
	Frosted hips	Roan or flecked areas over hips
	Varnish roan	Roan with dark areas over bony prominences
	Marble	Veins of color and white interlacing
	Buttermilk roan	Patchy roan
	Spotted blanket	White centered over hips, with **leopard spots**
	Snow cap blanket	White centered over hips, lacks **leopard spots**
	Leopard	Largely white with **leopard spots**
	Few spot leopard	Largely white with few or no **leopard spots**
	Leopard spots	Dark round or oval spots in white regions
	Lightning strikes	White on legs, usually with colored coronary bands
Manchado		White dorsally and in middle of body, roundish dark spots in white areas
Classic roan		Mix of white hairs into body, sparing points and head. Specific names for different base coats are as follows
	Blue roan	Roan on a black base
	Purple roan	Roan on a brown base
	Red roan	Roan on a bay base
	Lilac roan	Roan on a dark chestnut base

(continued)

Table 13.2 (*Continued*)

Pattern	Subtype	Defining characteristics
	Strawberry roan	Roan on a medium chestnut or sorrel base
	Honey roan	Roan on a light sorrel base
Roaned		Light sprinkling of white hairs, distinct from **classic roan**
Sabino		White on feet, head. Speckled, roan, or spotted body, variations described as follows
	Calico	Synonym for **sabino**
	Flecked	Synonym for **sabino**
	Buttermilk roan	Synonym for **sabino**
	Particolor	Used for Arabians with **sabino** patterns
	Spanish roan	Synonym for **sabino**
	Lightning strikes	Irregular white marks on legs
Splashed white		Crisp white on head, legs, lower body
Tobiano		Crisp white on legs, vertically on body, not on head
	Calico tobiano	**Tobiano** with yellow and red patches
White		White or nearly so
White lacing		Network of connected white lines on back
White ticking		Roan in flanks and base of tail; synonyms as follows
	Skunk tail	Roan tail
	Rabicano	Synonym for **white ticking**
	Coon tail	Roan tail

genotypes that are crossed (homozygous versus heterozygous). Because specific geno-types are rarely known, exact percentages of foal colors are not given in the table because they will be misleading in most cases. Accurate identification of parental colors is assumed. For example, no **smoky** horses are misidentified as **black**.

Table 13.7 is divided into different categories of offspring color. Some offspring colors are consistently produced, assuming that parental colors are homozygous for all dominant genes they possess. These are noted in the "Always" column, and these colors can always be expected as a percentage of the foal crop from the specific cross.

Other colors are expected to occur frequently in most breeds if certain fairly common recessives are present in the parents. These colors are in the "Common" column.

Colors in the "Occasional" column are those that will appear in most breeds, but are due to recessives that are fairly rare or are produced only occasionally due to the specific crosses made.

Colors in the "Rare" column will appear in some crosses, but are caused by alleles that are very rare in most breeds and therefore are not to be routinely expected. It must always be remembered that some rare colors are indeed likely or even assured as a result of specific crosses when rare genotypes are present as both sire and dam.

Table 13.3 Loci affecting color, with their alleles and the effects of the alleles.

Locus	Allele	Symbol	Action	Comment	Molecular mechanism	DNA test
Agouti signaling protein (ASIP)						
Agouti	*wild*	A^+ (?)	Dominant	Causes **wild bay**		No
	bay	A^A	Intermediate	Causes **bay**	Considered *wild type* by most	Yes
	black and tan	A^t	Intermediate	Causes **seal brown**	Not reported	Not currently
	black	A^a	Recessive	Causes **black**	11 bp deletion	Yes
Arabian dilution	?	?	Recessive	Lightens base color, skin, eyes	Unknown	No
Dominant black (*Extension* or *Beta defensin*)	*dominant black*	?	Dominant	Epistatic to *Agouti*; results in **black** or **brown-black**	Unknown	No
Flaxen	?	?	Polygenic	Varies the mane and tail color on the colors based on **chestnut**	Unknown	No
Membrane-associated transport protein (MATP)						
Cream	*wild*	C^+	Intermediate	Allows intense color	Reference type	No
	cremello	C^{Cr}	Intermediate	Heterozygotes: red diluted to yellow, black unaffected Homozygotes: red and black diluted to cream, pink skin, blue eyes	G457A missense mutation	Yes
	pearl	C^{pr}	Recessive	Mimics *champagne*	Not reported	Yes
Membrane-bound transcription factor peptidase, site 2 (MBPTS2)	*wild*			Normal color	Reference type	
brindle 1	*brindle-1*	*Br1*	X-linked dominant	Causes vertical striping with contrasting color and texture, sparse mane and tail	c.1437+4T>C (intron mutation)	Yes
Melanocortin receptor 1 (MC1R)	*dominant black*	E^D (?)	Dominant	Epistatic to *Agouti*; results in **black** or **brown-black**	Undocumented	No
Extension	*brown*	E^B (?)	Intermediate	Modifies *Agouti* to have sooty countershading	Undocumented	No

(continued)

Table 13.3 (Continued)

Locus	Allele	Symbol	Action	Comment	Molecular mechanism	DNA test
	wild	E^+	Intermediate	Allows *Agouti* colors	Reference type	No
	chestnut	E^e	Recessive	Epistatic to *Agouti*; results in **chestnut**	C901T (missense)	Yes
	chestnut	E^a	Recessive	Epistatic to *Agouti*; results in **chestnut**	codon 84 (GAC>AAC) (missense)	Yes
Mushroom	wild	Mu^+	Dominant	Allows intense colors	Unreported	No
	mushroom	Mu^M	Recessive	Changes **chestnut** to **mushroom**	Unreported	No
Pangaré	wild	Pa^+	Dominant	Causes **mealy** effect	Unreported	No
	non-pangaré	Pa^{np}	Recessive	Colors without the **mealy** effect	Unreported	No
Premelanosomal protein 17 (PMEL) Silver	silver	Z^Z	Dominant	Dilutes black to chocolate brown or flaxen; does not affect red	C1457T (missense)	Yes
	wild	Z^+	Recessive	Allows **nonsilver** colors	Reference type	No
Shade	?	?	Polygenic?	Varies the relative shade of body color from light to dark; polygenic	Unreported	No
Solute carrier family 36 Member 1 (SLC36A1) Champagne	champagne	Ch^C	Dominant	Black changed to light brown, red to yellow	C188G (missense)	Yes
	wild	Ch^+	Recessive	Wild type, black, and red fully expressed	Reference type	Yes
Sooty	?	?	?	Likely a single gene for *Agouti* locus colors, but polygenic on E^eE^e colors	Undocumented	No
T-Box 3 (TBX3) Dun	wild	Dn^+	Dominnt	Causes **linebacked duns**	Reference type	Yes
	non-dun 1	Dn^{d1}	Recessive	Allows nondun colors, with primitive marks	G to T single base change (regulatory)	Yes
	non-dun 2	Dn^{d2}	Recessive	Allows nondun colors, lacking primitive marks	1.6 kilobase pair deletion	Yes

Table 13.4 Loci and alleles controlling patterns of white.

Locus	Allele	Symbol	Action	Comment	Molecular Mechanism	DNA test
Birdcatcher spots	?	?	Unknown	Genetic mechanism not documented	Not documented	No
Calico	*calico tobiano*	*Cal^C*	Dominant	Causes **calico tobiano** on **buckskin** or **palomino tobianos**	Not documented	No
Endothelin receptor b (EDNRB) Frame	*frame*	*Fr^F*	Dominant	**Frame** spotting, homozygous lethal. Test available	TC353-354G dinucleotide missense mutation	Yes
Frosty roan	?	?	Dominant	Roaning in mane, tail, and over bony prominences	Not documented	No
KIT (Dominant white, Sabino 1) (Roan and Tobiano are close by)	*wild*	+	Recessive	Wild type, no pattern	Reference type	Yes
	Tobiano	*To^To*	Dominant	**Tobiano**, homozygotes have "bear paws." Near this locus	Inversion on ECA3q near *KIT*	Yes
	Roan	*Rn^Rn*	Dominant	**Roan** (near this locus)	Exact change is unknown	Yes
	Sabino 1	*Sb1^Sb1*	Intermediate	**Sabino** spotting, homozygotes whiter than heterozygotes	KI16+1037 T>A (intron mutation)	Yes
	Dominant white W1 to W24	*W1 to W24*	Dominant	**Dominant white**	Various; see Table 7.1 for details	Yes, for some
Lacing	?	?	Dominant?	White lacing over back of horse	Unknown	No
Manchado	?	?	Recessive?	Causes **manchado** pattern,	Unknown	No
Microphthalmia-associated transcription factor (MITF) Splashed white-1 and -3	*Splashed white-1*	*SW1*	Dominant	**Splashed white 1** pattern	Insertion of 11 base pairs into promoter region	Yes
	Splashed white-3	*SW3*	Dominant	**Splashed white 3** pattern	c.837_841delGTGTC	Yes
Paired Box 3 (PAX3)	*Spalshed white-2*	*SW2*	Dominant	**Splashed white 2** pattern	c.209G>missense mutation	Yes
Splashed white (3 and 4)	*Splashed white-4*	*SW4*	Dominant	**Splashed white** in some Appaloosas	c.95C>G missense mutation	Yes

(continued)

Table 13.4 (*Continued*)

Locus	Allele	Symbol	Action	Comment	Molecular Mechanism	DNA test
Ring Finger And WD Repeat Domain 3 (RFWD3) Pattern-1	*Pattern-1*	*PATN1*[P]	Dominant	Increases extent of **leopard** white pattern	ECA3:23 658 447T>G thought to be regulatory	Yes
Roaned	?	?	Unknown	Minor white hairs in coat	Unknown	No
Syntaxin 17 (STX17) Grey	*grey*	*STX17*[G]	Dominant	Causes progressive greying	4.6 kilobase duplication into intron 6	Yes
Transient Receptor Potential Cation Channel Subfamily M Member 1 (TRPM1) Leopard complex	*leopard*	*Lp*[Lp]	Intermediate	**Leopard** complex spotting, homozygotes often whiter than heterozygotes and lacking dark spots	1378 base pair insertion into intron 1 of gene	Yes
	wild	*Lp*[+]	Recessive	Wild type, no pattern	Reference type	Yes
White marks	?	?	Polygenic	White face and leg marks on any base color	*KIT* and *MITF* are thought to be involved	No
White ticking	?	?	Dominant?	Roaning in flanks and at base of tail	Unknown	No

Table 13.5 Usual genotypes of major colors.

Color group	Details	Alleles responsible for phenotype
Bay	Usual	$A^A,C^+C^+,Ch^+,Dn^{d2},E^+,Mu^m,Pa^{np},Z^+$
	Linebacked	$A^A,C^+C^+,Ch^+,Dn^{d1},E^+,Mu^m,Pa^{np},Z^+$
	Mealy	$A^A,C^+C^+,Ch^+,Dn^{d2},E^+,Mu^m,Pa^+,Z^+$
	Wild	$A^+,C^+C^+,Ch^+,Dn^{d2},E^+,Mu^m,Pa^{np},Z^+$
	Wild, mealy	$A^+,C^+C^+,Ch^+,Dn^{d2},E^+,Mu^m,Pa^+,Z^+$
Black	Usual	$A^a,C^+C^+,Ch^+,Dn^{d2},E^+,Mu^m,Pa^{np},Z^+$
	Sooty	$A^a,C^+C^+,Ch^+,Dn^{d2},E^B,Mu^m,Pa^{np},Z^+$
	Rare	$A^a,C^+C^+,Ch^+,Dn^{d2},E^D,Mu^m,Pa^{np},Z^+$
	Brown black	$A^+,C^+C^+,Ch^+,Dn^{d2},E^D,Mu^m,Pa^{np},Z^+$
	Brown black	$A^A,C^+C^+,Ch^+,Dn^{d2},E^D,Mu^m,Pa^{np},Z^+$
Brown	Sooty	Any **bay** with E^B added
	Brown-black	Any **bay** with E^D added, but only on some horses, not all
	Seal brown	$A^t,C^+C^+,Ch^+,Dn^{d2},E^+,Mu^m,Pa^{np},Z^+$ or $A^a,C^+C^+,Ch^+,Dn^{d2},E^B,Mu^m,Pa^{np},Z^+$ or any **black** plus Pa^+
Chestnut	Chestnut	$—,C^+C^+,Ch^+,Dn^{d2},E^e,Mu^+\ Pa^{np},—$
	Linebacked	$—,C^+C^+,Ch^+,Dn^{d1},E^e,Mu^+\ Pa^{np},—$
	Sorrel	$—,C^+C^+,Ch^+,Dn^{d2},E^e,Mu^+,Pa^+,—$
Dun	Grullo	Any **black** or **seal brown** with Dn^+ but without E^B
	Lobo dun	Any **black** or **seal brown** with Dn^+ and E^B
	Zebra dun	Any **bay** with Dn^+
	Gold dun	Any **bay** with Dn^+ and dark **shade**
	Coyote dun	Any **bay** with Dn^+ and EB
	Red dun	Any **chestnut** with Dn^+
	Apricot dun	Any **sorrel** with Dn^+
Cream-based	Buckskin, usual	Any **bay** plus C^+C^{Cr}
	Buckskin, sooty	Any **sooty** type **brown** with C^+C^{Cr}
	Palomino	**Chestnut** or **sorrel** with C^+C^{Cr}
	Linebacked palomino	**Chestnut** or **sorrel** with Dn^+,C^+C^{Cr}
	Smoky	Any **black** with C^+C^{Cr}
	Smoky seal brown	Any **seal brown** with C^+C^{Cr}
	Cremello	**Chestnut** or **sorrel** with $C^{cr}C^{Cr}$
	Perlino	Any **bay** or **brown** with $C^{cr}C^{Cr}$
	Smoky cream	Any **black** with $C^{Cr}C^{Cr}$
Champagne	Classic	Any **black** with Ch^C
	Sable	**Brown** or **seal brown** with Ch^C
	Amber	Any **bay** with Ch^C
	Gold	Any **chestnut** or **sorrel** with Ch^C
	Pale	Any **black**, **brown**, or **bay** with Ch^C and C^+C^{cr}

(continued)

Table 13.5 (*Continued*)

Color group	Details	Alleles responsible for phenotype
	Pale linebacked	Any **black, brown,** or **bay** with Ch^C, and Dn^+, with or without C^+C^{Cr}
	Ivory	Any **chestnut** or **sorrel** with Ch^C and C^+C^{cr}
Pearl	Classic	Any **black** with $C^{pr}C^{pr}$
	Sable	**Brown** or **seal brown** with $C^{pr}C^{pr}$
	Amber	Any **bay** with $C^{pr}C^{pr}$
	Gold	Any **chestnut** or **sorrel** with $C^{pr}C^{pr}$
	Pale	Any **black, brown,** or **bay** with $C^{Cr}C^{pr}$
	Pale linebacked	Any **black, brown,** or **bay** with $C^{pr}C^{pr}$, or $C^{Cr}C^{pr}$, and Dn^+
	Ivory	Any **chestnut** or **sorrel** with $C^{Cr}C^{pr}$
Silver	Blue, black, chocolate	Any **black** with Z^Z
	Brown	Any **brown** with Z^Z
	Red	Any **bay** with Z^Z
	Yellow silver	Any **brown** or **bay** with Z^Z, with C^+C^{Cr}
	Linebacked yellow silver	Any **brown** or **bay** with Z^Z, with Dn^+, and can also have C^+C^{cr}
	Pale	Any **brown** or **bay** with Z^Z, plus any of C^+C^{Cr}, $C^{Cr}C^{pr}$, $C^{pr}C^{pr}$, Ch^C

In general, the most useful columns will be the "Always" and the "Common" columns. The "Occasional" and "Rare" columns are included for completeness, and are extremely important when considering matings in which horses do indeed have rare alleles.

It is assumed that the relative frequency of alleles at each locus is as follows:

$$A^A >> A^a > A^t > A^+$$

$$C^+ >> C^{Cr} >>>> C^{pr}$$

$$Ch^+ >>> Ch^C$$

$$Dn^{d2} >> Dn^+ >> Dn^{d1}$$

$$E^+ > E^e > E^B >> E^D \quad \left(\begin{array}{l} \text{assuming that } \textbf{dominant black} \text{ resides here,} \\ \text{which it may well not} \end{array} \right)$$

$$Mu^+ >>>> Mu^m$$

$$Pa^{np} >> Pa^+$$

$$Z^+ >>> Z^Z.$$

Some obvious breed differences can change the expectations. In breeds based on Spanish breeding the A^a allele is relatively common, and in the Rocky Mountain Horse (and related breeds) A^a is common, as well as Z^Z. In the Fjord horse Dn^+ is uniform throughout the breed, at the expense of Dn^{d1} and Dn^{d2}. In any breed with an unusual frequency of color genes, colors that are rare in most breeds are expected more frequently.

Table 13.6   Alleles present in representative breeds in the USA.

Breed	Usual color alleles	Unusual color alleles
Akhal Teke	A^A, A^a, C^{Cr}, E^+, E^B, E^e, $Sb1^{Sb1}$, G^G	Dn^+
Albino	$W4$ (most likely), masking many others. C^{Cr}	
American Cream Draft	Ch^C, C^{Cr}, E^e	
American Quarter Horse	Most color alleles	$Sb1^{Sb1}$, Fr^F, Lp^{Lp} persist in low frequencies
American Saddlebred	A^A, A^a, C^{Cr}, Ch^C, E^+, E^B, E^e, $Sb1^{Sb1}$, ToT, G^G	splashed white, uncertain which specific allele
Andalusian	G^G, A^A, A^a	Dn^+, Rn^R, Lp^{Lp}, E^e, C^{Cr}, C^{pr}
Appaloosa	Lp^{Lp} and $PATN1^P$ are common. They determine breed character. Most base color alleles are present, also $PAX3^{SW4}$ in some horses	**Paint** alleles are discouraged, as is G^G
Arabian	A^A, A^a, E^D, E^B, E^+, E^e, G^G	Z^Z, $W3$, $W1$, $W19$, Arabian dilute
Belgian	A^A, A^a, E^e, E^+, E^B, Pa^+, Rn^{Rn}	Some **sabino** pattern
Buckskin	Many. Dn^+ determines breed character. White patterns rarely	
Cleveland Bay	A^A, E^B, E^+	E^e
Clydesdale	A^A, A^a, E^+, E^B, E^e, polygenic sabino	
Colorado Ranger	Lp^{Lp} is widespread because it determines breed character	
Connemara Pony	A^A, A^a, E^+, E^B, E^e, C^{Cr}, Dn^+, G^G	$Sb1^{Sb1}$, Lp^{Lp}, $PATN1^P$
Fjord	Dn^+ as a part of breed character. Also A^A, A^a, E^+, E^e, C^{Cr}	
Florida Cracker	A^A, A^a, E^+, E^B, E^e, C^{Cr}, Dn^+, G^G	
Friesian	A^a, E^+	E^e, Z^Z, Rn^{Rn}
Gotland	A^A, A^a, E^e, E^+, C^{Cr}	Some splashed white
Gypsy Cob	Nearly all, with A^a, $Sb1^{Sb1}$, To^T very common	C^{Cr}, C^{pr}, Rn^{Rn}, Lp^{Lp}, $PATN1^P$
Hackney	A^A, A^a, E^+, E^B, E^e, $Sb1^{Sb1}$	Lp^{Lp}, Rn^{Rn}, **manchado**
Haflinger	E^e, Pa^+, Pa^{np}, Z^Z	
Icelandic	All, except possibly Ch^C, C^{pr}, Lp^{Lp}, Fr^F	$W21$
Knabstrupper	Dark colors plus Lp^{Lp} and $PATN1^P$ because they determine breed character	
Lipizzan	A^A, A^a, G^G	Others rarely
Miniature	All	
Missouri Fox Trotter	All	

(continued)

Table 13.6 (*Continued*)

Breed	Usual color alleles	Unusual color alleles
Morgan	A^A, A^a, E^+, E^B, E^e	C^{Cr}, Dn^+, G^G, Rn^{Rn}, $Sb1^{Sb1}$
Mulassier	A^A, A^a, E^+, E^e, Dn^+, C^{Cr}, Z^Z, G^G, Rn^{Rn}	
Paint	All color alleles, plus To^T, Fr^F, $Sb1^{Sb1}$, $MITF^{SW1}$, $MITF^{SW3}$, PAX^{SW2} as part of breed character; not Lp^{Lp}	
Paso Fino	Most	Rare or nonexistent: Lp^{Lp}, Fr^F, rare **splashed white**
Percheron	A^a, E^+, E^e, G^G	Rn^{Rn}
Peruvian Paso	A^A, A^a, E^+, E^B, E^e, C^{Cr}, G^G, Rn^{Rn}	Many others rarely
Pinto	All color alleles, plus To^{To}, Fr^F, $Sb1^{Sb1}$, $MITF^{SW1}$, $MITF^{SW3}$, PAX^{SW2} as part of breed character; not Lp^{Lp}	
Pony of the Americas	Most color alleles. Lp^{Lp} is widespread because it determines breed character, as is $PATN1^P$	**Paint** pattern alleles are discouraged, as are Rn^{Rn}, G^G, and *dominant white*
Rocky Mountain Horse, Mountain Pleasure Horse	A^A, A^a, E^+, E^e, C^{Cr}, Dn^+, Z^Z, Rn^{Rn}, G^G	$Sb1^{Sb1}$
Shetland Pony	Nearly all, possible exceptions include *dominant white*, Lp^{Lp}, Fr^F	Mu^{mu} is rare
Shire	A^A, A^a, E^+, E^B, E^e, $Sb1^{Sb1}$, G^G	
Spanish Mustang, Spanish Barb	All color and pattern alleles	
Standardbred	A^A, A^a, E^+, E^B, E^e, G^G, Rn^{Rn}	Sb^S, **white** rarely
Suffolk	E^e, Pa^+, Pa^{np}	
Tennesse Walking Horse	A^A, A^a, E^+, E^B, E^e, C^{Cr}, Ch^C, $Sb1^{Sb1}$, Rn^{Rn}	
Thoroughbred	A^A, A^a, E^+, E^B, E^e, G^G	C^{Cr}, $W2$, $W5$, $W6$, $W7$, $W12$, $W14$, polygenic **sabino**, Fr^F, Rn^{Rn}
Warmbloods (includes many breeds)	A^A, A^a, E^+, E^B, E^e, C^{Cr}, G^G, Sb^S, To^T	Lp^{Lp}, Dn^+
Welsh Pony	Nearly all; patterns other than G^G and Rn^{Rn} are penalized, but persist	$Sb1^S$, Lp^{Lp}, $PATN1^P$, or one of the **splashed whites** as rare surprises

Table 13.7 Expected results of crossing various colors.

Parent color	Parent color	Foal colors with relative frequency that is expected			
		Always	Common	Occasional	Rare
Amber champagne	**Amber champagne**	**Amber champagne**	**Bay**	Champagne Black Gold champagne Chestnut	Mushroom Pearl
Amber champagne	**Bay**	**Amber champagne**	**Bay**	Champagne Black Gold champagne Chestnut	Mushroom Pearl
Amber champagne	**Black**	**Amber champagne**	**Bay**	Champagne Black Gold champagne Chestnut	Mushroom Pearl
Amber champagne	**Blue silver**	**Amber champagne** **Pale silver**	**Red silver** **Bay**	Champagne Black Blue silver Gold champagne Chestnut	Mushroom Pearl
Amber champagne	**Buckskin**	**Amber champagne** **Pale champagne**	**Bay** **Buckskin**	Champagne Smoky Black Gold champagne Palomino Ivory champagne Chestnut	Mushroom Pearl Ivory pearl
Amber champagne	**Champagne**	**Amber champagne**	**Bay**	Champagne Black Gold champagne Chestnut	Mushroom Pearl
Amber champagne	**Chestnut**	**Amber champagne**	**Bay**	Champagne Black Gold champagne Chestnut	Red silver Blue silver Mushroom Pale silver Pearl
Amber champagne	**Cream**	**Pale champagne**	**Buckskin**	Smoky Palomino Ivory champagne	Yellow silver Blue silver Zebra dun Grullo Pale silver Mushroom Ivory Pearl

(continued)

Table 13.7 (*Continued*)

Parent color	Parent color	Foal colors with relative frequency that is expected			
		Always	Common	Occasional	Rare
Amber champagne	Gold champagne	Amber champagne	Bay	Champagne Black Gold champagne Chestnut	Red silver Blue silver Pale silver Mushroom Pearl
Amber champagne	Grullo	Amber champagne Pale champagne	Bay Zebra dun	Champagne Black Grullo Gold champagne Red dun Chestnut	Mushroom Pearl
Amber champagne	Mushroom	Amber champagne	Bay	Champagne Black Gold Champagne Chestnut	Mushroom Pearl
Amber champagne	Palomino	Amber champagne Pale champagne	Bay Buckskin	Champagne Black Smoky Gold champagne Palomino Ivory champagne Chestnut	Red silver Blue silver Yellow silver Pale silver Mushroom Pearl Ivory pearl
Amber champagne	Pearl	Amber champagne	Bay	Champagne Black Gold Champagne Chestnut	Pearl Mushroom
Amber champagne	Red dun	Amber champagne Pale champagne	Bay Zebra dun	Champagne Black Grullo Gold champagne Red dun Chestnut	Red silver Blue silver Yellow silver Pale silver Mushroom Pearl
Amber champagne	Red silver	Amber champagne Pale silver	Red silver Bay	Champagne Black Blue silver Gold champagne Chestnut	Mushroom Pearl

Table 13.7 (*Continued*)

Parent color	Parent color	Foal colors with relative frequency that is expected			
		Always	Common	Occasional	Rare
Amber champagne	**Smoky**	**Amber champagne Pale champagne**	**Bay Buckskin**	**Champagne Black Smoky Gold champagne Palomino Ivory champagne Chestnut**	**Mushroom Pearl Ivory Pearl**
Amber champagne	**Zebra dun**	**Amber champagne**	**Bay Zebra dun**	**Champagne Black Grullo Gold champagne Red dun Chestnut Ivory champagne Pale champagne**	**Mushroom Pearl Ivory Pearl**
Bay	**Bay**	**Bay**		**Chestnut Black**	**Mushroom Pearl**
Bay	**Black**	**Bay**		**Chestnut Black**	**Mushroom Pearl**
Bay	**Blue silver**	**Red silver**	**Bay**	**Chestnut Blue silver Black**	**Mushroom Pearl**
Bay	**Buckskin**	**Buckskin Bay**		**Palomino Chestnut Smoky Black**	**Mushroom Pearl Ivory pearl**
Bay	**Champagne**	**Amber champagne**	**Bay**	**Champagne Black Chestnut Gold champagne**	**Mushroom Pearl**
Bay	**Chestnut**	**Bay**	**Chestnut**	**Black**	**Red silver Blue silver Mushroom Pearl**

(*continued*)

Table 13.7 (*Continued*)

Parent color	Parent color	Foal colors with relative frequency that is expected			
		Always	Common	Occasional	Rare
Bay	Cream	Buckskin		Palomino Smoky	Zebra dun Grullo Yellow silver Pale silver Ivory champagne Pale champagne Mushroom Ivory pearl
Bay	Gold champagne	Amber champagne	Bay	Champagne Black Gold champagne Chestnut	Red silver Blue silver Pale silver Mushroom Pearl
Bay	Grullo	Zebra dun	Bay	Red dun Chestnut Grullo Black	Buckskin Palomino Smoky Mushroom Pearl
Bay	Mushroom	Bay	Black Chestnut		Mushroom
Bay	Palomino	Buckskin Bay	Palomino Chestnut	Smoky Black	Yellow silver Red silver Blue silver Pale silver Mushroom Pearl Ivory pearl
Bay	Pearl	Bay	Black Chestnut		Mushroom Pearl
Bay	Red dun	Zebra dun	Bay Red dun Chestnut	Grullo Black	Yellow silver Red silver Blue silver Mushroom Pearl
Bay	Red silver	Red silver	Bay	Chestnut Blue silver Black	Mushroom Pearl
Bay	Smoky	Buckskin Bay		Palomino Chestnut Smoky Black	Mushroom Pearl Ivory pearl
Bay	Zebra dun	Zebra dun	Bay	Red dun Chestnut Grullo Black	Palomino Buckskin Smoky Mushroom Pearl Ivory pearl

Table 13.7 (*Continued*)

Parent color	Parent color	Foal colors with relative frequency that is expected			
		Always	Common	Occasional	Rare
Black	Black	Black		Chestnut	Bay Mushroom Pearl
Black	Blue silver	Blue silver	Black	Chestnut	Red silver Bay Mushroom Pearl
Black	Buckskin	Buckskin Bay		Palomino Chestnut Black Smoky	Mushroom Pearl Ivory pearl
Black	Champagne	Champagne	Black	Gold champagne Chestnut	Amber champagne Bay Mushroom Pearl
Black	Chestnut		Bay Chestnut	Black	Red silver Blue silver Mushroom Pearl
Black	Cream		Buckskin	Palomino Smoky	Zebra dun Grullo Red dun Yellow silver Pale silver Pale champagne Mushroom Ivory pearl
Black	Gold champagne		Amber champagne Bay Champagne Black Gold champagne Chestnut		Red silver Blue silver Pale silver Mushroom Pearl
Black	Grullo	Grullo	Black	Red dun Chestnut	Palomino Smoky Zebra dun Bay Buckskin Mushroom Pearl Ivory pearl
Black	Mushroom		Bay Black Chestnut		Mushroom Pearl

(*continued*)

Table 13.7 (*Continued*)

Parent color	Parent color	Foal colors with relative frequency that is expected			
		Always	Common	Occasional	Rare
Black	Palomino		Buckskin Bay Palomino Chestnut	Smoky Black	Zebra dun Red dun Grullo Red silver Yellow silver Blue silver Pale silver Mushroom Pearl Ivory pearl
Black	Pearl		Bay Black Chestnut		Mushroom Pearl
Black	Red dun		Zebra dun Bay Red dun Chestnut	Grullo Black	Yellow silver Red silver Blue silver Pale silver Mushroom Pearl
Black	Red silver	Red silver	Bay	Chestnut Blue silver Black	Mushroom Pearl
Black	Smoky	Smoky Black		Palomino Chestnut	Buckskin Bay Mushroom Pearl Ivory pearl
Black	Zebra dun	Zebra dun	Bay	Red dun Chestnut Grullo Black	Buckskin Palomino Smoky Mushroom Pearl
Blue silver	Blue silver	Blue silver	Black	Chestnut	Red silver Bay Mushroom Pearl
Blue silver	Buckskin	Yellow silver Red silver Pale silver	Buckskin Bay	Palomino Chestnut Blue silver Smoky Black	Zebra dun Red dun Grullo Mushroom Pearl
Blue silver	Cream		Yellow silver Buckskin Pale silver	Palomino Smoky	Zebra dun Grullo Ivory champagne Pale champagne Mushroom Ivory Pearl

Table 13.7 (*Continued*)

Parent color	Parent color	Foal colors with relative frequency that is expected			
		Always	Common	Occasional	Rare
Blue silver	Gold champagne	Pale silver	Amber champagne Bay Red silver	Champagne Blue silver Black Gold champagne Chestnut	Mushroom Pearl
Blue silver	Grullo	Blue silver Pale silver	Black Grullo	Red dun Chestnut	Palomino Smoky Cream Red silver Yellow silver Bay Zebra dun Buckskin Mushroom Pearl Ivory pearl
Blue Silver	Mushroom		Red Silver Bay Blue silver Black Chestnut		Mushroom Pearl
Blue silver	Palomino		Yellow silver Red silver Pale silver Buckskin Bay Palomino Chestnut	Blue silver Smoky Black	Zebra dun Red dun Grullo Mushroom Pearl Ivory pearl
Blue Silver	Pearl		Red Silver Bay Blue silver Black Chestnut		Mushroom Pearl
Blue silver	Red dun		Yellow silver Zebra dun Red silver Bay Red dun Chestnut	Blue silver Grullo Black	Mushroom Pearl
Blue silver	Red silver	Red silver	Bay	Chestnut Blue silver Black	Mushroom Pearl

(*continued*)

Table 13.7 (*Continued*)

Parent color	Parent color	Foal colors with relative frequency that is expected			
		Always	Common	Occasional	Rare
Blue silver	**Smoky**	**Blue silver** **Pale silver**	**Black** **Smoky**	**Chestnut** **Palomino**	**Buckskin** **Red silver** **Yellow silver** **Bay** **Zebra dun** **Grullo** **Red dun** **Mushroom** **Pearl** **Ivory pearl**
Blue silver	**Zebra dun**	**Yellow silver** **Pale silver**	**Red silver** **Zebra dun** **Bay**	**Red dun** **Chestnut** **Blue silver** **Grullo** **Black**	**Buckskin** **Palomino** **Smoky** **Mushroom** **Pearl** **Ivory pearl**
Buckskin	**Buckskin**	**Buckskin** **Bay** **Cream**		**Palomino** **Chestnut** **Smoky** **Black**	**Mushroom**
Buckskin	**Champagne**		**Buckskin** **Amber** **champagne** **Bay** **Pale** **champagne**	**Gold** **champagne** **Ivory** **champagne** **Palomino** **Chestnut** **Champagne** **Smoky** **Black**	**Mushroom** **Pearl**
Buckskin	**Chestnut**	**Buckskin** **Bay**	**Palomino** **Chestnut**	**Smoky** **Black**	**Yellow silver** **Red silver** **Blue silver** **Mushroom** **Pearl** **Ivory pearl**
Buckskin	**Cream**	**Buckskin** **Cream**		**Palomino** **Smoky**	**Zebra dun** **Yellow silver** **Pale silver** **Grullo** **Pale** **champagne**
Buckskin	**Gold** **champagne**	**Amber** **champagne** **Pale** **champagne**	**Bay** **Buckskin**	**Champagne** **Smoky** **Black** **Gold** **champagne** **Ivory** **champagne** **Palomino** **Chestnut**	**Blue silver** **Red silver** **Yellow silver** **Pale silver** **Mushroom** **Pearl** **Ivory pearl**

Table 13.7 (*Continued*)

Parent color	Parent color	Foal colors with relative frequency that is expected			
		Always	Common	Occasional	Rare
Buckskin	Grullo	Zebra dun	Buckskin Bay	Red dun Chestnut Palomino Grullo Black Smoky	Cream Mushroom Pearl Ivory pearl
Buckskin	Mushroom	Bay Buckskin	Black Smoky Chestnut Palomino		Mushroom Pearl Ivory pearl
Buckskin	Palomino	Buckskin Bay Cream	Palomino Chestnut	Smoky Black	Yellow silver Red silver Blue silver Zebra dun Red dun Grullo Mushroom
Buckskin	Pearl	Bay Buckskin Ivory Pearl	Black Smoky Chestnut Palomino		Mushroom
Buckskin	Red dun	Zebra dun	Buckskin Bay Palomino Red dun Chestnut	Grullo Smoky Black	Yellow silver Red silver Blue silver Mushroom Pearl Ivory pearl
Buckskin	Red silver	Yellow silver Red silver Pale silver	Buckskin Bay	Chestnut Palomino Smoky Black Blue silver	Mushroom Pearl Ivory pearl
Buckskin	Smoky	Buckskin Bay Cream		Palomino Chestnut Smoky Black	Mushroom
Buckskin	Zebra dun	Zebra dun	Bay Buckskin	Palomino Red dun Chestnut Grullo Smoky Black	Cream Mushroom Pearl Ivory pearl
Champagne	Champagne	Champagne		Black Chestnut Gold champagne	Amber champagne Bay Mushroom

(continued)

Table 13.7 (*Continued*)

Parent color	Parent color	Foal colors with relative frequency that is expected			
		Always	Common	Occasional	Rare
Champagne	Chestnut	Champagne		Black Bay Amber champagne Chestnut Gold champagne	Pearl Red silver Blue silver Pale silver Mushroom Pearl
Champagne	Blue silver	Champagne Pale silver	Blue silver	Black Chestnut	Bay Red silver Mushroom Pearl
Champagne	Cream	Pale champagne	Cream	Palomino Ivory champagne Smoky Buckskin	Zebra dun Grullo Yellow silver Pale silver Mushroom Ivory pearl
Champagne	Gold champagne		Amber champ	Bay Champagne Black Gold champagne Chestnut	Red silver Blue silver Pale silver Mushroom Pearl
Champagne	Grullo	Champagne Pale champagne	Grullo Black	Gold champagne Red dun Chestnut	Palomino Smoky Amber champagne Buckskin Zebra dun Bay Mushroom Pearl
Champagne	Mushroom		Bay Amber champagne Black Champagne Chestnut Gold champagne		Mushroom Pearl
Champagne	Palomino	Champagne Pale champagne	Buckskin Bay Amber champagne	Palomino Gold champagne Chestnut Black Smoky	Red silver Blue silver Yellow silver Pale silver Mushroom Pearl Ivory pearl

Table 13.7 (*Continued*)

Parent color	Parent color	Foal colors with relative frequency that is expected			
		Always	Common	Occasional	Rare
Champagne	Pearl		Amber champagne Bay Champagne Black Gold champagne Chestnut		Mushroom Pearl
Champagne	Red dun		Amber champagne Zebra dun	Bay Champagne Grullo Black Gold champagne Red dun Chestnut	Blue silver Red silver Pale silver Mushroom Pearl
Champagne	Red silver	Amber champagne	Red silver Pale silver	Bay Champagne Black Gold champagne Chestnut Blue silver	Mushroom Pearl
Champagne	Smoky	Champagne Pale champagne	Smoky Black	Ivory champagne Gold champagne Palomino Chestnut	Amber champagne Buckskin Bay Mushroom Pearl Ivory pearl
Champagne	Zebra dun	Amber champagne Pale champagne	Zebra dun	Bay Champagne Gold champagne Red dun Chestnut Grullo Black	Ivory champagne Buckskin Smoky Palomino Mushroom Pearl Ivory pearl
Chestnut	Chestnut	Chestnut			Mushroom Pearl
Chestnut	Blue silver		Red silver Bay Chestnut	Blue silver Black	Mushroom Pearl

(*continued*)

Table 13.7 (*Continued*)

Parent color	Parent color	Always	Common	Occasional	Rare
		Foal colors with relative frequency that is expected			
Chestnut	**Cream**		**Buckskin** **Palomino**	**Smoky**	**Zebra dun** **Grullo** **Yellow silver** **Pale silver** **Ivory** **champagne** **Pale** **champagne** **Mushroom** **Ivory pearl**
Chestnut	**Gold** **champagne**	**Gold** **champagne**	**Chestnut**		**Mushroom** **Pearl**
Chestnut	**Grullo**		**Zebra dun** **Bay** **Red dun** **Chestnut**	**Grullo** **Black**	**Buckskin** **Palomino** **Smoky** **Red silver** **Yellow silver** **Blue silver** **Pale silver** **Mushroom** **Pearl**
Chestnut	**Mushroom**	**Chestnut**			**Mushroom** **Pearl (gold)**
Chestnut	**Palomino**	**Palomino** **Chestnut**			**Red dun** **Mushroom** **Pearl** **Ivory pearl**
Chestnut	**Pearl**		**Bay** **Black** **Chestnut**		**Mushroom** **Pearl**
Chestnut	**Red dun**	**Red dun**	**Chestnut**		**Mushroom** **Pearl**
Chestnut	**Red silver**	**Red silver**	**Bay** **Chestnut**	**Blue silver** **Black**	**Mushroom** **Pearl**
Chestnut	**Smoky**		**Buckskin** **Bay** **Palomino** **Chestnut**	**Smoky** **Black**	**Yellow silver** **Red silver** **Blue silver** **Pale silver** **Mushroom** **Pearl** **Ivory pearl**

Table 13.7 (Continued)

Parent color	Parent color	Foal colors with relative frequency that is expected			
		Always	Common	Occasional	Rare
Chestnut	Zebra dun	Zebra dun	Bay Red dun Chestnut	Grullo Black	Buckskin Palomino Smoky Yellow silver Red silver Blue silver Pale silver Mushroom Pearl Ivory pearl
Cream	Cream	Cream			
Cream	Gold champagne		Pale champagne Ivory champagne	Buckskin Smoky Palomino	Grullo Zebra dun Pale silver Mushroom Ivory pearl
Cream	Grullo		Zebra dun Buckskin	Palomino Smoky Grullo	Yellow silver Pale silver Cream Pale champagne Ivory champagne Mushroom Ivory pearl
Cream	Mushroom		Palomino	Buckskin Smoky	Mushroom Ivory pearl
Cream	Palomino	Cream	Buckskin Palomino	Smoky	Zebra dun Grullo Yellow silver Pale champagne Ivory champagne Mushroom
Cream	Pearl	Ivory pearl			Mushroom
Cream	Red dun		Zebra dun Palomino Buckskin	Smoky Grullo	Yellow silver Pale silver Pale champagne Ivory champagne Mushroom Ivory pearl

(continued)

Table 13.7 (*Continued*)

Parent color	Parent color	Foal colors with relative frequency that is expected			
		Always	Common	Occasional	Rare
Cream	Red silver	Yellow silver	Buckskin	Palomino Smoky	Zebra dun Grullo Pale silver Pale champagne Ivory champagne Mushroom Ivory pearl
Cream	Smoky	Cream	Buckskin	Palomino Smoky	Yellow silver Zebra dun Grullo Pale champagne Ivory champagne Mushroom
Cream	Zebra dun	Zebra dun	Buckskin	Palomino Grullo Smoky	Yellow silver Pale silver Cream Pale champagne Ivory champagne Mushroom Ivory pearl
Gold champagne	Gold champagne	Gold champagne	Chestnut		Mushroom Pearl
Gold champagne	Grullo	Amber champagne	Bay Zebra dun	Champagne Grullo Black Gold champagne Red dun Chestnut	Buckskin Palomino Smoky Ivory champagne Pale champagne Blue silver Red silver Yellow silver Pale silver Mushroom Pearl
Gold champagne	Mushroom	Gold champagne	Chestnut		Mushroom Pearl
Gold champagne	Palomino	Gold champagne Ivory champagne	Palomino Chestnut		Mushroom Pearl Ivory pearl

Table 13.7 (*Continued*)

Parent color	Parent color	Foal colors with relative frequency that is expected			
		Always	Common	Occasional	Rare
Gold champagne	Pearl		Gold champagne Amber champagne Champagne Bay Black Chestnut		Mushroom Pearl
Gold champagne	Red dun	Gold champagne	Red dun Chestnut		Mushroom Pearl
Gold champagne	Red silver	Amber champagne Pale silver	Bay Red silver	Blue silver Champagne Black Gold champagne Chestnut	Mushroom Pearl
Gold champagne	Smoky	Pale champagne	Amber champagne Buckskin Bay	Champagne Smoky Black Gold champagne Palomino Chestnut	Blue silver Red silver Yellow silver Pale silver Mushroom Pearl Ivory pearl
Gold champagne	Zebra dun		Zebra dun Amber champagne Bay	Champagne Grullo Black Gold champagne Red dun Chestnut	Pale champagne Palomino Smoky Buckskin Mushroom Pearl Ivory pearl
Grullo	Grullo	Grullo	Black	Red dun Chestnut	Palomino Smoky Cream Buckskin Mushroom Pearl Ivory pearl
Grullo	Mushroom		Zebra dun Grullo Red dun Bay Black Chestnut		Buckskin Palomino Smoky Mushroom Pearl

(*continued*)

Table 13.7 (*Continued*)

Parent color	Parent color	Foal colors with relative frequency that is expected			
		Always	Common	Occasional	Rare
Grullo	Palomino		Zebra dun Buckskin Bay Palomino Chestnut Red dun	Grullo Smoky Black	Blue silver Yellow silver Red silver Pale silver Cream Mushroom Pearl Ivory pearl
Grullo	Pearl		Zebra dun Grullo Red dun Bay Black Chestnut		Buckskin Smoky Palomino Mushroom Pearl Ivory pearl
Grullo	Red dun		Zebra dun Red dun Bay	Chestnut Grullo Black	Palomino Buckskin Smoky Yellow silver Red silver Blue silver Pale silver Mushroom Pearl
Grullo	Red silver	Yellow silver	Red silver Zebra dun Bay	Red dun Chestnut Grullo Blue silver Black	Buckskin Palomino Smoky Pale silver Mushroom Pearl
Grullo	Smoky	Grullo	Smoky Black	Palomino Chestnut Red dun	Cream Mushroom Pearl Ivory pearl
Grullo	Zebra dun	Zebra dun	Bay	Red dun Chestnut Grullo Black	Buckskin Palomino Smoky Cream Mushroom Pearl Ivory pearl
Mushroom	Mushroom	Mushroom			Pearl
Mushroom	Palomino		Palomino Chestnut		Mushroom Pearl
Mushroom	Pearl		Bay Black Chestnut		Mushroom Pearl

Table 13.7 (*Continued*)

Parent color	Parent color	Always	Common	Occasional	Rare
Mushroom	Red Dun		Red Dun Chestnut		Mushroom Pearl
Mushroom	Red silver		Red silver Bay Blue silver Black Chestnut		Mushroom Pearl
Mushroom	Smoky		Buckskin Palomino Smoky Bay Chestnut Black		Mushroom Pearl
Mushroom	Zebra dun		Zebra dun Grullo Red dun Bay Chestnut Black	Buckskin Palomino Smoky	Mushroom Pearl Ivory pearl
Palomino	Palomino	Palomino Chestnut Cream			Red dun Mushroom
Palomino	Pearl		Ivory pearl Chestnut Palomino Buckskin Bay Smoky Black		Mushroom
Palomino	Red dun	Palomino Red dun	Chestnut		Mushroom Pearl Ivory pearl
Palomino	Red silver	Yellow silver Red silver Pale silver	Buckskin Bay Palomino Chestnut	Blue silver Smoky Black	Zebra dun Grullo Red dun Mushroom Pearl Ivory pearl
Palomino	Smoky	Cream	Buckskin Bay Palomino Chestnut	Smoky Black	Yellow silver Red silver Blue silver Pale silver Zebra dun Red dun Grullo Mushroom Pearl Ivory pearl

(continued)

Table 13.7 *(Continued)*

Parent color	Parent color	Foal colors with relative frequency that is expected			
		Always	Common	Occasional	Rare
Palomino	**Zebra dun**	**Zebra dun**	**Buckskin**	**Grullo**	**Yellow silver**
			Bay	**Smoky**	**Red silver**
			Palomino	**Black**	**Blue silver**
			Chestnut		**Pale silver**
			Red dun		**Cream**
					Mushroom
					Pearl
					Ivory pearl
Pearl	**Pearl**	**Pearl**			**Mushroom**
Pearl	**Red dun**		**Zebra dun**		**Mushroom**
			Red dun		**Pearl**
			Grullo		
			Bay		
			Chestnut		
			Black		
Pearl	**Red silver**		**Red silver**	**Blue silver**	**Mushroom**
			Bay	**Black**	**Pearl**
			Chestnut		
Pearl	**Smoky**	**Ivory pearl**	**Bay**	**Black**	**Mushroom**
			Chestnut		
Pearl	**Zebra dun**		**Zebra dun**	**Grullo**	**Buckskin**
			Bay	**Black**	**Palomino**
			Red dun		**Smoky**
			Chestnut		**Mushroom**
					Pearl
					Ivory pearl
Red dun	**Red dun**	**Red dun**	**Chestnut**		**Mushroom**
					Pearl
Red dun	**Red silver**	**Yellow silver**	**Zebra dun**	**Grullo**	**Mushroom**
			Bay	**Blue silver**	**Pearl**
			Red dun	**Black**	
			Chestnut		
Red dun	**Smoky**		**Zebra dun**	**Grullo**	**Yellow silver**
			Buckskin	**Smoky**	**Red silver**
			Bay	**Black**	**Blue silver**
			Red dun		**Pale silver**
			Palomino		**Mushroom**
			Chestnut		**Pearl**
					Ivory pearl
Red dun	**Zebra dun**	**Zebra dun**	**Red dun**	**Grullo**	**Yellow silver**
			Bay	**Black**	**Red silver**
			Chestnut		**Blue silver**
					Pale silver
					Buckskin
					Palomino
					Smoky
					Mushroom
					Pearl
					Ivory pearl

Table 13.7 (*Continued*)

Parent color	Parent color	Foal colors with relative frequency that is expected			
		Always	Common	Occasional	Rare
Red silver	Red silver	Red silver	Bay	Chestnut Blue silver Black	Mushroom Pearl
Red silver	Smoky	Yellow silver Red silver	Buckskin Bay	Palomino Chestnut Blue silver Smoky Black	Mushroom Pearl Ivory pearl
Red silver	Zebra dun	Yellow silver	Zebra dun Red silver Bay	Red dun Chestnut Blue silver Grullo Black	Buckskin Palomino Smoky Mushroom Pearl Ivory pearl
Smoky	Smoky	Smoky Black Cream		Palomino Chestnut	Buckskin Bay Mushroom
Smoky	Zebra dun	Zebra dun	Buckskin Bay	Palomino Red dun Chestnut Grullo Smoky Black	Cream Mushroom Pearl Ivory pearl
Zebra dun	Zebra dun	Zebra dun	Bay	Red dun Chestnut Grullo Black	Buckskin Palomino Smoky Cream Mushroom Pearl Ivory pearl

Table 13.7 is arranged alphabetically for ease of use, and colors are lumped together rather than split. The order of the parental colors is as follows: **amber champagne**, **bay** (including **sooty** type **brown** and **seal brown** for simplicity), **black**, **blue silver** (including **chocolate silver** and **silver dapple**), **buckskin** (including **sooty buckskin**), **champagne**, **chestnut** (including **sorrel**), **cream** (including **cremello**, **perlino**, and **smoky cream** as well as **linebacked cream**), **gold champagne**, **grullo** (including **lobo dun** and **olive dun**, as well as types with C^{Cr}), **mushroom**, **palomino** (including **linebacked palomino**), **pearl** (including all **pearl** shades) **red dun** (including **apricot dun**), **red silver** (including **brown silver**), **smoky**, and **zebra dun** (including **coyote dun**, as well as compounds with the *cremello* allele). In order to look up a cross it is important to remember that the list is alphabetical. So, the **red dun** × **black** mating is listed under **black** × **red dun** and not under **red dun** × **black**, because information would be needlessly repeated in what is already a very long table.

Very few of the "compound dilutes" are included as separate parental colors. Details of crosses involving these colors can be determined by adding the results of the components. In this manner, **ivory champagne** can be determined by looking up the results for **palomino** and **gold champagne** and adding these together for a complete array of colors that are possible from the mating of **ivory champagne** to other specific colors. Other important compound dilutes include **yellow silver** (usually **buckskin** plus **red silver**, although sometimes **zebra dun** plus **red silver**). Other combinations of C^{Cr}, C^{pr}, Ch^C, Dn^+, and Z^Z are difficult to identify accurately as distinctly recognizable colors. Pale horses with light brown points could by any of several combinations of these alleles. These are identified under foal colors as **pale silver** (**silver** plus **champagne**) and **pale champagne** (**champagne** plus **cream**-related colors or the *dun* allele) where appropriate.

The illustrations for this book would have been impossible without the generosity of many people that provided photographs. Horse photography is tricky at the best of times, so that good photographs of even the most common colors are often difficult to access. For rare colors the challenge becomes even more steep. Table 13.8 lists the names, breeds, owners, and photographers of horses where this information is known, and provides a location to thank these many people for their contributions to this work.

Table 13.8 Sources of photographs.

Figure	Horse name	Breed	Owner	Image credit
1.1	Bay B Doll	Arabian	Dyan Westvang	Dyan Westvang
1.2	Foxvangen's Pagan	Missouri Fox Trotter	Dyan Westvang	Dyan Westvang
1.3	Paterson Banjo	Pryor Mountain Mustang		Nancy Cerroni
1.4		Clydesdale	Larry Barnes	Jeannette Beranger
1.5	Maya FVF	Missouri Fox Trotter	Dyan Westvang	Dyan Westvang
1.6	Maya FVF	Missouri Fox Trotter	Dyan Westvang	Dyan Westvang
1.7				Dr Teri Lear
1.8				Francesca Gianino
1.9				Dr Teri Lear
1.10				Francesca Gianino
1.11				Francesca Gianino
1.12		Choctaw Spanish Mustang	Darlene and Bryant Rickman	Jeannette Beranger
1.13				Francesca Gianino
2.1	Icky's Miss Camper	Choctaw Spanish Mustang	Mary McConnell	D. Phillip Sponenberg
2.2	Spring Lake Thistle	Morgan	Niven Owings	Laura Hornick Behning

Table 13.8 *(Continued)*

Figure	Horse name	Breed	Owner	Image credit
2.3	Black Camp	Choctaw Spanish Mustang	Darlene and Bryant Rickman	Jeannette Beranger
2.4				Francesca Gianino
2.5				Francesca Gianino
2.6				Francesca Gianino
2.7	Tabac	Cherokee Spanish	Mary Carter McConnell	D. Phillip Sponenberg
2.8	Kleary's M&M	Irish Draught	Kleary Field	Kleary Field
2.9		Brabant		Laurent Rottiers
2.10	Foxvangen's Black Sonya	Missouri Fox Trotter	Dyan Westvang	Dyan Westvang
2.11	Foxvangen's Black Sonya	Missouri Fox Trotter	Dyan Westvang	Dyan Westvang
3.1		Mustang		Dan Elkins
3.2	London	Pryor Mountain		Nancy Cerroni
3.3		Mustang		Dan Elkins
3.4		Choctaw Spanish Mustang	Darlene and Bryant Rickman	Jeannette Beranger
3.5	Charli Girl	Morgan	Lucy Ray	Laura Hornick Behning
3.6	Foxvangen's Ruby Slippers	Missouri Fox Trotter	Dyan Westvang	Dyan Westvang
3.7	P.C.'s Sheer Bliss	Missouri Fox Trotter	Dyan Westvang	Dyan Westvang
3.8	Foxvangen's Sasha	Missouri Fox Trotter	Dyan Westvang	Dyan Westvang
3.9	W A R Adikyrie	Morgan	Laura Hornick Behning	Laura Hornick Behning
3.10	Onyx	Choctaw Spanish	Mary Carter McConnell	D. Phillip Sponenberg
3.11	Coin's Touch of Magic	Missouri Fox Trotter	Dyan Westvang	Dyan Westvang
3.12		Mustang		Dan Elkins
3.13				Francesca Gianino
3.14	Notable WBF	Haflinger	Donna Kuck	Ruth Schwab
3.15	Notorio	Wilbur-Cruce Colonial Spanish	Robin Collins	Robin Collins
3.16	Barton of Nonesuch	Exmoor Pony	Exmoor Ponies of North America	Exmoor Ponies of North America
3.17	Enoha Tan	Gypsy Cob	Laurence Viala	Laurence Viala
		Choctaw Spanish Mustang	Darlene and Bryant Rickman	Neil Chapman
3.18	Marquis MJW Woodward	Haflinger	Mike and Jacque Woodward	Ruth Schwab

(continued)

Table 13.8 (*Continued*)

Figure	Horse name	Breed	Owner	Image credit
3.19		American Belgian	Larry Barnes	Jeannette Beranger
3.20	Torreno	Wilbur-Cruce Colonial Spanish	Robin Collins	Robin Collins
3.21	Foxvangen's Chica Mia	Missouri Fox Trotter	Dyan Westvang	Dyan Westvang
3.22	Foxvangen's Noble Ambassador	Missouri Fox Trotter	Dyan Westvang	Dyan Westvang
3.23	Montera	Santa Cruz Spanish Mustang	Christine Nooner	Jeannette Beranger
3.24	Quietude Calais	Morgan	Lucy Ray	Laura Hornick Behning
3.25	Hofrat	Haflinger		© Evelyn Simak
3.26		Noriker		© Evelyn Simak
3.27	Inshalla	Santa Cruz Spanish Mustang	Christine Nooner	D. Phillip Sponenberg
3.28		Noriker		© Evelyn Simak
3.29	Country Charm Maxs Rare Tresor	Miniature Horse	Chanel Bradley	Chanel Bradley
3.30	Sharp Trilogy Sharp One Sharp Too		Denise Charpilloz	Denise Charpilloz
3.31	Stars Stripes of Kala	American Paint Horse	Janelle Osborne	Janelle Osborne
3.32	Tri A Brindle	Quarter Horse	Elyse Morano	Janelle Osborne
3.33	Hershey	Mustang		Fran Ackley
3.34		Choctaw Spanish Mustang	Darlene and Bryant Rickman	Neil Chapman
3.35	Madre Mia	Puerto Rican Paso Fino		Jo-Ann Ferré Crossley
3.36		Choctaw Spanish Mustang	Darlene and Bryant Rickman	Neil Chapman
3.37		Choctaw Spanish Mustang	Darlene and Bryant Rickman	Neil Chapman
3.38		Choctaw Spanish Mustang	Darlene and Bryant Rickman	Neil Chapman
3.39		Marsh Tacky	Marion Gohagan	Jeannette Beranger
3.40	Dynasty	Tennessee Walking Horse	Vonda Hamilton	Vonda Hamilton
3.41		Mustang		Dan Elkins
4.1	Hataali and Oracle	Pryor Mountain Mustang		Nancy Cerroni
4.2		Pryor Mountain Mustang	Daphne and Dale Hartmann	D. Phillip Sponenberg
4.3		Choctaw Spanish Mustang	Darlene and Bryant Rickman	Neil Chapman

Table 13.8 (*Continued*)

Figure	Horse name	Breed	Owner	Image credit
4.4	Pax	Pryor Mountain Mustang		Nancy Cerroni
4.5	Mirabella's Mesmerized	Morgan	Cindy Dietz	Cindy Dietz
4.6		Pryor Mountain Mustang		Dan Elkins
4.7		Pryor Mountain Mustang		Dan Elkins
4.8	Jackson	Pryor Mountain Mustang		D. Phillip Sponenberg
4.9		Pryor Mountain Mustang		Dan Elkins
4.10		Criollo Paraguayo	Eduardo Prayones	D. Phillip Sponenberg
4.11		Sulphur Spanish Mustang		D. Phillip Sponenberg
4.12	Moment Light Begins	Choctaw Spanish Mustang	Mary Carter McConnell	D. Phillip Sponenberg
4.13	Lancelot and Durango	Pryor Mountain Mustang		D. Phillip Sponenberg
4.14		Spanish Mustang	Roeliff Annon	D. Phillip Sponenberg
4.15	Milton's Chickasaw Penny	Choctaw Spanish Mustang	Mary Carter McConnell	D. Phillip Sponenberg
4.16	Kiamichi True Gold	Choctaw Spanish Mustang	Mary Carter McConnell	D. Phillip Sponenberg
4.17		Choctaw Spanish Mustang	Darlene and Bryant Rickman	D. Phillip Sponenberg
4.18	Ynskje	Fjord	Anouk Schurink	Anouk Schurink
4.19	Lena and Lila	Fjord	Joyce Concklin	JoAnn Bellone
4.20	Multiple Fjords	Fjord	Line Shøn Nielsen	Line Shøn Nielsen
4.21				Francesca Gianino
4.22		Criollo Paraguayo	Eduardo Prayones	D. Phillip Sponenberg
4.23		Criollo Venezolano	Agropecuaria Florestal	D. Phillip Sponenberg
4.24	PKR Primavera Brio	Morgan	John Hutcheson	Laura Hornick Behning
4.25	Foxvangen's Aysha	Missouri Fox Trotter	Dyan Westvang	Dyan Westvang
4.26	Gab Creek Golden Vaquero	Morgan	John Hutcheson	Laura Hornick Behning
4.27	Coral Forest	Morgan	Laura Hornick Behning	Laura Hornick Behning
4.28	Donegreagh An Pearla Dubh	Connemara	Finola Mulholland	Finola Mulholland
4.29	SFG Infinity and Beyond	Morgan	Patty Clark	Laura Hornick Behning
4.30		Pine Tacky	Bill Brown	Jeannette Beranger

(*continued*)

Table 13.8 (*Continued*)

Figure	Horse name	Breed	Owner	Image credit
4.31	Benvarden Camille/ Benvarden Karma	Connemara	Finola Mulholland	Finola Mulholland
4.32	Apollo	Andalusian	Suzan Sommer	Suzan Sommer
4.33	Oso de Oro	Andalusian	Suzan Sommer	Suzan Sommer
	Majodero	Lusitano	Ginger Vosburg	Ginger Vosburg
4.34	Hy Color Champagne Diva	7/8 Friesian and 1/8 Saddlebred	Aimee Ziller/Bryan Ludens	Aimee Ziller
4.35		Choctaw Spanish Mustang	Darlene and Bryant Rickman	Neil Chapman
4.36	Ebony's Rocky Boy	Tennessee Walking Horse	Midge McGoldrick	Midge McGoldrick
4.37		Tennessee Walking Horse		Liz Nutter
4.38	Windcrest's High Voltage	Tennessee Walking Horse	Midge McGoldrick	Midge McGoldrick
4.39	St. Clarins	Gypsy Cob	Celeste Huston	Celeste Huston
4.40	Positively Charmed	Morgan	Laura Hornick Behning	Laura Hornick Behning
4.41	Unconventional	Morgan	Lyle and Cindy Dietz	Cindy Dietz
4.42	Ali from Dalalif	Icelandic	Lucinda Nold	Lucinda Nold
4.43	Coulee Bend Talisman	Morgan	Lyle and Cindy Dietz	Cindy Dietz
4.44	Kella's Windfaerie with foal	Shetland Pony	Elisabeth Mead	Elisabeth Mead
4.45	Bayhall Magic	Shetland Pony	Elisabeth Mead	Elisabeth Mead
4.46	Mireyenion Tos	Arabian	Becky Huffman	Dan Stanfield
4.47	Foxvangen's Duncan	Missouri Fox Trotter	Dyan Westvang	Dyan Westvang
4.48	Foxvangen's Duncan	Missouri Fox Trotter	Dyan Westvang	Dyan Westvang
4.49	Shadows at Dusk	Quarter Horse	Jennifer R. Kuipers	Jennifer R. Kuipers
5.1				Francesca Gianino
5.2				D. Phillip Sponenberg
6.1	Richochet's Grey Chief	Choctaw Spanish Mustang	John Fusco	Return to Freedom Sanctuary
6.2		Percheron	Providence RI Police Department	Jeannette Beranger
6.3		Shire	Ayrshire Farm	Jeannette Beranger
6.4		Mount Taylor	Dan Elkins	Dan Elkins
6.5		Lipizzan	Colonial Williamsburg	D. Phillip Sponenberg
6.6		Dales Pony	Debbie Hamilton	Jeannette Beranger
6.7		Criollo Venezolano		D. Phillip Sponenberg

Table 13.8 (*Continued*)

Figure	Horse name	Breed	Owner	Image credit
6.8		Criollo Venezolano		D. Phillip Sponenberg
6.9	Portos	Westphalian	Lyndsey Marsh	Lyndsey Marsh
6.10		Criollo Venezolano		D. Phillip Sponenberg
6.11		Percheron		© Evelyn Simak
6.12	Simba du Pont de Tournay	Ardennes	Joyce Concklin	JoAnn Bellone
6.13	Cadiz	Mustang	Joan Smith	Joan Smith
6.14	Cadiz	Mustang	Joan Smith	Joan Smith
6.15	Cadiz	Mustang	Joan Smith	Joan Smith
6.16		Pryor Mountain Mustang		Dan Elkins
6.17	Simba du Pont de Tournay	Ardennes	Joyce Concklin	JoAnn Bellone
6.18		Choctaw Spanish Mustang	Darlene and Bryant Rickman	Neil Chapman
6.19		Spanish Mustang	Marye Ann Thompson	D. Phillip Sponenberg
6.20	Custer	Pryor Mountain Mustang		Dan Elkins
6.21	Cottonwood Cassidy	Percheron	Marie Winn	Diane Blanzy
6.22	Katy de Chevemont and Clover Oaks Alexandra	Ardennes	Joyce Concklin	JoAnn Bellone
6.23	Jasoorah	Arabian	Alyssa Viera	Alyssa Viera
6.24	Chickasaw Sunrise	Choctaw Spanish Mustang	Mary Carter McConnell	D. Phillip Sponenberg
6.25	Pinta	Warmblood		© Evelyn Simak
6.26	Santiago	Wilbur-Cruce Spanish Mustang	Janie and Steve Dobrott	D. Phillip Sponenberg
6.27	Tamliora	Arabian	Michelle Stephens	Tom Sayvetz
6.28	Riley	Mustang	Sandi Claypool	Sandi Claypool
6.29	Miss Ternura	Paso Fino	Claire Hodgin	Dr Deb Bennett
6.30		Shagya Arab		© Evelyn Simak
6.31	Cimmetry	Arabian	Mary Collins	Mary Collins
7.1				Francesca Gianino
7.2				Francesca Gianino
7.3				D. Phillip Sponenberg
7.4				D. Phillip Sponenberg
7.5	Go Boy's Zorro I.A.	Missouri Fox Trotter	Dyan Westvang	Dyan Westvang
7.6		Jicarilla Apache		Dan Elkins

(*continued*)

Table 13.8 (*Continued*)

Figure	Horse name	Breed	Owner	Image credit
7.7	Foxvangen's Bracken	Missouri Fox Trotter	Dyan Westvang	Dyan Westvang
7.8		Choctaw Spanish Mustang	Darlene and Bryant Rickman	Neil Chapman
7.9	Desert Jewel Fenella	Gypsy Cob	Jennifer Gilson	Jennifer Gilson
7.10		American Paint	Jim Edwards	D. Phillip Sponenberg
7.11	Bandit's Ultimate Progression	Choctaw Spanish Mustang	Darlene and Bryant Rickman	Jeannette Beranger
7.12		Choctaw Spanish	Bryant Rickman	D. Phillip Sponenberg
7.13	Takara	Half Arabian	Sarah Murray	Sarah Murray
7.14				D. Phillip Sponenberg
7.15	Tambourine Man	Spanish Mustang	Vicki Ives	Gretchen Patterson
7.16		Nokota Horse	Leo Kuntz	D. Phillip Sponenberg
7.17		Choctaw Spanish Mustang	Darlene and Bryant Rickman	Neil Chapman
7.18		Rocky Mountain Horse	Rea Swan	D. Phillip Sponenberg
7.19	Foxvangen's Celestial Event	Missouri Fox Trotter	Dyan Westvang	Dyan Westvang
7.20		Welsh Pony	Joan Dunning	D. Phillip Sponenberg
7.21	Foxvangen's High Cotton Lass	Missouri Fox Trotter	Dyan Westvang	Dyan Westvang
7.22	Gwenog Tan	Gypsy Cob	Laurence Viala	Laurence Viala
		Clydesdale		D. Phillip Sponenberg
7.23	Comes From Dream	Spanish Mustang	Cindy Torres	Marye Ann Thompson
7.24		Choctaw Spanish Mustang	Darlene and Bryant Rickman	Neil Chapman
7.25	Foxvangen's Casper	Missouri Fox Trotter	Dyan Westvang	Dyan Westvang
7.26				D. Phillip Sponenberg
7.27				D. Phillip Sponenberg
7.28				D. Phillip Sponenberg
7.29				D. Phillip Sponenberg
7.30	Gloria frá Litla-Bergi (mare), Hlér frá Sóleyjarkoti (foal)	Icelandic	Henriette Smit-Arriens	Henriette Smit-Arriens
7.31	Journey's Made to Order	Morgan	Judith Dexter	Laura Hornick Behning
7.32	Skrámur frá Hurdaraki, Kappi frá Laugaboli, Engill frá Refsstödum	Icelandic	Henriette Smit-Arriens	Henriette Smit-Arriens
7.33				D. Phillip Sponenberg
7.34		Criollo Argentino		Luis Flores

Table 13.8 (*Continued*)

Figure	Horse name	Breed	Owner	Image credit
7.35		Thoroughbred		Luis Flores
7.36	Wind Is Red	Choctaw Spanish Mustang	Mary Carter McConnell	D. Phillip Sponenberg
7.37	Medicine Springs	Choctaw Spanish Mustang	Mary Carter McConnell	D. Phillip Sponenberg
7.38		Choctaw Spanish Mustang	Debbie Hamilton	D. Phillip Sponenberg
7.39	Big Medicine	Wilbur-Cruce Spanish Mustang	Eva Cruce	D. Phillip Sponenberg
7.40	Betsy Ross	Gypsy Cob	Debbi Jenson	Debbi Jenson
8.1	Sartor's Supermodel	Knabstrupper	Samantha McAuliffe	Petra Davidson
8.2				Sheila Archer
8.3	Don't Doubt I'm Sweet	Appaloosa	Sherry Byrd	Sherry Byrd
8.4	Taylored by Moolah	Appaloosa	Palisades Appaloosas (Lisa Estridge)	Lisa Estridge
8.5	Cayuse Song of Joy	Knabstrupper cross	Samantha McAuliffe	Petra Davidson
8.6	APS Sweet Dreams Honey	Appaloosa	Aanuka Park Stud	Petra Davidson
8.7	Florabelle	Knabstrupper cross	Judy Allen	Petra Davidson
8.8	Cayuse Iron Duke	Appaloosa	Karen Bates	Petra Davidson
8.9	Momentarily Zipped	Appaloosa cross	Petra Davidson	Petra Davidson
8.10	QAR Last Chocolate Bar	Appaloosa	Joanne and Bill Greenwood	Sheila Archer
8.11	Goer's Poco Bar	Appaloosa	Felicity Taylor	Petra Davidson
8.12	J.D.	Appaloosa	Rebecca Bellone	Rebecca Bellone
8.13	Skipelletta	Appaloosa	Palisades Appaloosas (Lisa Estridge)	Lisa Estridge
8.14	Nuggets Super Shado	Appaloosa	Palisades Appaloosas (Lisa Estridge)	Lisa Estridge
8.15	Sandys Picture	Appaloosa	Double M Bar Ranch	Cassidy Cobarr
8.16	Ambition's Copper Totem	Appaloosa	Sheila Kaminski	Sheila Kaminski
8.17	Leopardo	Andalusian × Appaloosa	Joanne and Bill Greenwood	Sheila Archer
8.18	Contessa	Knabstrupper	Sartor Stud	Sheila Archer
8.19	Nicole	Knabstrupper	Sartor Stud	Sheila Archer
8.20	Stonewall Firefly	Appaloosa	Pat Bowles	Rebecca Bellone
8.21	Cayuse Confewsion	Appaloosa	Ann and Warren Lewis	Petra Davidson
8.22	CTR Smokin Hot Eagle	Appaloosa	Cheryl Wood	Cheryl Wood

(*continued*)

Table 13.8 (*Continued*)

Figure	Horse name	Breed	Owner	Image credit
8.23	Leopardo	Andalusian × Appaloosa	Joanne and Bill Greenwood	Sheila Archer
8.24	Twilight Reemarkable	Appaloosa	Palisades Appaloosas (Lisa Estridge)	Lisa Estridge
8.25		Appaloosa		D. Phillip Sponenberg
8.26				Sheila Archer
8.27				Francesca Gianino
8.28				Sheila Archer
8.29				Sheila Archer
8.30				Francesca Gianino
8.31	Hermits Ghost Elza	Gypsy Cob	Diane Butterfield	Diane Butterfield
8.32	Mighty Incandescent	Knabstrupper cross	Robyn Payne	Petra Davidson
9.1	Stars and Stripes	Choctaw Spanish Mustang	Mary McConnell	D. Phillip Sponenberg
9.2				Francesca Gianino
11.1	Limerick Lady	Gypsy Cob	Debbi Jenson	Debbi Jenson
11.2	Curly Bess		Dyan Westvang	Dyan Westvang
11.3	Stag Creek Nabesna Dove	American Bashkir Curly	Barbara Carroll	Barbara Carroll
11.4	Stag Creek Solen	American Bashkir Curly	Barbara Carroll	Barbara Carroll
12.1		Standard	Jess Brown	D. Phillip Sponenberg
12.2		Standard	Jess Brown	D. Phillip Sponenberg
12.3	Hollyfield Magic Flower	American Mammoth	Mary Ellen Nicholas	Mary Ellen Nicholas
12.4		Poitou	Hamilton Rare Breed Foundation	D. Phillip Sponenberg
12.5	Hollyfield Irish Rose	American Mammoth	Mary Ellen Nicholas	Mary Ellen Nicholas
12.6	Front: Rebecca of Hollyfield Farm Next: Hollyfield Josie Rear: Hollyfield Magic Moonlight	American Mammoth	Mary Ellen Nicholas	Mary Ellen Nicholas
12.7		American Mammoth	Mary Ellen Nicholas	Mary Ellen Nicholas
12.8		Miniature Donkey	Marlene Clark	Marlene Clark
12.9	Honey		Good Samaritan Donkey Sanctuary Inc.	BNA Photography
12.10	Li'l Angels Brave Heart	Miniature Donkey	Deb Mix	Deb Mix
12.11	Hollyfield Oxford	American Mammoth	Mary Ellen Nicholas	Mary Ellen Nicholas

Table 13.8   *(Continued)*

Figure	Horse name	Breed	Owner	Image credit
12.12	Takota	Miniature Donkey	Connie Bonczek	Connie Bonczek
12.13	Cabinwood Farm Alexandria	Miniature Donkey	Lori Wargo	Lori Wargo
12.14		Miniature Donkey	Joan Young, Joy Miniature Donkeys	Bianca Haase
12.15	Harley	Australian	Lyn Micallef	Lyn Micallef
12.16				D. Phillip Sponenberg drawing
12.17		Andalusian	Spanish Military	D. Phillip Sponenberg
12.18	Polly		Good Samaritan Donkey Sanctuary Inc.	BNA Photography
12.19				D. Phillip Sponenberg
12.20	Hollyfield Sophie with Hollyfield Joseph	American Mammoth	Mary Ellen Nicholas	Mary Ellen Nicholas
12.21				D. Phillip Sponenberg drawing
12.22		American Mammoth	Mary Ellen Nicholas	Jeannette Beranger
12.23		Miniature Donkey	Joan Young	Bianca Haase
12.24	Carousel Farms Houston	American Mammoth	Mary Ellen Nicholas	Mary Ellen Nicholas
12.25		Miniature Donkey	Joan Young	Bianca Haase
12.26	Kit Kat	Miniature Donkey	Joan Young	Bianca Haase
12.27		Miniature Donkey	Joan Young	Bianca Haase
12.28				D. Phillip Sponenberg drawing
12.29	Wee Ones Lots of Dots	Miniature Donkey	L.J. and Deb Mix	L.J. and Deb Mix
12.30		Asinara Donkey		Valerio Joe Utzeri

Bibliography

This bibliography, while extensive, is probably not exhaustive. An attempt has been made to include most of the scientific, data-based works. To those have been added more anecdotal works if they involve the rarer colors and patterns.

Abeles, H.M.-S. 1979. A coat of many colors. *Equus* **17**: 30–38.

Abitbol, M., Legrand, R., and Tiret, L. 2014. A missense mutation in *melanocortin 1 receptor* is associated with the red coat colour in donkeys. *Immunogenetics, Molecular Genetics, and Functional Genomics* **45**: 878–880.

Abitbol, M., Legrand, R., and Tiret, L. 2015. A missense mutation in the *agouti signaling protein* gene (*ASIP*) is associated with the no light points coat phenotype in donkeys. *Genetics, Selection, Evolution* **47**: 28.

Adalsteinsson, S. 1974a. Color inheritance in farm animals and its application in selection. In *First World Congress on Genetics in Relation to Animal Breeding*, October 7–11, Madrid; pp. 29–37.

Adalsteinsson, S. 1974b. Inheritance of the palomino color in Icelandic horses. *Journal of Heredity* **65**: 15–20.

Adalsteinsson, S. 1976. Colour inheritance in Icelandic Ponies. In *First International Symposium on Genetics and Horse Breeding, Royal Dublin Society*, September 17–18, 1975, Dublin; pp. 42–49.

Adalsteinsson, S. 1978a. Inheritance of yellow dun and blue dun in the Icelandic Toelter horse. *Journal of Heredity* **69**: 146–148.

Adalsteinsson, S. 1978b. A new interpretation of the inheritance of the horse colors dun and Isabella in a Russian stud during the period 1854–1894. *Journal of Heredity* **69**: 426–429.

Adalsteinsson, S. 1978c. Vindóttur litur (Silver dapple colour). *Hesturinn okkar* **19**(1): 40.

Adalsteinsson, S. 1979a. Erfdir á litum hrossa (Inheritance of horse colours). In *Hesturinn Minn, Handbók Hestamanna*. National Association of Riding Clubs, Reykjavik.

Adalsteinsson, S. 1979b. Inheritance of colour in the Icelandic Toelter horse. In *National Seminar on Coat Colours in Horses*. Ministry of Agriculture and Fisheries.

Adalsteinsson, S. 1979c. Inheritance of colour in the Icelandic Toelter horse. In *Hoof and Horns Prospects*, May; pp. 82–86.

Adalsteinsson, S. 1979d. Inheritance of colour in the Icelandic Toelter horse. *Palomino* **24**(3): 7–10.

Equine Color Genetics, Fourth Edition. D. Phillip Sponenberg and Rebecca Bellone.
© 2017 John Wiley & Sons, Inc. Published 2017 by John Wiley & Sons, Inc.

Adalsteinsson, S. and Thorkelsson, F. 1991. *Íslenski hesturinn, litaerfdir (The Icelandic Horse, Colour Inheritance).* Islandsmyndir, Kópavógur, Iceland.

Al-Diwan, M.A. and Al-Jassim, A.F. 1988. Morphological aspects of Arab horses in Iraq. *Indian Journal of Animal Sciences* **58**: 396–398.

Almen, M.S., Imsland, F., Mikko, S., and Rubin, C.J. 2015. Whole genome reseqeucnig of ten breed specific DNA pools and 34 individual horses-selective sweep screens and comprehensive analyses of genetic variation. In *Eleventh Dorothy Russell Havemeyer Foundation International Equine Genome Mapping Workshop,* Hannover, Germany, July 22–25.

Andersson, L. 2003. Melanocortin receptor variants with phenotypic effects in horse, pig, and chicken. *Annals of the New York Academy of Sciences* **994**: 313–318.

Andersson, L. and Sandberg, K. 1982. A linkage group composed of three coat color genes and three protein loci in horses. *Journal of Heredity* **73**: 91–94.

Andersson, L.S., Axelsson, J., Dubielzig, R.R., *et al.* 2011. Multiple congenital ocular abnormalities in Icelandic horses. *BMC Veterinary Research* **7**: 21.

Arabian Horse Registry of America. 1970. *Identifying the Arabian.* Arabian Horse Registry of America, Englewood, CO.

Bellone, R., Lawson, S., Hunter, N., *et al.* 2006a. Analysis of a SNP found in exon 7 of equine OCA2 and its exclusion as a cause for Appaloosa spotting. *Animal Genetics* **37**: 525.

Bellone, R., Lear, T., Adelson, D., and Bailey, E. 2006b. Comparative mapping of oculocutaneous albinism type II (*OCA2*), transient receptor potential cation channel, subfamily M member 1 (*TRPM1*) and two equine microsatellites, *ASB08* and *1CA43*, among four equid species by in situ hybridization. *Cytogenetic and Genome Research* **114**: 93A. doi: 10.1159/000091935.

Bellone, R., Brooks, S.A., Sandmeyer, L., *et al.* 2008. Differential gene expression of *TRPM1*, the potential cause of congenital stationary night blindness and coat spotting patterns (*LP*) in the Appaloosa horse (*Equus caballus*). *Genetics* **179**: 1861–1870.

Bellone, R.R., Holl, H., Setaluri, V., *et al.* 2013. Evidence for a retroviral insertion in *TRPM1* as the cause of congenital stationary night blindness and leopard complex spotting in the horse. *PLoS One* **8**(10): e78220. doi: 10.1371/journal.pone.0078280.

Bennett, D. 1987. Genetic alchemy, true colors. *Modern Horse Breeding* **4**(2): 21–25.

Berge, S. 1963. Heste fargenes Genetikk. *Tidsskrift for det Norske Landbruk* **70**: 359–410.

Bin, B.-H., Bhin, J., Yang, S.H., *et al.* 2015. Membrane-associated transporter protein (MATP) regulates melanosomal pH and influences tyrosinase activity. *PLoS One* **10**(6): e0129273. doi: 10.1371/journal.pone.0129273.

Blakeslee, L.H., Huston, R.S., and Hunt, H.R. 1943. Curly coat in horses. *Journal of Heredity* **34**: 115–118.

Blunn, C. and Howell, C. 1936. The inheritance of white facial markings in Arab horses. *Journal of Heredity* **27**: 293–299.

Bogart, R. 1978. Color changes with age. *Appaloosa News* (April): 134–135.

Bowling, A.T. 1987. Equine linkage group II: phase conservation of *To* with *Al^B* and *Gc^{S.}* *Journal of Heredity* **78**: 248–250.

Bowling, A.T. 1994. Dominant inheritance of overo spotting in Paint horses. *Journal of Heredity* **85**: 222–224.

Brandsch, H. and Gerber, J. 1987a. The inheritance of hair colour in Hafling horses. *Archiv für Tierzucht* **30**: 55–62.

Brandsch, H. and Gerber, J. 1987b. Inheritance of markings in horses. 1. Objective and description of statistical studies. *Archiv für Tierzucht* **30**: 451–457.

Brandsch, H. and Gerber, J. 1987c. The inheritance of markings in horses. 2. Segregation in different mating groups. *Archiv für Tierzucht* **30**: 517–521.

Brandsch, H. and Gerber, J. 1988a. The inheritance of markings in horses. 3. Relationships between colour, markings, and sex. *Archiv für Tierzucht* **31**: 73–81.

Brandsch, H. and Gerber, J. 1988b. The inheritance of markings in horses. 4. Working hypothesis to explain the relationship between inheritance of colour and markings. *Archiv für Tierzucht* **31**: 385–390.

Briquet, R., Jr. 1957. So-called "albino horses". *Boletim de Indústria Animal* **16**: 243.

Briquet, R., Jr. 1959a. Investigations on the Relationship between Markings on the Face and Limbs in Horses. *Revista de Ramonta Veterinaria* **19**. (whole issue).

Briquet, R., Jr. 1959b. The genetics of pangaré. *Anais da Escola de Fluminense Medicina Veterinaria (Niteroi)* **2**: 93–96.

Brooks, S.A. and Bailey, E. 2005. Exon skipping in the *KIT* gene casues a sabino spotting pattern in horses. *Mammalian Genome* **16**: 893–902.

Brooks, S.A., Terry, R.B., and Bailey, E. 2002. A PCR–RFLP for *KIT* associated with tobiano spotting pattern in horses. *Animal Genetics* **33**: 301–303.

Brooks, S.A., Lear, T.L., Anderson, D.L., and Bailey, E. 2007. A chromosome inverstion near the *KIT* gene and the tobiano spotting pattern in horses. *Cytogenetic and Genome Research* **119**: 225–230.

Brooks, S.A., Gabreski, N., Miller, D., *et al.* 2010. Whole-genome SNP association in the horse: identification of a deletion in myosin Va responsible for lavender foal syndrome. *PLoS Genetics* **6**(4): e1000909. doi: 10.1371/journal.pgen.1000909.

Brunberg, E., Andersson, L., Cothran, G., *et al.* 2006. A missense mutation in PMEL17 is associated with the silver color in the horse. *BMC Genetics* **7**: 46.

Butaye, R. 1974. Inheritance of coat colors in Belgian horses. *Vlaams Diergeneeskundig Tijdschrift* **43**: 464–486.

Cabrera, A. 1933. Curiosidades sobre los pelajes overos. *Anales de la Asociación de Criadores del Criollo* **8**: 29–37.

Caldeira, R.M. and Portas, M.C.P. 1999. Contributo para a classificaçao dos tipos de pelagens de equinos. *Veterinária Técnica* **9**(4): 18–32.

Carr, G. 1972. Few spotted leopards—a possible key to high color production. *Appaloosa News* (Nov–Dec): 18–20.

Carr, G. 1973. Few spotted leopards—a study in increasing Appaloosa foal percentage. *Pony of the Americas Magazine* 12–14.

Castle, W. 1940a. *Mammalian Genetics*. Harvard University Press, Cambridge, MA.

Castle, W. 1940b. The genetics of coat color in horses. *Journal of Heredity* **31**: 127–128.

Castle, W. 1942. The ABC of color inheritance in horses. *Journal of Heredity* **33**: 23–25.

Castle, W. 1946. Genetics of the palomino horse. *Journal of Heredity* **37**: 35–38.

Castle, W. 1951a. Dominant and recessive black in mammals. *Journal of Heredity* **42**: 48–50.

Castle, W. 1951b. Genetics of the color variety of horses. *Journal of Heredity* **42**: 297.

Castle, W. 1952. The eumelanin horse: black or brown. *Journal of Heredity* **43**: 68.

Castle, W. 1953. Note on the silver dapple mutation of Shetland Ponies. *Journal of Heredity* **44**: 224.

Castle, W. 1954. Coat colour inheritance in horses and in other animals. *Genetics* **39**: 35–44.

Castle, W. 1960. Fashion in the color of Shetland ponies and its genetic basis. *Journal of Heredity* **51**: 247.

Castle, W. 1961. The genetics of the claybank-dun horse. *Journal of Heredity* **52**: 121–122.

Castle, W. and King, F. 1951. New evidence of the genetics of the palomino horse. *Journal of Heredity* **42**: 61–64.

Castle, W. and Singleton, W. 1960. Genetics of the brown horse. *Journal of Heredity* **51**: 127–131.

Castle, W. and Smith, F. 1953. Silver dapple, a unique color variety among Shetland Ponies. *Journal of Heredity* **44**: 139–146.

Cook, D., Brooks, S., Bellone, R., and Bailey, E. 2008. Missense mutation in exon 2 of SLC36A1 responsible for champagne dilution in horses. *PLoS Genetics* **4**(9): e1000195. doi: 10.1371/journal.pgen.1000195.

Craig, L. and Van Vleck, L.D. 1985. Evidence for inheritance of the red dun dilution in the horse. *Journal of Heredity* **76**: 138–139.

Crew, F. and Smith, B.A. 1930. The genetics of the horse. *Bibliographica Genetica* **6**: 123–170.

Curik, I., Seltenhammer, M., and Sölkner, J. 2002. Quantitative genetic analysis of melanoma and grey level in Lipizzan horses. In *Proceedings of the 7th World Congress on Genetics Applied to Livestock Production*, Montpellier, France, August, Session 5, pp. 0–4.

Curik, I., Druml, T., Seltenhammer, M., *et al.* 2013. Complex inheritance of melanoma and pigmentation of coat and skin in grey horses. *PLoS Genetics* **9**(2): e1003248. doi: 10.1371/journal.pgen.1003248.

Denhardt, R.M. 1948. What color is he? *Western Horseman* (Jan–Feb): 19–62.

Denhardt, R.M. 1975. *The Horse of the Americas*, 2nd edn. University of Oklahoma Press, Norman, OK.

Dobie, J.F. 1952. *The Mustangs*. Little, Brown, Boston, MA.

Domanski, A. and Prawochenski, R. 1948. Dun coat colours in horses. *Journal of Heredity* **39**: 367–371.

Dowdall, R.C. 1935. Overos y tobianos—su diferenciación. *Anales de la Asociación de Criadores del Criollo* **10**: 46–61.

Dowdall, R.C. 1937. Overos y tobianos (continuación). *Anales de la Asociación de Criadores del Criollo* **11**: 23–33.

Dowdall, R.C. 1963. *Ensayo de Clasificación de las Pelajes de Caballo*. Author, Buenos Aires.

Dreux, P. 1966. Contribution a l'étude du gène *E* chez le cheval domestique. *Annales de Génétique* **9**(4): 168–170.

Dreux, P. 1970. The degree of expression on limited piebaldness in the domestic horse. *Annales de Génétique et de Sélection Animale* **2**: 119.

Dring, L.A., Hintz, H.F., and Van Vleck, L.D. 1981. Coat color and gestation length in Thoroughbred mares. *Journal of Heredity* **72**: 65–66.

Evans, C.C. 1979. The celestial heritage of a few-spotted leopard. *Appaloosa News* **36**: 58–61.

Ewart, S.L., Ramsey, D.T., Xu, J., and Meyers, D. 2000. The horse homolog of congenital aniridia conforms to codominant inheritance. *Journal of Heredity* **91**: 93–98.

Gallardo, R.C. 1923. *La Equitación Mexicana*. Havana.

Gallardo, R.C. 1936. *El Libro del Charro Mexicano*. Mexico City.

García Martínez, A., Valera Córdoba, M., Molina Alcalá, A., and Rodero Franganillo, A. 1998. Genetic study of coat color in the characterization of horse breeds. *Archivos de Zootecnia* 47: 247–253.

Geurts, R. 1977. *Hair Colour in the Horse*. J.A. Allen and Co., London.

Gower, J. 1999. *Horse Colour Explained: A Breeder's Perspective*. Kangaroo Press, East Roseville, NSW, Australia.

Green, B.K. 1974. *The Color of Horses*. Northland Press, Flagstaff, AZ.

Gremmel, F. 1939. Coat colors in horses. *Journal of Heredity* 30: 437–445.

Haase, B., Brooks, S.A., Schlumbaum, A., *et al.* 2007. Allelic heterogeneity at the equine *Kit* locus in dominant white (*W*) horses. *PloS Genetics* 3: 2101–2108.

Haase, B., Jude, R., Brooks, S.A., and Leeb, T. 2008. An equine chromosome 3 inversion is associated with the tobiano spotting pattern in German horse breeds. *Animal Genetics* 39: 306–309.

Haase, B., Brooks, S.A., Tozaki, T., *et al.* 2009. Seven novel *KIT* mutations in horses with white coat colour phenotypes. *Animal Genetics* 40(5): 623–629. doi: 10.1111/j.1365-2052.2009.01893.x.

Haase, B., Signer-Hasler, H., Binns, M.M., *et al.* 2013. Accumulating mutations in series of haplotypes at the *KIT* and *MITF* loci are major determinants of white markings in Franches-Montagnes horses. *PLoS One* 8(9): e75071. doi: 10.1371/journal.pone.0075071.

Haase, B., Rieder, S., and Leeb, T. 2015. Two variants in the *KIT* gene as candidate causative mutations for a dominant white and a white spotting phenotype in the donkey. *Immunogenetics, Molecular Genetics, and Functional Genomics* 46: 321–324.

Hadwen, S. 1931. The melanomata of gray and white horses. *Canadian Medical Association Journal* 21: 519.

Haines, F. 1963. *Appaloosa, the Spotted Horse in Art and History*. University of Texas Press, Austin, TX.

Halvorson, J. 1977. The leopard that didn't get his spots. *Appaloosa News* (Dec): 62–64.

Hatley, G.B. 1962. Crosses that will kill your color. *Appaloosa News* 19(Feb) (available as an eight-page reprint).

Hauswirth, R., Haase, B., Blatter, M., *et al.* 2012. Mutations in *MITF* and *PAX3* cause "splashed white" and other white spotting phenotypes in horses. *PLoS Genetics* 8(4): e1002653. doi: 10.1371/journal/pgen.1002653.

Hauswirth, R., Jude, R., Haase, B., *et al.* 2013. Novel variants in the *KIT* and *PAX3* genes in horses with white-spotted coat colour phenotypes. *Animal Genetics* 44(6): 763–765. doi: 10.1111/age.12057.

Hawkins, R. 1965. *The Appaloosa: Breed Characteristics*. Hawkins & Hubbell, Riverside, CA.

Hemmer, H. 1990. *Domestication: The Decline of Environmental Appreciation*. Cambridge University Press, Cambridge.

Henner, J., Poncet, P.A., Aebi, L., *et al.* 2002a. Horse breeding: genetic tests for coat colors chestnut, bay, and black. Results from a first study in the Swiss Franches-Montagnes horse breed. *Schweizer Archiv für Tierheilkunde* 144: 405–412.

Henner, J., Poncet, P.A., Guérin, G., *et al.* 2002b. Genetic mapping of the (*G*) locus, responsible for the coat colour phenotype progressive greying with age in horses (*Equus caballus*). *Mammalian Genome* 13: 535–537.

Hintz, H.F. and Van Vleck, L.D. 1979. Lethal dominant roan in horses. *Journal of Heredity* **70**: 145–146.

Holl, H., Brooks, S., and Bailey, E. 2010. De novo mutation of KIT discovered as a result of a non-hereditary white coat colour pattern. *Animal Genetics* **41**: 196–198.

Holl, H., Brooks, S., Archer, A., *et al.* 2016. Variant in the *RFWD3* gene associated with *PATN1*, a modifier of leopard complex spotting. *Animal Genetics* **47**: 91–101. doi: 10.1111/age.12375.

Huitema, H. 1964. Archaic pattern in the horse and its relation to colour genes. *Zeitschrift für Säugetierkunde* **29**: 42–46.

Hultgren, B.D. 1982. Ileocolonic aganglionosis in white progeny of overo spotted horses. *Journal of the American Veterinary Medicine Association* **180**: 289–292.

Hultgren, B.D. 1985. Lethal whites, the problem that won't go away. *Paint Horse Journal* (Jan): 38–39.

Hultgren, B.D. and Duffield, D. 1986. Spotted horse research, an update. *Paint Horse Journal* (Mar): 116.

Hultgren, B.D., Appell, L.H., Wagner, P.C., *et al.* 1987. Current research topics in equine genetics. *I. Equine Practice* **9**(10): 38–43.

Imsland, F., McGowan, K., Rubin, C.-J., *et al.* 2016. Regulatory mutations in *TBX3* disrupt asymmetric hair pigmentation that underlies Dun camouflage color in horses. *Nature Genetics* **48**: 152–158. doi: 10.1038/ng.3475.

Jacobs, L.N., Staiger, E.A., Albright, J.D., and Brooks, S.A. 2015. "A sorrel is hot . . .": a genetic investigation of the horseman's myth. *Journal of Equine Veterinary Science* **35**: 383. doi: http://dx.doi.org/10.1016/j.jevs.2015.03.009.

Jones, W. 1971. Appaloosa color inheritance. *Appaloosa News* **28**(1): 26–30.

Jones, W.E. 1979. Overo white foal syndrome. *Journal of Equine Medicine and Surgery* **3**: 54.

Jones, W.E. 1982. *Genetics and Horse Breeding.* Lee and Febiger, Philadelphia, PA.

Jones, W. and Bogart, R. 1971. *Genetics of the Horse.* Caballus Publications, East Lansing, MI.

Kaseda, Y. 1988. Fourteen pedigrees and their purity in Misaki feral horses. *Bulletin of the Faculty of Agriculture, Miyazaki University* **35**: 171–185.

Kathman, L. 2014. *The Equine Tapestry: An Introduction to Colors and Patterns.* Blackberry Lane Press.

Kilby, E. 1984. Visible differences: when coat color counts. *Equus* **81**: 37–84.

Klemola, V. 1933. The pied and splashed white patterns in horses and ponies. *Journal of Heredity* **24**: 65–69.

Knowles-Pfeiffer, C. 2000. *Horse and Pony Coat Colours.* Allen Photographic Guides, Number 30. J.A. Allen, London.

Kowalski, E.J.A. and Bellone, R.R. 2011. Investigation of *HERC2* and *OCA2* SNP for iris color variation in Puerto Rican Paso Fino horses. *Journal of Equine Veterinary Science* **31**(5): 319.

Kräusslich, H. 1996. On the genetics of point and body color loci in horses in comparison to molecular analyses of colour loci in mice. *Züchtungskunde* **63**: 1–11.

Kriegesmann, B., Jansen, S., Bishop, M., and Brenig, B. 1996. The equine MSH-R TaqI RFLP is not informative for hair colour in Arabian horses. *Animal Genetics* **27**: 64.

Labiano, A.M. 1977. *Tres Ensayos Sobre Pelajes: El Bayo, El Moro, y El Tordillo.* Editorial Hemisferio Sur, Buenos Aires.

Labiano, A.M. 1999. *Overos Manchados*. Editorial Dunken, Buenos Aires.

Lauvergne, J.J., Silvestrelli, M., Langlois, B., *et al.* 1991. A new scheme for describing horse coat colour. *Livestock Production Science* **27**: 219–229.

LeFevre, A.A. 1989. La robe du cheval: nomenclature et determinisme génétique. Thesis, Toulouse Veterinary School, Toulouse, France.

Legrand, R., Tiret, L., and Abitbol, M. 2014. Two recessive mutations in *FGF5* are associated with long-hair phenotype in donkeys. *Genetics, Selection, Evolution* **46**: 65.

Lieberman, B. 1982. Speckles, splashes, and spots. *Equus* **62**: 40–45.

Llewellyn, R. 1963. A theory on Appaloosa coat markings. *Appaloosa News* (Apr): 16–18.

Locke, M.M., Rugh, L.S., Millon, L.V., *et al.* 2001. The cream dilution gene, responsible for the palomino and buckskin coat colours, maps to horse chromosome 21. *Animal Genetics* **32**: 340–343.

Locke, M.M., Penedo, M.C.T., Bricker, S.J., *et al.* 2002. Linkage of the grey coat colour locus to microsatellites on horse chromosome 25. *Animal Genetics* **33**: 329–337.

Loen, J. 1939. Fargenedarvinga hos Vestlandshesten (Fjordhesten) (Color inheritance in the Norwegian Fjord Horse). *Stambok over Vestlandshesten*. II. Band 1–52, Oslo, Norway.

Lubas, G. and Bertani, P. 1988. Historical and morphological review of the Appaloosa breed of horse, with consideration of colour inheritance. *Annali della Facoltà di Medicina Veterinaria di Pisa* **41**: 348–355.

Ludwig, A., Pruvost, M., Reissman, M., *et al.* 2009. Coat Color variation at the beginning of horse domestication. *Science* **324**: 485.

Ludwig, A., Reissmann, M., Benecke, N., *et al.* 2015. Twenty-five thousand years of fluctuating selection on leopard complex spotting and congenital night blindness in horses. *Philosophical Transactions of the Royal Society B* **370**: 20130386. doi: http://dx.doi.org/10.1098/rstb.2013.0386.

Mariat, D., Taourit, S., and Guérin, G. 2003. A mutation in the *MATP* gene causes cream coat colour in the horse. *Genetics, Selection, Evolution* **35**: 119–133.

Marklund, S., Moller M., Sandberg, K., and Andersson, L. 1996. A missense mutation in the gene for melanocyte-stimulating hormone receptor (*MC1R*) is associated with the chestnut coat colour in horses. *Mammalian Genome* **7**: 895–899.

Marklund, S., Moller, M., Sandberg, K., and Andersson, L. 1999. Close association between sequence polymorphism in the *KIT* gene and the roan coat colour in horses. *Mammalian Genome* **10**: 283–288.

Marrero y Galindez, A. 1945. *Cromohipologia*. Author, Buenos Aires.

Mau, C., Poncet, P.A., Bucher, B., *et al.* 2004. Genetic mapping of dominant white (*W*) a homozygous lethal condition in the horse (*Equus caballus*). *Journal of Animal Breeding and Genetics* **11**: 374–383.

McCabe, L., Griffin, L.D., Kinzer, A., *et al.* 1990. Overo lethal white foal syndrome: equine model of aganglionic megacolon (Hirschsprung disease). *American Journal of Medical Genetics* **36**: 336–340.

McCann, L. 1916. Sorrel color in horses. *Journal of Heredity* **7**: 370–72.

Merkens, J. 1953. De Vererving van de Kleuren Bij Paarden. *Tijd. voor Diergeneeskunde* **78**: 189–216.

Metallinos, D.L., Bowling, A.T., and Rine, J. 1998 A missense mutation in the endothelin-B receptor gene is associated with lethal white foal syndrome: an equine version of Hirschsprung disease. *Mammalian Genome* **9**: 426–431.

Meyer, E., von Kumn, U., and Dencker, C. 1981. *Farbe und Abzeichen bei Pferden*. M&H Schaper, Hannover.

Miller, R.W. n.d. *Appaloosa Coat Color Inheritance*. The Appaloosa Horse Club, Inc., Moscow, ID.

Mills, D.S., Alston, R.D., Rogers, V., and Longford, N.T. 2002. Factors associated with the prevalence of stereotypic behaviour amongst Thoroughbred horses passing through auctioneer sales. *Applied Animal Behaviour Science* **78**: 115–124.

Morgenthaler, C., Gilles, M., Cothran, E.G., *et al.* 2015. Caratérisation de l'hypoallergenie du cheval Curly et analyse du lien avac la frisure. *Journée de la Recherche Équine* **41**: 150–153.

Murgiano, L., Waluk, D., Towers, R., *et al.* 2017. An intronic *MBTPS2* variant results in a splicing defect in horses with brindle coat texture. *Genes Genomes Genetics*. doi: 10.1534/g3.116.032433.

Nebe, H.D. 1984. Colour inheritance in the horse with special reference to white markings. Thesis, Justus-Liebig-Universität Giessen.

Neto, A.P.L. 1990. The inheritance of coat color in saddle horses. *Revista Portuguesa de Ciencia Veterinarias* **35**: 214–218.

Norton, D. 1949. *The Palomino Horse*. Bordon, Los Angeles, CA.

Ochsner, V. 1980. At the end of a rainbow. *The Pony Journal* (Oct–Nov): 25–52.

Odriozola, M. 1948. *Agouti* color in horses: change of dominance in equine hybrids. In *Proceedings of the Eighth International Congress of Genetics*; p. 635.

Odriozola, M. 1951. *A los Colores del Caballo*. Publicaciones del Sindicato Nacional de Ganadería, Madrid.

Odriozola, M. 1952. The eumelanin horse: black or brown? *Journal of Heredity* **43**: 76–77.

Pielberg, G., Mikko, S., Sandberg, K., and Andersson, L. 2005. Comparative linkage mapping of the grey coat colour gene in horses. *Animal Genetics* **36**: 390–395.

Pielberg, G.S., Golovko, A., Sundström, E., *et al.* 2008. A *cis*-acting regulatory mutation causes premature hair graying and susceptibility to melanoma in the horse. *Nature Genetics* **40**: 1004–1009. doi: 10.1038/ng.185.

Pinna, W., Cappio Borlino, A., Vacca, G.M., and Lai, G. 1993. Morphology of adult white donkeys of Asinara. *Bollettino della Societa Italiana di Biologia Sperimentale* **69**: 595–600.

Porte F., Garibaldi, E., and Garibaldi, M.G. 1987. A study of some biological traits in Chilean Criollo horses. 2. Coat colour. *Avances en Producción Animal* **12**: 203–208.

Pulos, W. and Hutt, F. 1969. Lethal dominant white in horses. *Journal of Heredity* **60**: 59–64.

Reissman, M., Bierwolf, B., and Brockman, G.A. 2007. Two SNPs in the *SILV* gene are associated with silver coat colour in ponies. *Animal Genetics* **38**: 1–6.

Rieder, S. 2009. Molecular tests for coat colours in horses. *Journal of Animal Breeding and Genetics* **126**(6): 415–424. doi: 10.1111/j.1439-0388.2009.00832.x.

Rieder, S., Taourit, S., Mariat, D., *et al.* 2001. Mutations in the agouti (*ASIP*), the extension (*MCIR*) and the brown (*TYRP1*) loci and their association to coat color phenotypes in the horses (*Equus caballus*). *Mammalian Genome* **12**: 450–455.

Rieder, S., Hagger, C., Obexer-Ruff, G., *et al.* 2008. Genetic analysis of white facial and leg markings in the Swiss Franches-Montagnes horse breed. *Journal of Heredity* **99**: 130–136.

Rogers, L. 1972. Inheritance of coat color and markings in the Tennessee Walking Horse. *Voice of the Tennessee Walking Horse* (Feb): 32–34.

Royal College of Veterinary Surgeons. 1954. *Colors and Markings of Horses.* Royal College of Veterinary Surgeons, London.

Salisbury, G. and Britton, J. 1914a. The inheritance of equine coat color. I. The basic colors and patterns. *Journal of Heredity* **32**: 235–240.

Salisbury, G. and Britton, J. 1914b. The inheritance of equine coat color. II. The dilutes. *Journal of Heredity* **32**: 255–260.

Sánchez-Belda A. 1995. Pied coat colour in horses and a censure of its veto in the Andalusian breed. *Avances en Alimentación y Mejora Animal* **35**: 13–24.

Sánchez-Belda, A. 1997. The veto against chestnut coat color in Andalusian horses. *Avances en Alimentación y Mejora Animal* **37**: 3–25.

Sanders, I.M. and Wiersema, J.K. 1963. Het Hippisch Kleurenpalet. *Veeteelt en Zuivel Berichten* **6**: 54–58.

Sandmeyer, L.S., Breaux, C.B., Archer, S., and Grahn, B.H. 2007. Clinical and electroretinographic characteristics of congenital stationary night blindness in the Appaloosa and the association with the leopard complex. *Veterinary Ophthalmology* **10**: 368–375.

Sandmeyer, L.S., Bellone, R.R., Archer, S., *et al.* 2012. Congenital stationary night blindness is associated with the leopard complex in the miniature horse. *Veterinary Ophthalmology* **15**(1): 18–22.

Santschi, E.M., Purdy, A.K., Valberg, S.J., *et al.* 1998. Endothelin receptor B polymorphism associated with lethal white foal syndrome in horses. *Mammalian Genome* **9**: 306–309.

Santschi, E.M., Vrotsos, P.D., Purdy, A.K., and Mickelson, J.R. 2001. Incidence of the lethal white foal endothelin receptor B mutation in white patterned horses. *American Journal of Veterinary Research* **62**: 96–102.

Schneider, G.W. and Leipold, H.W. 1978. Recessive lethal white in two foals. *Journal of Equine Medicine and Surgery* **2**: 479–482.

Shchkein, V.A. and Kalaev, V.V. 1941. Inheritance of curliness in horses. *Comptes Rendus de l'Académie des Sciences de l'URSS* **26**: 262–263.

Shephard, C. 2002. The barlink factor. *Champagne Horse Journal* **1**(3): 10.

Searle, A. 1968. *Comparative Genetics of Coat Colour in Mammals.* Logos, London.

Sigre, B. 1984. *Pelajes del Caballo.* Editorial Albatross, Buenos Aires.

Singleton, R. 1969. The genetics of mammalian coat color. *Journal of Heredity* **60**: 25–26.

Singleton, R. and Bond, Q. 1966. A allele necessary for dilute coat color in horses. *Journal of Heredity* **57**: 75–77.

Skorkowski, E. 1966. The derivation of domestic horses from the wild ones. *World Review of Animal Production* **2**(4): 59–64.

Skorkowski, E. 1972. Colour and constitutional peculiarities go together (Darwin, 1859). *World Review of Animal Production* **8**(4): 70–75.

Skorkowski, E. 1976. Colour, types, and shapes and the principles of horse breeding. *World Review of Animal Production* **12**(1): 45–50.

Smith, A. 1925. A study of the inheritance of certain color characters in the Shorthorn breed. *Journal of Heredity* **16**: 73–84.

Spence, S.E. 1967. Can you tell tobiano from overo? *Paint Horse Journal* **1**: 17.

Sponenberg, D.P. 1982. The inheritance of leopard spotting in the Noriker horse. *Journal of Heredity* **73**: 357–359.

Sponenberg, D.P. 1990. Dominant curly coat in horses. *Genetics Selection Evolution* **22**: 257–260.

Sponenberg, D.P. 1996. *Equine Color Genetics*, 1st edn. Iowa State University Press, Ames, IA.

Sponenberg, D.P. and Beaver, B.V. 1983. *Horse Color.* Texas A&M University Press, College Station, TX.

Sponenberg, D.P. and Weise, M.C. 1997. Dominant black in horses. *Genetics, Selection, and Evolution* **29**: 405–410.

Sponenberg, D.P., Harper, H.T., and Harper, A.L. 1984. Direct evidence for linkage of roan and extension loci in Belgian horses. *Journal of Heredity* **75**: 413–414.

Sponenberg, D.P., Ito, S., Eng, L.A., and Schwink, K. 1988. Pigment types of various color genotypes of horses. *Pigment Cell Research* **1**: 410–413.

Sponenberg, D.P., Carr, G., Simak, E., and Schwink, K. 1990. The inheritance of the leopard complex of spotting patterns in horses. *Journal of Heredity* **81**: 323–331.

Stachurska, A., and Jansen, P. 2015. Crypto-tobiano horses in Hucul breed. *Czech Journal of Animal Science* **60**(1): 1–9. doi: 10.17221/7905-CJAS.

Stachurksa, A. and Pieta, M. 2006. Is there a relationship between coat colour, age, and racing performance in horses? *Annals of Animal Science* **6**: 249–255.

Stachurska, A., Ussing, A.P., and Kolstrung, R. 2005. Tobiano and leopard alleles in Felin Pony population. *Electronic Journal of Polish Agricultural Universities* **5**(1): 04. http://www.ejpau.media.pl/volume5/issue1/animal/art-04.html (accessed February 15, 2017).

Sturtevant, A.H. 1910. On the inheritance of color in the American harness horse. *Biological Bulletin* **19**(3): 204–216.

Sturtevant, A.H. 1912. A critical examination of recent studies on color inheritance in horses. *Journal of Genetics* **2**(1): 41–51.

Sundström, E., Imsland, F., Mikko, S., *et al.* 2012a. Copy number expansion of the *STX17* duplication in melanoma tissue from Grey horses. *BMC Genomics* **13**, 1–14.

Sundström, E., Komisarczuk, A.Z., Jiang, L., *et al.* 2012b. Identification of a melanocyte-specific, microphthalmia-associated transcription factor-dependent regulatory element in the intronic duplication causing hair greying and melanoma in horses. *Pigment Cell & Melanoma Research* **25**(1): 28–36.

Swinburne, J.E., Hopkins, A., and Binns, M.M. 2002. Assignment of the horse grey coat colour gene to *ECA25* using whole genome scanning. *Animal Genetics* **33**: 338–342.

Terry, R.B., Bailey, E., Lear, T., and Cothran, E.G. 2002. Rejection of *MITF* and *MGF* as the genes responsible for Appaloosa coat colour patterns in horses. *Animal Genetics* **33**: 82–84.

Terry, R.B., Archer, S., Brooks, S., *et al.* 2004. Assignment of the Appaloosa coat colour gene (*LP*) to equine chromosome 1. *Animal Genetics* **35**: 134–137.

Terry, R.R., Bailey, E., Bernoco, D., and Cothran, E.G. 2001. Linked markers exclude *KIT* as the gene responsible for Appaloosa coat color spotting patterns in horses. *Animal Genetics* **32**: 98–101.

Teixeira, R.B.C., Rendahl, A.K., Anderson, S.M., *et al.* 2013. Coat color genotypes and risk and severity of melanoma in gray quarter horses. *Journal of Veterinary Internal Medicine* **27**: 1201–1208.

Towers, R.E., Murgiano, L., Millar, D.S., *et al.* 2013. A nonsense mutation in the *IKBKG* gene in mares with incontinentia pigmenti. *PloS One* **8**(12): e81625. doi: 10.1371/journal.pone.0081625.

Trommershausen-Smith, A. 1972. Inheritance of chin spot markings in horses. *Journal of Heredity* **63**: 100.

Trommershausen-Smith, A. 1977. Lethal white foals in matings of overo spotted horses. *Theriogenology* **8**: 303–311.

Trommershausen-Smith, A. 1978. Linkage of tobiano coat spotting and albumin markers in a pony family. *Journal of Heredity* **69**: 214–216.

Trommershausen-Smith, A. 1979. Positive horse identification. 3. Coat color genetics. *Equine Practice* **1**: 24–35.

Trommershausen-Smith, A., Suzuki, Y., and Stormont, C. 1976. Use of blood typing to confirm principles of coat color genetics in horses. *Journal of Heredity* **67**: 6–10.

Tuff, P. 1933. Genetiske undersøkelser over hestefarver. In Nordiska Veterinärmöt— Kongressberättelse (Helsingfors), pp. 689–716.

Ussing, A.P. 2000. *Hestenes Farver*. Nucleus Forlag, Aarhus.

Utzeri, V.J., Bertolini, F., Ribani, A., *et al.* 2015. The albinism of feral Asinara white donkeys (*Equus asinus*) is determined by a missense mutation in a highly conserved position of the tyrosinase (*TYR*) gene deduced protein. *Animal Genetics* **47**: 120–124.

VanVleck, L.D. and Davitt, M. 1977. Confirmation of a gene for dominant dilution of horse color. *Journal of Heredity* **68**: 280–282.

Vecchioto, G.G. 1991. A note on the inheritance of coat colour in the Haflinger breed. 1. Flaxen mane and tail. *Ippologia* **2**: 61–63.

Von Lehmann, E. 1975. Zur Farbgenetik des Pferdes unter besonderer Berücksichtigung der Wildformen. *Zeitschrift für Tierzüchtung und Züchtungsbiologie* **92**: 106–117.

Von Lehmann, E. 1981. Zur Genetik eines abgestuften Farbmerkmales (Tigerung) beim Pferd (*Equus caballus* L.) und Hauskaninchen (Oryctolagus cuniculus L.). *Bonner Zoologische Beiträge* **32** (1–2): 46–66.

Von Lehmann, E. 1989. Dappling in coats of horses. *Journal of Animal Breeding and Genetics* **106**: 237–239.

Von Tscharner, C., Kunkle, G., and Yager, J. (eds) 2000. Stannard's Illustrated Equine Dermatology Notes. *Veterinary Dermatology* **11**. (3).

Vonerfecht, S.L., Bowling, A.T., and Cohen, M. 1983. Congenital intestinal aganglionosis in white foals. *Veterinary Pathology* **20**: 65–70.

Wagner, H.-J. and Reissmann, M. 2000. New polymorphism detected in the horse *MC1R* gene. *Animal Genetics* **31**: 290–291.

Walther, A. 1912. *Beiträge zur Kenntnis de Vererberung der Pferdefarben*. Schaper, Hannover.

Wentworth, E. 1914. Color inheritance in the horse. *Zeitschrift fur Induktive Abstammungs- und Vererbungslehre* **2**: 10–17.

Wiersema, J.K. 1977. *Het Paard in Zijn Kleurenrijkdoom*. Zuidgroep B.V. Uitgevers, The Hague.

Wilson, J. 1910. The inheritance of coat colour in horses. *Proceedings of the Royal Dublin Society* **12**: 341–348.

Wilson, J. 1912. The inheritance of the dun coat colour in horses. *Proceedings of the Royal Irish Academy* **13**: 184–201.

Woolf, C.M. 1989. Multifactorial inheritance of white facial markings in the Arabian horse. *Journal of Heredity* **80**: 173–178.

Woolf, C.M. 1990. Multifactorial inheritance of common white markings in the Arabian horse. *Journal of Heredity* **81**: 250–256.

Woolf, C.M. 1991. Common white facial markings in bay and chestnut Arabian horses and their hybrids. *Journal of Heredity* **82**: 167–169.

Woolf, C.M. 1992. Common white facial markings in Arabian horses that are homozygous and heterozygous for alleles at the A and E loci. *Journal of Heredity* **83**: 73–77.

Woolf, C.M. 1993. Does homozygosity contribute to the asymmetry of common white leg markings in Arabian horse? *Genetica* **89**: 25–33.

Woolf, C.M. 1995. Influence of stochastic events on the phenotypic variation of common white leg markings in the Arabian horse: implications for various genetic disorders in humans. *Journal of Heredity* **86**: 129–135.

Woolf, C.M. 1998. Directional and anteroposterior asymmetry of common white markings in the legs of the Arabian horse: response to selection. *Genetica* **101**: 199–208.

Woolf, C.M. and Swafford, J.R. 1988. Evidence for eumelanin and pheomelanin producing genotypes in the Arabian horse. *Journal of Heredity* **79**: 100–106.

Wriedt, C. 1918. Albinisme i hester (Albinism in horses). *Tidsskrift for det Norske Landbruk* **25**: 396–404.

Wright, S. 1917. Color inheritance in mammals VII: the horse. *Journal of Heredity* **8**: 560–564.

Yokohama, M. and Nozawa, K. 2004. An additional analysis on lethality of roan allele in Hokkaido native horses. *Journal of Agricultural Science, Tokyo University of Agriculture* **49**(3): 147–149.

Yokohama, M., Nomura, H., Yasuhara, T., and Nozawa, K. 2002. Lethal dominant roan is not found in Hokkaido native horses. *Journal of Agricultural Science, Tokyo University of Agriculture* **47**(2): 98–101.

Index

Equine Color Genetics, Fourth Edition. D. Phillip Sponenberg and Rebecca Bellone.
© 2017 John Wiley & Sons, Inc. Published 2017 by John Wiley & Sons, Inc.

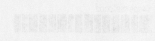

Printed and bound by CPI Group (UK) Ltd, Croydon, CR0 4YY

16/04/2025

14658459-0002

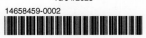